Advances in the Management of HIV

Editors

DANIEL A. SOLOMON
PAUL E. SAX

INFECTIOUS DISEASE CLINICS OF NORTH AMERICA

www.id.theclinics.com

Consulting Editor
HELEN W. BOUCHER

September 2024 • Volume 38 • Number 3

ELSEVIER

1600 John F. Kennedy Boulevard • Suite 1800 • Philadelphia, Pennsylvania, 19103-2899.
http://www.theclinics.com

INFECTIOUS DISEASE CLINICS OF NORTH AMERICA Volume 38, Number 3
September 2024 ISSN 0891–5520, ISBN-13: 978-0-443-29314-6

Editor: Kerry Holland
Developmental Editor: Varun Gopal

Infectious Disease Clinics of North America (ISSN 0891–5520) is published in March, June, September, and December by Elsevier Inc., 360 Park Avenue South, New York, NY 10010-1710. Periodicals postage paid at New York, NY and additional mailing offices. Subscription prices are $379.00 per year for US individuals, $100.00 per year for US students, $432.00 per year for Canadian individuals, $472.00 per year for international individuals, $100.00 per year for Canadian students, and $200.00 per year for international students. For institutional access pricing please contact Customer Service via the contact information below. To receive student rate, orders must be accompanied by name of affiliated institution, date of term, and the *signature* of program/residency coordinator on institution letterhead. Orders will be billed at individual rate until proof of status is received. Foreign air speed delivery is included in all *Clinics* subscription prices. All prices are subject to change without notice. Orders, claims, and journal inquiries: Please visit our Support Hub page https://service.elsevier.com for assistance.

Infectious Disease Clinics of North America is also published in Spanish by Editorial Inter-Médica, Junin 917, 1er A 1113, Buenos Aires, Argentina.

Reprints. For copies of 100 or more, of articles in this publication, please contact the Commercial Reprints Department, Elsevier Inc., 360 Park Avenue South, New York, New York 10010-1710. Tel. 212-633-3874, Fax: 212-633-3820, E-mail: reprints@elsevier.com.

Infectious Disease Clinics of North America is covered in *MEDLINE/PubMed (Index Medicus), Current Contents/ Clinical Medicine, Science Citation Alert, SCISEARCH,* and *Research Alert.*

Contributors

CONSULTING EDITOR

HELEN W. BOUCHER, MD, FACP, FIDSA
Dean and Professor of Medicine, Tufts University School of Medicine, Chief Academic
Officer, Tufts Medicine, Boston, Massachusetts, USA

EDITORS

DANIEL A. SOLOMON, MD
Assistant Professor of Medicine, Harvard Medical School, Physician, Infectious Diseases
Division, Brigham and Women's Hospital, Associate Program Director, Massachusetts
General Brigham ID Fellowship, Boston, Massachusetts, USA

PAUL E. SAX, MD
Clinical Director, Division of Infectious Diseases, Brigham and Women's Hospital,
Professor of Medicine, Harvard Medical School, Boston, Massachusetts, USA

AUTHORS

WENDY S. ARMSTRONG, MD
Professor, Division of Infectious Diseases, Department of Medicine, Emory University
School of Medicine; Ponce de Leon Center, Grady Health System, Atlanta, Georgia, USA

DANILO BACIC LIMA, MD
Clinical Fellow in Infectious Diseases, Massachusetts General Hospital, Brigham;
Women's Hospital, HIV Fellow, Infectious Diseases Division, Brigham and Women's
Hospital, Boston, Massachusetts, USA

SAMUEL S. BAILIN, MD, MSCI
Assistant Professor, Division of Infectious Diseases, Vanderbilt University Medical Center,
Nashville, Tennessee, USA

MADHU CHOUDHARY, MD
Associate Professor, Department of Medicine, University of Pittsburgh, Pittsburgh,
Pennsylvania, USA

CONSTANCE DELAUGERRE, PharmD, PhD
Professor, Virology Department, Assistance Publique - Hôpitaux de Paris, Hôpital Saint
Louis, Paris Cité University, Paris, France

DANA DUNNE, MD, MHS
Associate Professor, Department of Internal Medicine (Infectious Diseases), Yale School
of Medicine, New Haven, Connecticut, USA

MATTHEW S. DURSTENFELD, MD, MAS
Assistant Professor, Division of Cardiology, Department of Medicine, University of
California, Zuckerberg San Francisco General, San Francisco, California, USA

MARIANA ESPINAL, MD
Fellow, Division of Maternal-Fetal Medicine, Department of Obstetrics and Gynecology, Northwestern University Feinberg School of Medicine, Chicago, Illinois, USA

VALERIA FINK, MD
Director, Innovation and Translational Research Research Department, Fundación Huésped, Buenos Aires, Argentina

STEPHANIE A. FISHER, MD, MPH
Assistant Professor, Division of Maternal-Fetal Medicine, Department of Obstetrics and Gynecology, Northwestern University Feinberg School of Medicine, Chicago, Illinois, USA

MORGAN M. GOHEEN, MD, PhD
Post-Doctoral Fellow, Department of Internal Medicine (Infectious Diseases), Yale School of Medicine, New Haven, Connecticut, USA

SATISH GOPAL, MD, MPH
Director, Center for Global Health, National Cancer Institute, Rockville, Maryland, USA

DANIEL S. GRACIAA, MD, MPH, MSc
Assistant Professor, Division of Infectious Diseases, Department of Medicine, Emory University School of Medicine, Atlanta; Hope Clinic of Emory Vaccine Center, Decatur, Georgia, USA

PRISCILLA Y. HSUE, MD
Professor, Division of Cardiology, Department of Medicine, University of California, Zuckerberg San Francisco General, San Francisco, California, USA

JOHN R. KOETHE, MD, MSCI
Associate Professor, Division of Infectious Diseases, Vanderbilt University Medical Center, Nashville, Tennessee, USA

IRENE KUO, PhD, MPH
Associate Research Professor, Department of Epidemiology, The George Washington University, Milken Institute School of Public Health, Washington, DC, USA

YIJIA LI, MD
Assistant Professor, Department of Medicine, University of Pittsburgh, Pittsburgh, Pennsylvania, USA

GEOFFROY LIEGEON, MD, PhD
Post-Doctoral Fellow, Department of Infectious Diseases and Global Health, University of Chicago Medicine, Chicago, Illinois, USA

AUDUN J. LIER, MD, MPH
Assistant Professor of Clinical Medicine, Renaissance School of Medicine at Stony Brook University, Stony Brook; Northport VA Medical Center, Northport, New York, USA

DAVID M. MARGOLIS, MD
Sarah Graham Keenan Distinguished Professor of Medicine, Medicine, Microbiology and Immunology, Epidemiology; Director, UNC HIV Cure Center; University of North Carolina at Chapel Hill, Chapel Hill, North Carolina, USA

JOHN W. MELLORS, MD
Professor, Department of Medicine, University of Pittsburgh, Pittsburgh, Pennsylvania, USA

JEAN-MICHEL MOLINA, MD, PhD
Professor, Department of Infectious Diseases, Assistance Publique - Hôpitaux de Paris, Hôpitaux Saint Louis et Lariboisière, Paris, France

MAZVITA MUCHENGETI, PhD, MSc (Epidemiology & Biostatistics)
Senior Lecturer, School of Public Health, University of the Witwatersrand, Johannesburg; South African DSI-NRF Centre of Excellence in Epidemiological Modelling and Analysis, Stellenbosch University, Stellenbosch, South Africa

NATHANIAL S. NOLAN, MD, MPH, MHPE
Instructor in Medicine, Division of Infectious Disease, Washington University School of Medicine; Division of Infectious Disease, VA St. Louis Health Care, St Louis, Missouri, USA

THOMAS A. ODENY, MD, MPH, PhD
Assistant Professor, Division of Oncology, Department of Medicine, Washington University School of Medicine, St Louis, Missouri, USA

KATHERINE PROMER, MD
Associate Physician, Division of Infectious Diseases and Global Public Health, University of California, San Diego, San Diego, California, USA

NADINE ROUPHAEL, MD, MSc
Professor, Division of Infectious Diseases, Department of Medicine, Emory University School of Medicine, Atlanta; Hope Clinic of Emory Vaccine Center, Decatur, Georgia, USA

CARLOS S. SALDANA, MD
Assistant Professor, Division of Infectious Diseases, Department of Medicine, Emory University School of Medicine; Ponce de Leon Center, Grady Health System, Atlanta, Georgia, USA

RUCHI VYOMESH SHAH, DO
Physician, Boston Medical Center, Grayken Center for Addiction, Boston, Massachusetts, USA

SHEELA V. SHENOI, MD, MPH
Associate Professor of Medicine and Public Health, Yale School of Medicine; Veterans Administration Connecticut Healthcare System, West Haven, Connecticut, USA

DANIEL A. SOLOMON, MD
Assistant Professor of Medicine, Harvard Medical School, Physician, Infectious Diseases Division, Brigham and Women's Hospital, Associate Program Director, Massachusetts General Brigham ID Fellowship, Boston, Massachusetts, USA

SANDRA A. SPRINGER, MD
Professor of Medicine, Yale University School of Medicine, New Haven; Veterans Administration Connecticut Healthcare System, West Haven, Connecticut, USA

MICHAEL TANG, MD
Assistant Professor, Division of Infectious Diseases and Global Public Health, University of California, San Diego, San Diego, California, USA

ADATI TARFA, PharmD, MS, PhD
Postdoctoral Associate, Yale University School of Medicine, New Haven, Connecticut, USA

WILLIAM TREBELCOCK, MD
Resident Physician, Yale New Haven Hospital, New Haven, Connecticut, USA

JESSICA TUAN, MD, MS
Assistant Professor, Department of Internal Medicine (Infectious Diseases), Yale School of Medicine, New Haven, Connecticut, USA

STEPHEN R. WALSH, MDCM
Assistant Professor, Division of Infectious Diseases, Brigham and Women's Hospital; Harvard Medical School, Boston, Massachusetts, USA

DARCY WOOTEN, MD, MS
Professor, Division of Infectious Diseases and Global Public Health, University of California, San Diego, San Diego, California, USA

ALYSSE G. WURCEL, MD, MS
Physician, Division of Infectious Diseases and Geographic Medicine, Tufts Medicine, Boston, Massachusetts, USA

LYNN M. YEE, MD, MPH
Associate Professor, Division of Maternal-Fetal Medicine, Department of Obstetrics and Gynecology, Northwestern University Feinberg School of Medicine, Chicago, Illinois, USA

Contents

Highly effective antiretroviral therapy (ART) has transformed human immunodeficiency virus (HIV) care in the past 3 decades. 30 years ago, how many would have imagined that a single-tablet daily ART regimen containing different drug classes could achieve sustained HIV-1 suppression and halt disease progression to acquired immunodeficiency syndrome (AIDS)? Despite this remarkable achievement, challenges in HIV care remain that require further innovation for ART. In this review, we focus on newly approved antiretroviral agents and those undergoing phase 2/3 clinical trials. These new antiretrovirals hold great promise to expand treatment options and fill gaps in HIV care.

The number of options for effective antiretroviral therapy (ART) is steadily increasing. Although older regimens may achieve the goal of virologic suppression, newer options can offer advantages in safety, tolerability, and convenience. In this article, we offer guiding principles for switching ART, highlighting reasons to pursue a switch and key factors to consider when selecting a new regimen.

Recent advances in human immunodeficiency virus (HIV) management during pregnancy and infant feeding encompass several key elements: expanded HIV testing guidance; growing evidence of safety, efficacy, and pharmacokinetic data favoring the use of preferred antiretroviral therapy (ART) during pregnancy and breastfeeding; increasing advocacy for the inclusion of pregnant individuals with HIV in clinical trials to expedite access to new ART; and updated guidelines supporting shared decision-making for choice of infant feeding methods in people with HIV.

Pre-exposure prophylaxis (PrEP) of human immunodeficiency virus (HIV) represents the most significant breakthrough in the HIV prevention field over the past decade. PrEP is an effective strategy in preventing the transmission of HIV across all populations, providing high adherence. The current PrEP options include oral daily and on-demand tenofovir-based regimens, long-acting injections of cabotegravir, and a 1-month dapivirine vaginal ring. As a component of a multifaceted prevention approach, extensive deployment of PrEP holds the promise to significantly reduce the global HIV epidemic. Nonetheless, barriers still exist in terms of uptake, adherence, and persistence, while disparities in PrEP accessibility remain a concern.

We review the intersection of human immunodeficiency virus (HIV) and cancer globally, including the complex interplay of oncogenic infections, chronic inflammation, and behavioral and other factors in increasing cancer risk among people with HIV (PWH). We discuss current cancer screening, prevention, and treatment recommendations for PWH. Specific interventions include vaccination, behavioral risk reduction, timely HIV diagnosis and treatment, screening for specific cancer sites, and multifaceted treatment considerations unique to PWH including supportive care and drug interactions. Finally, the potential of novel therapies and the need for inclusive cancer clinical trials are highlighted. Collaborative multidisciplinary efforts are critical for continued progress against cancer among PWH.

Sexually transmitted infections (STIs) are more commonly seen in patients with human immunodeficiency virus (PWH). Routine sexual history taking and appropriate multisite screening practices support prompt identification and treatment of patients, which in turn reduces morbidity and spread of STIs including HIV. Nucleic acid amplification testing has high accuracy for diagnosing many of the major STIs. Diagnosis of syphilis remains complex, requiring 2 stage serologic testing, along with provider awareness of the myriad symptoms that can be attributable to this disease. Prevention through mechanisms such as vaccines and postexposure prophylaxis hold promise to reduce the burden of STIs in PWH.

The authors examine the HIV epidemic in the Southern United States, emphasizing its severe impact on minority and young populations. The authors highlight challenges including limited health care access, systemic racism influencing social determinants of health, and lesbian, gay, bisexual, transgender, and queer+ stigma. The South faces a critical human immunodeficiency virus (HIV) workforce shortage, especially in rural areas, and struggles with coexisting syndemics like other sexually transmitted infections and substance-use disorders. The authors describe comprehensive strategies such as Medicaid expansion, workforce enhancement, stigma reduction, and policy reforms to improve HIV prevention and treatment, emphasizing the need for a multifaceted approach to improve health outcomes for those with HIV in the South.

Over 1.2 million Americans aged 13 years and older have been diagnosed with human immunodeficiency virus (HIV). While HIV incidence has been declining since 2017, the risk of HIV acquisition and transmission persists among persons who use drugs via injection drug use and unprotected

INFECTIOUS DISEASE CLINICS OF NORTH AMERICA

Preface

Advances in the Management of HIV

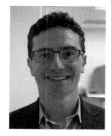 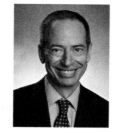

Daniel A. Solomon, MD   Paul E. Sax, MD
Editors

In 2021, one of us (P.E.S.) received an invitation to give a talk on the history of HIV. Entitled "A Medical Miracle: 40 Years of HIV Care and Research," the talk covered the remarkable progress from the first report of pneumocystis pneumonia in *Morbidity and Mortality Weekly Report* in 1981[1] to the modern era of antiretroviral therapy (ART) for treatment and prevention of HIV. The final slide both celebrated how far we have come and recognized the many unsolved and emerging challenges in HIV research and clinical care.

This special issue of *Infectious Disease Clinics* picks up where the talk left off: what is the current state of HIV medicine, and what challenges and advances are on the frontier? We designed this collection to include four broad categories of topics. The first group of articles focuses on HIV treatment and prevention. There are four topics in this section, including a review of investigational ART, a practical guide on how to approach ART switches (the most common treatment decision in clinical practice), an update on management of HIV in pregnancy, and finally, a review of HIV preexposure prophylaxis. The second group of articles includes reviews of the two most challenging fields in HIV basic and clinical research: development of an HIV vaccine and an HIV cure. The next set of articles focuses on the common medical complications and comorbidities in people with HIV, including weight gain related to ART, cardiovascular disease, malignancy, and sexually transmitted infections. The last group of articles addresses key populations impacted by HIV. These topics include a review of the unique HIV epidemic in the United States South, HIV among people with substance use disorders, and challenges in treatment and prevention of HIV for people in jails and prisons. Having examined the opportunities and challenges we face, we conclude with a final article on how we should address the HIV workforce needs of the future.

Infect Dis Clin N Am 38 (2024) xiii–xiv
https://doi.org/10.1016/j.idc.2024.06.006
0891-5520/24/© 2024 Published by Elsevier Inc.

We are grateful to the group of national and international experts who contributed to this collection, and are hopeful that by selecting a range of topics, it will reach a broad readership. More than forty years on, the field of HIV remains dynamic and exciting. There is much work to be done.

Daniel A. Solomon, MD
Harvard Medical School
75 Francis Street
Boston, MA 02115, USA

Paul E. Sax, MD
Harvard Medical School
75 Francis Street
Boston, MA 02115, USA

E-mail addresses:
DASOLOMON@bwh.harvard.edu (D.A. Solomon)
PSAX@bwh.harvard.edu (P.E. Sax)

REFERENCE

1. Centers for Disease Control and Prevention (CDC). Pneumocystis pneumonia—Los Angeles. MMWR Morb Mortal Wkly Rep 1981;30(21):250–2. PMID: 6265753.

The Current Pipeline of Antiretroviral Therapy

Expanding Options and Filling Gaps

Yijia Li, MD*, Madhu Choudhary, MD, John W. Mellors, MD

KEYWORDS

- HIV-1 • Antiretrovirals • Antiretroviral therapy (ART) • Clinical trials • Drug resistance
- Long-acting ART

KEY POINTS

- Despite great advances in antiretroviral therapy, there are still unmet needs in human immunodeficiency virus (HIV) care, especially related to the requirement for daily medication adherence and for activity against multi-drug resistant (MDR) HIV-1.
- Small molecules targeting different steps in HIV-1 life cycle provide new options for MDR HIV-1 therapy.
- New chemical entities and formulations of small molecules extend the duration of drug exposure allowing less frequent dosing.
- HIV-neutralizing and HIV coreceptor-targeting monoclonal antibodies, with or without combinations of small molecules, provide long-acting non-pill (parenteral) options for HIV treatment.

INTRODUCTION

Since its introduction, antiretroviral therapy (ART) has been constantly evolving[1,2] and has remarkably transformed the landscape of human immunodeficiency virus (HIV) medicine, significantly improving the lifespan of people with HIV (PWH)[3] and reducing transmission of the virus.[4] It was estimated that over 20 million acquired immunodeficiency syndrome (AIDS)-related deaths have been averted since the introduction of combination ART in 1996.[5] Despite this tremendous achievement, there remain numerous challenges in HIV care, including the requirement for daily adherence to ART, emergence of multi-drug resistant (MDR) HIV-1, barriers to treatment access, and the persistence of stigma. These challenges continue to pose significant obstacles to optimal HIV management. Globally, in 2022, only 71% of PWH were estimated to achieve viral suppression[5] as a consequence of the challenges. Shockingly, among PWH in the United States in 2021, only 66% achieved viral suppression and 54% were

Department of Medicine, University of Pittsburgh, Pittsburgh, PA, USA
* Corresponding author. 3601 Fifth Avenue, Floor 7, Pittsburgh, PA 15213.
E-mail address: liy33@upmc.edu

Infect Dis Clin N Am 38 (2024) 395–408
https://doi.org/10.1016/j.idc.2024.04.001

id.theclinics.com

retained in care.[6] In this review, we aim to highlight unmet needs and examine how the next generation of antiretrovirals (ARVs) and combination ART may fill persisting gaps in HIV care. This review focuses on HIV treatment; therapeutic approaches focused on HIV cure including latency reversing agents and vaccines are covered elsewhere in this issue.

CHALLENGES IN MODERN HUMAN IMMUNODEFICIENCY VIRUS CARE

Multiple unmet needs continue to pose challenges in achieving better HIV suppression at both population and individual levels (**Fig. 1**A). First, despite improved adherence to ART since the introduction of single-tablet regimens,[1] many PWH still have difficulty taking daily medication for a myriad of reasons, ranging from pill aversion, stigma, certain medical conditions (eg, dysphagia), work schedule, unstable housing, substance use disorder, and other social or psychologic factors. Second, MDR HIV-1, albeit infrequent, remains an unsolved challenge in HIV care. MDR HIV-1 is most frequent in heavily treatment-experienced individuals who have limited treatment options.[7] Even when options exist, they usually involve complex combinations of multiple ARVs with associated adverse effects and adherence challenges. In addition, current long-acting, injectable ART, consisting of cabotegravir (CAB) and rilpivirine (RPV), developed to reduce drug administration frequency and improve adherence,[8] do not prevent hepatitis B virus (HBV) infection or provide antiviral activity against HBV (prevalence ~7% of PWH[9]). Metabolic side effects associated with current

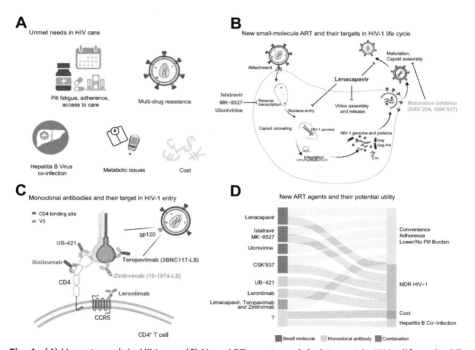

Fig. 1. (*A*) Unmet needs in HIV care. (*B*) New ART agents and their target in HIV-1 life cycle. (*C*) New monoclonal antibody regimens and their target in HIV-1 entry. gp120, glycoprotein 120; LS, Methionine428Leucine and Asparagine434Serine modification at the antibody Fc region. (*D*) New ART agents and their potential utility. HBV, hepatitis B virus; MDR, multi-drug resistance. (Panel (A–C) created with BioRender.com.)

ART, especially weight gain, hyperlipidemia, and other associated cardiometabolic adverse effects, can impact the quality of life and overall health of PWH on ART.[10] Finally, newly developed therapies are inevitably associated with high cost. Addressing these unmet needs is crucial to improve HIV treatment outcomes and enhance the healthy life span of PWH. In the following sections, we will introduce ARVs that are newly approved or in the pipeline and discuss their potential advantages for future HIV care.

SMALL MOLECULES DIRECTLY TARGETING THE HUMAN IMMUNODEFICIENCY VIRUS-1 REPLICATION CYCLE
Capsid Inhibitor: Lenacapavir

Lenacapavir (LEN) is a first-in-class capsid inhibitor (**Fig. 1**B) with antiviral activity against both wild-type virus and variants resistant to current antiretroviral agents. It also achieves unprecedented duration of therapeutic activity after 3 oral loading doses and single subcutaneous administration, sufficient for dosing every 6 months.[11] It was approved by the European Commission on August 22, 2022, followed by the U.S Food and Drug Administration (FDA) on December 22, 2022, for treatment of HIV-1 infection in heavily treatment-experienced adults with MDR infection who are taking a failing ART regimen due to resistance, intolerance, or adverse effects.[12] The approvals were based on a phase 3 study (CAPELLA) in which a decrease of at least $0.5 \log_{10}$ copies/mL in plasma HIV-1 RNA by day 15 was observed in 21 of 24 (88%) when LEN was added to the failing regimen, compared to 2 of 12 (17%) in the placebo group (absolute difference, 71%).[13] At week 26, plasma HIV-1 RNA of less than 50 copies/mL was observed in 29 of 36 participants (81%) and less than 200 copies/mL in 32 of 36 participants (89%).[13] At week 52 using the FDA snapshot criteria, 78% (56 of 72 participants) achieved HIV-1 RNA suppression less than 50 copies/mL and 82% (59 of 72 participants) less than 200 copies/mL.[14]

Because of its ultra-long half-life, the possibility of either 6-monthly subcutaneous dosing or weekly oral dosing allows exploration of LEN as an appealing option for ART initiation in the treatment-naïve population or as part of a simplification regimen. An open label phase 2 study (CALIBRATE) in treatment-naïve PWH who received LEN in combination with various agents (**Table 1**), demonstrated virological suppression less than 50 copies/mL at week 52 ranging from 85% to 92% in different treatment groups.[15] Mild to moderate injection site reactions were the most common adverse reactions.[15] Further exploration of LEN in combination with other ARVs is ongoing, including nucleoside reverse transcriptase translocation inhibitors (NRTTI) as weekly dosing (LEN/ISL switch study, week 24 results available, **Table 1**),[16] cabotegravir, and with broadly HIV-1 neutralizing antibodies (bNAb) as 6-monthly dosing.

For subcutaneous dosing, LEN injection requires 2 of 1.5 mL subcutaneous injections for a complete dose of 927 mg every 6 months. Due to slow-release kinetics of subcutaneous formulation, oral lead-in dosing is required for treatment initiation. LEN is a moderate inhibitor of CYP3A and there is potential for increased exposure of drugs primarily metabolized by CYP3A if initiated within 9 months of the last dose administered. Oral bridging dosing (300 mg weekly) in the setting of subcutaneous treatment interruption is safe and associated with high rates of viral suppression in the CAPELLA and CALIBRATE studies subanalysis.[17]

In summary, LEN has broad potential for use in PWH with MDR HIV-1 and in those who desire extended dosing to enhance adherence and lower pill burden. For the latter indication, companion ARVs with equally long half-lives are under investigation as discussed in the following section.

Table 1
Lenacapavir (LEN) clinical trials

Target Population	Phase	ClinicalTrials.gov Identifier	Short Title	Study Design	Status as of May 2024	Reference
Treatment-experienced, multidrug-resistant HIV-1 infection ART switch/salvage therapy	Phase 3	NCT04150068	CAPELLA	Cohort 1: Randomization 2:1 to receive LEN (oral) vs placebo + failing ART for 14 d (lead-in). Then from day 15, active LEN group received LEN (SC) every 6 mo; at day 15 placebo group started to receive oral LEN lead-in followed by LEN (SC) every 6 mo. Both groups also received optimized background ART. Cohort 2: Open-label LEN (oral) + optimized background ART lead-in (14-d course) followed by SC LEN every 6 mo starting on day 15+ optimized background ART	Day 1–15 Cohort 1: decrease of ≥ 0.5 $\log_{10}$ copies/mL in HIV-1 RNA by day 15 • LEN: 88% (21/24) • Placebo: 17% (2/12) Week 26 HIV-1 RNA<50 copies/mL • Cohort 1: 81% (29/36) • Cohort 2: 83% (30/36) Week 52 HIV-1 RNA<50 copies/mL • Cohort 1: 83% (30/36) • Cohort 2: 72% (26/36)	Segal-Maurer et al,[13] 2022; Ogbuagu et al,[14] 2023
Treatment naive ART initiation	Phase 2	NCT04143594	CALIBRATE	Open-label, randomized: Oral LEN + TAF/FTC lead in followed by Group1: SC LEN every 26 week; also daily TAF/FTC then daily TAF from week 28 Group 2: SC LEN every 26 week; also daily TAF/FTC then daily BIC from week 28	Week 54 HIV-1 RNA<50 copies/mL • Group 1: 90% (47/52) • Group 2: 85% (45/53) • Group 3: 85% (44/52) • Group 4: 92% (23/25)	Gupta et al,[15] 2023

Indication	Phase	NCT Number	Trial Name	Regimen	Results/Status	Reference
Virologically suppressed ART switch: Simplification of complex regimen and an existing STR not possible due to drug resistance, intolerance etc.	Phase 2 Phase 3	NCT05502341	ARTISTRY-1	Open-label, randomized: Phase 2: • BIC + oral daily LEN 25 mg after loading dose • BIC/LEN (50 mg) FDC after loading dose • Current ART regimen Phase 3: • BIC/LEN FDC, dosage based on phase 2, after loading dose • Current ART regimen Group 3: Continue oral daily LEN + TAF/FTC Group 4: Active comparator TAF/FTC/BIC	Recruitment ongoing[a]	
Virologically suppressed. ART switch	Phase 2	NCT05052996		Open label randomization to immediate vs 48 week deferred oral weekly LEN and ISL after B/F/TAF	Week 24 HIV-1 RNA<50 copies/ml • LEN/ISL: 94.2% (49/52) • B/F/TAF: 94.2% (49/52)	Colson et al,[16], 2024
Virologically suppressed. ART switch	Phase 2	NCT05729568		Open label, bNAbs teropavimab and zinlirvimab in combination with SC LEN every 6 mo	Recruiting	

Abbreviations: ART, antiretroviral therapy; BIC, bictegravir; FTC, emtricitabine; ISL, islatravir; LEN, lenacapavir; SC, subcutaneous; TAF, tenofovir alafenamide.
[a] https://www.gileadclinicaltrials.com/study?id=GS-US-621-6289.

Nucleoside Reverse Transcriptase Translocation Inhibitor: Islatravir and Others

Islatravir (ISL; chemical name 4′-Ethynyl-2-fluoro-2′-deoxyadenosine, EFdA; previously known as MK-8591) is the first-in-class NRTTI in late-phase clinical trials (see **Fig. 1**B). It is an adenosine analogue[18] like tenofovir, but employs very different mechanisms to inhibit reverse transcription compared to other traditional nucleoside reverse transcriptase inhibitors (NRTI).[18] In addition, its very long half-life[19] allows less frequent dosing.

ISL has been evaluated in treatment-naïve individuals as part of initial ART. In a phase 2b randomized, double-blind, dose-ranging trial, treatment-naïve adult PWH were randomized to either a comparator group of tenofovir disoproxil fumarate (TDF) or one of the ISL daily dose groups (0.25 mg, 0.75 mg, or 2.25 mg) in combination with standard dose of doravirine (DOR) and lamivudine (3TC). Participants in the ISL groups who achieved plasma HIV-1 RNA less than 50 copies/mL after 24 weeks of treatment were then switched to DOR/ISL maintenance therapy. ISL groups had similar virologic outcomes compared to the TDF/3TC/DOR group FDA snapshot of week 48 viral suppression: 90%, 90%, 77% (numerically lower viral suppression rate likely due to higher rate of discontinuation than other groups) in 0.25 mg, 0.75 mg and 2.25 mg ISL groups versus 84% in TDF/3TC/DOR group[20] with viral suppression mostly maintained through week 96.[21] Another randomized, double-blind phase 3 trial (MK-8591A-020, NCT04233879) comparing DOR/ISL (100 mg/0.75 mg) with BIC/FTC/TAF in treatment naïve PWH demonstrated that rates of viral suppression at 48 weeks with DOR/ISL (88.9%) was non-inferior to BIC/TAF/FTC (88.3%).[22] The mean increase in CD4 + T-cell count was 182 cells/μL for DOR/ISL and 234 cells/μL for BIC/FTC/TAF. Of note, one participant did develop treatment-emerging drug resistance and virologic failure, with M184I and V106A + P225H mutations detected in the *reverse transcriptase* (*rt*) gene, along with an unquantifiable ISL level at the time of virologic failure.[22] Safety profiles were comparable in both groups. Of note, both groups had comparable lipid changes and weight gain,[22] despite the DOR/ISL regimen sparing both integrase strand transfer inhibitors (INSTIs) and TAF.[23]

Another focus for ISL development has been the potential for ART switch. In an open-labeled, randomized, non-inferiority phase 3 trial (MK-8591A-017, NCT04223778), adult PWH with at least 3 months of viral suppression on stable baseline ART were randomized to either DOR/ISL (100mg/0.75mg) or staying on baseline ART (bART). Week 48 FDA snapshot of HIV-1 RNA suppression less than 50 copies/mL was 95.2% and 94.3% in DOR/ISL versus bART groups, showing non-inferiority.[24] The safety profile was similar between 2 groups; however, the DOR/ISL group had a decline in CD4 + T cell count (mean change −30.3 cells/μL from baseline) compared to the bART group (+38.9 cells/μL), without increase in infection-related adverse effects.[24] Similarly, in another randomized, double-blind, non-inferiority phase 3 study, switching to DOR/ISL (100mg/0.75 mg) was non-inferior to continuing baseline BIC/FTC/TAF in virally-suppressed adult PWH (MK-8591A-018, NCT04223791) with 93.8% versus 94.4% viral suppression respectively at week 48[24]. This study also showed minor CD4 + T cell decline in DOR/ISL group (−19.7 cells/μL from baseline) compared to BIC/FTC/TAF group (+40.5 cells/μL) and weight change was again comparable between 2 groups.[25] Since development of the 0.75 mg daily dosing of ISL was halted for concerns about lymphocytopenia, the FDC DOR/ISL (0.25 mg) dosage was adopted for ongoing switch trials (switch from bART, MK-8591A-051, NCT05631093; switch from BIC/FTC/TAF, MK-8591A-052, NCT05630755).

ISL was also explored in heavily treatment experienced PWH with MDR HIV-1 infection in combination with DOR in a phase 3 study (MK-8591A-019, NCT04233216). In 35 heavily treatment-experienced PWH with MDR HIV-1, DOR/ISL (0.75 mg)+ failing ART was associated with higher rates of viral load reduction $\geq$1.0 log10 copies/mL (85.7%) compared to ISL + ART (14.3%), DOR + ART (50.0%), and placebo + ART (0%) at day 8[25]. All participants switched to DOR/ISL (0.75 mg) + optimized background ART after day 8 and 71% (22 out of 31 participants with available data) had HIV viral load less than 50 copies/mL at week 49.[26]

Beyond daily or weekly dosing, ISL pharmacokinetics would allow monthly dosing (oral administration) and potentially longer intervals with subcutaneous administration at higher doses. However, a dose/exposure-related decrease in total lymphocyte and CD4 + T cell count was observed across ISL clinical trials (both HIV prevention and HIV-1 treatment) with higher frequencies and magnitude of changes with higher-dose regimens including 20 mg weekly and 120 mg and 60 mg monthly dosing.[27] This effect is attributed to supratherapeutic concentrations of ISL-triphosphate in lymphocytes leading to apoptosis.[27] Pharmacokinetic/pharmacodynamic modeling with lower doses and exposure has led to revised oral dosing of 0.25 mg daily and 2 mg weekly.[28] Currently DOR/ISL 100/0.25 mg oral daily dosing and ISL 2 mg + LEN 300 mg oral weekly dosing have been resumed in clinical development.

ISL also shows a high genetic barrier to resistance.[29] Due to different mechanisms of action than approved NRTI, canonical NRTI-associated RT mutations including K65R, L74I, V90I and thymidine analog mutations (TAMs) have limited or no impact on ISL activity.[29] M184V and M184I, 2 classic 3TC/FTC (XTC) associated mutations, have the most impact on ISL activity; high intracellular concentrations can largely overcome the effect of these 2 mutations,[29,30] but only reliably when ISL is given at an oral dosage of 0.75mg daily or equivalent.[31] A combination of *rt* mutations A114S/M184V has been shown to confer high level resistance to ISL (24 to 35-fold increase in half maximal inhibitory concentration [IC_{50}][29,30]), but this combination of mutations is associated with reduced fitness[29] and increased sensitivity to tenofovir.[30] Another recent study showed that M184 V + V106I (a DOR selected mutation conferring low-level DOR resistance), is associated with 33.8-fold resistance.[32] This along with the treatment-emerging M184I + V106A (which confers high-level DOR resistance) reported in the phase 3 trial,[22] merits further evaluation.

MK-8527, a second NRTTI with very long intracellular half-life (118–211 hours[33]), is in early phase evaluation for HIV-1 treatment (NCT05494736). The risk of lymphocyte decrease remains unknown and no further information is available at the time of this review.

In summary, ISL if approved could be used for ART simplification, and have a potential role in management of MDR HIV-1 infection. It may also help with adherence especially if weekly, monthly, or even longer dosing interval can be achieved (eg, implant). Based on the available data, it does not appear that ISL would help with metabolic complications and/or weight gain when compared to TAF and/or INSTI containing regimens, but further studies are needed. Drug-resistance mutations to ISL, especially in the ISL/XTC and DOR/ISL combination, require further in-depth evaluation.

Non-nucleoside Reverse Transcriptase Inhibitor: Ulonivirine (MK-8507)

Ulonivirine is a new NNRTI with a long half-life that supports weekly oral dosing.[34] In a phase 1 open label trial, untreated PWH (HIV-1 RNA$\geq$10,000 copies/mL) received single dose of ulonivirine (40, 80 or 600 mg) orally and experienced a mean HIV viral load reduction of 1.2 to 1.5 $\log_{10}$ copies/mL across different dosage groups after 7 days.[34]

A phase 2b randomized, controlled, double-blind study was initiated to evaluate switching to an ISL/ulonivirine once weekly regimen versus continuing BIC/FTC/TAF, among virally suppressed PWH on BIC/FTC/TAF for greater than or equal to 6 months (NCT04564547; currently on hold). The utility of ulonivirine, other than potential once-weekly dosing, remains unclear at this time.

Maturation Inhibitors

Maturation inhibitors are a new group of ARV that block structural Gag polyproteins from being fully cleaved by HIV-1 protease by binding to the Gag protein.[35] Earlier generations of maturation initiators were found to have reduced activity against HIV-1 with several different *gag* polymorphisms, which ended their clinical development.[35,36] GSK3640254 (GSK'254) is a next-generation maturation inhibitor that was designed to overcome resistance from *gag* polymorphisms. In a phase 2a double-blinded, placebo-controlled, dose-ranging trial, treatment-naïve PWH (n = 34) were randomized to daily oral dosing of 10 mg, 40 mg, 80 mg, 140 mg, 200 mg, or placebo. At the end of an 8–10-day dosing period, any dosage greater than or equal to 40 mg daily was associated with a plasma viral load decline of greater than 1 $\log_{10}$ copies/mL.[37] GSK'254 was generally well tolerated. A *gag* A364V mutation in the 200 mg group was found to reduce the activity of GSK'254.[37] Despite its promising phase 2 results, GSK has stopped the development of GSK'254 for reasons other than safety or efficacy concerns,[38] while its analog GSK3739937 (GSK'937) that can be orally dosed once-weekly, is under early-phase trial.[39] Overall, maturation inhibitors have potential to improve management of MDR HIV-1 infection, and the newer generation agent GSK'937 may help with adherence with once-weekly dosing.

FURTHER TARGETING OF HUMAN IMMUNODEFICIENCY VIRUS-1 ENTRY: MONOCLONAL ANTIBODIES AND COMBINATIONS WITH SMALL MOLECULES
Broadly Neutralizing Antibodies (bNAbs): General Comments

bNAb have been a hot topic of HIV research over the past decade with potential roles in pre-exposure prophylaxis, HIV treatment, and HIV cure. However, they are still in the early phase for clinical development, and frequent virological failure (compared to current small molecule ART) and emergence of bNAb resistant HIV-1 have been observed in trials when bNAbs were used without small molecule ARVs.[40,41] This virologic failure and resistance is due to extensive diversity of HIV-1 *env* gene and variable post-translational glycosylation that can readily alter the glycoprotein surface and shift bNAb affinity.[42,43] There have been proof-of-concept, early-phase trials demonstrating prolonged viral suppression in a subset of PWH with bNAb-sensitive HIV-1.[41,44] However, baseline bNAb sensitivity testing in virologically-suppressed individuals cannot always be successfully performed, complicating patient selection for bNAb therapy.[40,44,45] In addition, improvements in potency, activity breadth, formulation, and half-life are needed to simplify pre-treatment testing and administration.[46] Long acting versions of 3BNC117 and 10–1074, 2 of the bNAbs that have been modified to prolong their half-lives (3BNC117-LS and 10–1074-LS), will be tested in the upcoming Phase 2 trials in acute HIV-1 infection, namely RHIVIERA-02 (small molecule ART + bNAbs followed by small molecule ART treatment interruption, NCT05300035) and RIO (small molecule ART + bNAbs followed by small molecule ART treatment interruption; NCT04319367). Alternatively, bNAbs have the potential to be approved in PWH with MDR HIV-1. Currently, a phase 2 trial enrolling highly treatment-experienced PWH with 3BNC117 + a long-acting fusion inhibitor albuvirtide is ongoing (NCT04560569).

Lenacapavir, Teropavimab, and Zinlirvimab

To overcome the low genetic barrier to resistance of bNAbs, a Phase 1b trial combined teropavimab (3BNC117-LS), zinlirvimab (10–1074-LS) (**Fig. 1C**) with lenacepavir (LEN). Of note, teropavimab and zinlirvimab have lysine-serine mutations in the crystallizable fragment (Fc) of the antibody that prolong the half-lives of the prototype bNAbs.[47] Participants in the trial were meticulously selected so that only those with greater than or equal to 18-month viral suppression and sensitive provirus to both bNAbs (based on the Monogram PhenoSense assay) were included (124 participants screened, 55 met bNAb susceptibility criteria, and 21 randomized to either a low or high dose of zinlirvimab arm plus teropavimab + LEN).[48] A single dose of the combination regimen plus LEN oral loading doses were given. Viral suppression was maintained for 90% of individuals in each arm at week 26, with 1 participant having viral rebound.[48] Reassuringly, both bNAbs and LEN remained well above therapeutic threshold concentration throughout 26 weeks of observation, and the safety profile was encouraging.[48] Low level anti-drug antibody against bNAbs was detected in 30% (6 out of 20) of participants but was not shown to have significant clinical impact.[48] This very long-acting combination ARVs represents a potential new paradigm for HIV treatment and its phase 2 trial is ongoing (NCT05729568). Another phase 2 trial enrolling virally suppressed PWH evaluating parenteral CAB + bNAb VRC07 to 523LS (NCT03739996) is also ongoing.

CD4-Targeting Monoclonal Antibodies

Instead of targeting gp120, there are other groups of monoclonal Antibodies (mAbs) targeting the HIV-1 receptor CD4 molecule without depleting CD4 + T cells or interfering with other CD4 functions.[49,50] Among them, ibalizumab was the first, approved in 2018, after meeting the primary virological endpoint in PWH with MDR HIV-1 infection on failing ART regimens.[49] It is a humanized IgG4 mAb derived from a murine mAb first described in 1992 as 5A8,[51] and represents a unique class of mAb that targets CD4 extracellular domain 2 (see **Fig. 1C**). Currently Ibalizumab is only approved for PWH with MDR HIV-1 as rescue therapy and there have been case reports on its role as a bridging therapy in PWH who need to stop boosted protease inhibitors to avoid drug-drug interactions.[52] The requirement for every-2-week intravenous dosing does not make ibalizumab attractive for therapeutic indications beyond MDR HIV-1 treatment unless its half-life can be prolonged.

UB-421 (Semzuvolimab)

UB-421 represents another group of mAb targeting CD4 instead of gp120. Unlike ibalizumab, UB-421 is a humanized IgG1 monoclonal antibody that binds to CD4 extracellular domain 1 and directly competes with HIV-1 gp120 binding.[50] In an open-label, nonrandomized, phase 2 trial, 29 virally-suppressed PWH received a total of 8 doses of UB-421 monotherapy at 2 different intravenous dosing frequencies: 10 mg/kg weekly and 25 mg/kg every 2 weeks. Viral suppression was maintained in all participants during monotherapy and no participants experienced virological failure.[50] Further clinical trials of UB-421 are planned to include subcutaneous administration (Phase 1 NCT04620291) and rescue therapy for MDR HIV-1 (Phase 3 NCT04406727).

C-C Motif Chemokine Receptor 5-Targeting Monoclonal Antibody: Leronlimab (PRO 140)

C-C motif chemokine receptor (CCR5)-targeting monoclonal antibody leronlimab (PRO 140) represents another class of therapeutic antibody that potentially prevents

HIV-1 entry. Similar to Maraviroc, a small-molecule CCR5 antagonist, leronlimab is only active against R5-tropic virus. However, leronlimab directly competes with gp120 binding to CCR5, whereas maraviroc induces allosteric changes in CCR5 to prevent gp120 binding.[53] Previous phase 2a trial demonstrated substantial plasma HIV-1 RNA reduction in PWH with HIV-1 RNA greater than 5000 copies/mL off of ART.[54] Phase 2/3 studies evaluating subcutaneous leronlimab at different dosages have shown promise in both as monotherapy in PWH with exclusively CCR5-tropic virus,[55] and as rescue therapy in PWH with MDR HIV-1 infection,[56] although these results are preliminary and yet to be published. It is currently under FDA partial clinical hold and its timeline for FDA approval remains unclear. If approved, it could be used in PWH with exclusively CCR5-tropic HIV-1 infection as a rescue therapy in the setting of MDR HIV-1. Once weekly subcutaneous dosing may potentially help with adherence and simplify treatment if companion ART with the same dosing interval could be included, although longer acting formulations would be preferred.

SUMMARY

Several innovative ARVs and combination ARVs targeting different steps in the HIV-1 life cycle have been recently approved or show promising results in clinical trials. The newly approved ART regimens have potential to improve HIV care by reducing or eliminating pill burden, decreasing the required frequency of dosing, or providing effective suppression of MDR HIV-1 infection. Nevertheless, there are still substantial barriers to overcome, especially the logistics of widespread implementation of parenteral drug administration, associated health care and drug costs, and simultaneous treatment of HBV co-infection, which are all significant issues for low or middle-income country as well as certain populations in high income countries (eg, the U.S.) with disadvantaged socioeconomic status (**Fig. 1**D). More importantly, current ARVs already have high efficacy and excellent safety profiles, making it somewhat challenging for these new regimens to be widely used. The effects of newer agents on metabolic profiles and longer-term adverse events also remain to be determined. Overall, the pipeline of new ARVs has several strong contenders to improve ART simplicity, convenience, adherence, and activity against multi-drug-resistant HIV-1.

CLINICS CARE POINTS

- Small-molecule ARVs with distinct mechanisms from current failing ARVs, provide new options for MDR HIV-1 therapy.
- Certain new ARVs (both small molecules and antibody-based regimen) with prolonged half-lives provide options for infrequent dosing, and hopefully promote adherence in certain populations.
- HIV-neutralizing and HIV coreceptor-targeting mAbs, with or without small-molecule ARVs, provide long-acting parenteral options for HIV treatment.

DISCLOSURE

The authors declared no potential conflicts of interest with respect to this article. Y. Li and M. Choudhary report no competing interests related to this work. J.W. Mellors is a consultant to Gilead Sciences, has received grant support to the University of

Pittsburgh from Gilead Sciences, United States, is a founder and share option holder of Infectious Disease Connect and owns shares of Galapagos, NV and MingMed, Inc, unrelated to the current work. Y. Li is supported by Rustbelt CFAR (Case Western Reserve University/University Hospitals Cleveland Medical Center and University of Pittsburgh, P30 AI036219). Y. Li is a topic editor for DynaMed.

REFERENCES

1. Choudhary MC, Mellors JW. The transformation of HIV therapy: One pill once a day. Antivir Ther 2022;27(2). 13596535211062396.
2. Markowitz M. Introduction: long-acting antiretrovirals for the treatment and prevention of HIV-1 infection: the future is now. Curr Opin HIV AIDS 2020;15(1):1–3.
3. Trickey A, Sabin CA, Burkholder G, et al. Life expectancy after 2015 of adults with HIV on long-term antiretroviral therapy in Europe and North America: a collaborative analysis of cohort studies. Lancet HIV 2023;10(5):e295–307.
4. Cohen MS, Chen YQ, McCauley M, et al. Prevention of HIV-1 infection with early antiretroviral therapy. N Engl J Med 2011;365(6):493–505.
5. UNAIDS. The Paths that Ends AIDS. 2023. Available at: https://www.unaids.org/sites/default/files/media_asset/2023-unaids-global-aids-update_en.pdf.   [Accessed 18 July 2023].
6. Centers for Disease Control and Prevention. Monitoring selected national HIV prevention and care objectives by using HIV surveillance data—United States and 6 dependent areas, 2021. HIV Surveillance Supplemental Report 2023; 28(4). Available at: https://www.cdc.gov/hiv/library/reports/hiv-surveillance.html. [Accessed 18 July 2023].
7. Dvory-Sobol H, Shaik N, Callebaut C, et al. Lenacapavir: a first-in-class HIV-1 capsid inhibitor. Curr Opin HIV AIDS 2022;17(1):15–21.
8. Gandhi M, Hickey M, Imbert E, et al. Demonstration project of long-acting antiretroviral therapy in a diverse population of people with HIV. Ann Intern Med 2023; 176(7):969–74.
9. Klein MB, Althoff KN, Jing Y, et al. Risk of end-stage liver disease in hiv-viral hepatitis coinfected persons in North America from the early to modern antiretroviral therapy eras. Clin Infect Dis 2016;63(9):1160–7.
10. Chandiwana NC, Siedner MJ, Marconi VC, et al. Weight gain after HIV therapy initiation: pathophysiology and implications. J Clin Endocrinol Metab 2023. https://doi.org/10.1210/clinem/dgad411.
11. Link JO, Rhee MS, Tse WC, et al. Clinical targeting of HIV capsid protein with a long-acting small molecule. Nature 2020;584(7822):614–8.
12. FDA. FDA Product Insert - Sunlenca (Lenacapavir). 2022. Available at: https://www.accessdata.fda.gov/drugsatfda_docs/label/2022/215973s000lbl.pdf.   [Accessed 24 September 2023].
13. Segal-Maurer S, DeJesus E, Stellbrink HJ, et al. Capsid Inhibition with Lenacapavir in Multidrug-Resistant HIV-1 Infection. N Engl J Med 2022;386(19):1793–803.
14. Ogbuagu O, Segal-Maurer S, Ratanasuwan W, et al. Efficacy and safety of the novel capsid inhibitor lenacapavir to treat multidrug-resistant HIV: week 52 results of a phase 2/3 trial. Lancet HIV 2023;10(8):e497–505.
15. Gupta SK, Berhe M, Crofoot G, et al. Lenacapavir administered every 26 weeks or daily in combination with oral daily antiretroviral therapy for initial treatment of HIV: a randomised, open-label, active-controlled, phase 2 trial. Lancet HIV 2023; 10(1):e15–23.

16. Colson A, Crofoot G, Ruane PJ, et al., Efficacy and Safety of Weekly Islatravir Plus Lenacapavir in PWH at 24 Weeks: A Phase II Study. Paper presented at: Conference on Retroviruses and Opportunistic Infections (CROI) 2024; Denver, CO.

17. Ogbuagu O, Avihingsanon A, Segal-Maurer S, et al. Lenacapavir oral bridging maintains efficacy with a similar safety profile when SC LEN cannot be administered. Brisbane, Australia: IAS; 2023.

18. Michailidis E, Huber AD, Ryan EM, et al. 4'-Ethynyl-2-fluoro-2'-deoxyadenosine (EFdA) inhibits HIV-1 reverse transcriptase with multiple mechanisms. J Biol Chem 2014;289(35):24533–48.

19. Schürmann D, Rudd DJ, Zhang S, et al. Safety, pharmacokinetics, and antiretroviral activity of islatravir (ISL, MK-8591), a novel nucleoside reverse transcriptase translocation inhibitor, following single-dose administration to treatment-naive adults infected with HIV-1: an open-label, phase 1b, consecutive-panel trial. Lancet HIV 2020;7(3):e164–72.

20. Molina JM, Yazdanpanah Y, Afani Saud A, et al. Islatravir in combination with doravirine for treatment-naive adults with HIV-1 infection receiving initial treatment with islatravir, doravirine, and lamivudine: a phase 2b, randomised, double-blind, dose-ranging trial. Lancet HIV 2021;8(6):e324–33.

21. Molina JM, Yazdanpanah Y, Afani Saud A, et al. Brief Report: Efficacy and Safety of Oral Islatravir Once Daily in Combination With Doravirine Through 96 Weeks for Treatment-Naive Adults With HIV-1 Infection Receiving Initial Treatment With Islatravir, Doravirine, and Lamivudine. J Acquir Immune Defic Syndr 2022;91(1):68–72.

22. Rockstroh J, Paredes R, Cahn P, et al. Doravirine/Islatravir (100mg/0.75mg) once daily compared to bictegravir/emtricitabine/tenofovir alafenamide (B/F/TAF) as Initial HIV-1 treatment: 48 week results from a double-blind phase 3 trial. Brisbane, Australia: Paper presented at: IAS; 2023.

23. Wood BR, Huhn GD. Excess weight gain with integrase inhibitors and tenofovir alafenamide: what is the mechanism and does it matter? Open Forum Infect Dis 2021;8(12):ofab542.

24. Molina JM, Rizzardini G, Orrell C, et al. Switch to fixed-dose doravirine (100 mg) with islatravir (0·75 mg) once daily in virologically suppressed adults with HIV-1 on antiretroviral therapy: 48-week results of a phase 3, randomised, open-label, non-inferiority trial. Lancet HIV 2024. S2352-3018(24)00031-6.

25. Mills AM, Rizzardini G, Ramgopal MN, et al. Switch to fixed-dose doravirine (100 mg) with islatravir (0·75 mg) once daily in virologically suppressed adults with HIV-1 on bictegravir, emtricitabine, and tenofovir alafenamide: 48-week results of a phase 3, randomised, controlled, double-blind, non-inferiority trial. Lancet HIV 2024. S2352-3018(24)00030-4.

26. Doravirine/Islatravir (DOR/ISL) in Heavily Treatment-Experienced (HTE) Participants for Human Immunodeficiency Virus Type 1 (HIV-1) Infection (MK-8591A-019). [Clinical trial registration]. 2023. Available at: https://clinicaltrials.gov/study/NCT04233216. [Accessed 11 February 2024].

27. Squires KE, Correll TA, Robertson MN, et al. Effect of Islatravir on total lymphocyte and lymphocyte subset counts. Seattle, WA: Paper presented at: Conference on Retroviruses and Opportunistic Infections (CROI); 2023.

28. Vargo R, Robey S, Zang X, et al. Modeling to optimize islatravir QW dose in HIV virologically supressed PWH. Seattle, WA: Paper presented at: Conference on Retroviruses and Opportunistic Infections (CROI); 2023.

29. Diamond TL, Ngo W, Xu M, et al. Islatravir has a high barrier to resistance and exhibits a differentiated resistance profile from approved nucleoside reverse

transcriptase inhibitors (NRTIs). Antimicrob Agents Chemother 2022;66(6): e0013322.

30. Cilento ME, Reeve AB, Michailidis E, et al. Development of human immunodeficiency virus type 1 resistance to 4'-ethynyl-2-fluoro-2'-deoxyadenosine starting with wild-type or nucleoside reverse transcriptase inhibitor-resistant strains. Antimicrob Agents Chemother 2021;65(12):e0116721.

31. Rudd DJ, Cao Y, Vaddady P, et al. Modeling-Supported Islatravir Dose Selection for Phase 3, 2020, Paper presented at: Conference on Retroviruses and Opportunistic Infections (CROI); Boston, MA.

32. Aulicino PC, Sharma S, Truong K, et al. Variable antiviral activity of islatravir against M184I/V mutant HIV-1 selected during antiretroviral therapy. J Antimicrob Chemother 2024;79(2):370–4.

33. A Study of MK-8527 in Human Immunodeficiency Type 1 Virus (HIV-1) Infected Participants (MK-8527-002). 2020. Available at: https://classic.clinicaltrials.gov/ct2/show/results/NCT03615183. [Accessed 11 February 2024].

34. Schürmann D, Jackson Rudd D, Schaeffer A, et al. Single Oral Doses of MK-8507, a Novel Non-Nucleoside Reverse Transcriptase Inhibitor, Suppress HIV-1 RNA for a Week. J Acquir Immune Defic Syndr 2022;89(2):191–8.

35. Wang D, Lu W, Li F. Pharmacological intervention of HIV-1 maturation. Acta Pharm Sin B 2015;5(6):493–9.

36. Regueiro-Ren A, Sit SY, Chen Y, et al. The Discovery of GSK3640254, a Next-Generation Inhibitor of HIV-1 Maturation. J Med Chem 2022;65(18):11927–48.

37. Spinner CD, Felizarta F, Rizzardini G, et al. Phase IIa proof-of-concept evaluation of the antiviral efficacy, safety, tolerability, and pharmacokinetics of the next-generation maturation inhibitor GSK3640254. Clin Infect Dis 2022;75(5):786–94.

38. A Clinical Trial of GSK3640254 + Dolutegravir (DTG) in Human Immunodeficiency Virus-1 Infected Treatment-naive Adults. 2023. Available at: https://clinicaltrials.gov/study/NCT04900038. [Accessed 11 February 2024].

39. Benn PD, Zhang Y, Kahl L, et al. A phase I, first-in-human study investigating the safety, tolerability, and pharmacokinetics of the maturation inhibitor GSK3739937. Pharmacol Res Perspect 2023;11(3):e01093.

40. Shapiro RL, Ajibola G, Maswabi K, et al. Broadly neutralizing antibody treatment maintained HIV suppression in children with favorable reservoir characteristics in Botswana. Sci Transl Med 2023;15(703):eadh0004.

41. Sneller MC, Blazkova J, Justement JS, et al. Combination anti-HIV antibodies provide sustained virological suppression. Nature 2022;606(7913):375–81.

42. Zhou T, Zheng A, Baxa U, et al. A neutralizing antibody recognizing primarily n-linked glycan targets the silent face of the HIV envelope. Immunity 2018; 48(3):500–13.e506.

43. Pancera M, Shahzad-Ul-Hussan S, Doria-Rose NA, et al. Structural basis for diverse N-glycan recognition by HIV-1-neutralizing V1-V2-directed antibody PG16. Nat Struct Mol Biol 2013;20(7):804–13.

44. Gaebler C, Nogueira L, Stoffel E, et al. Prolonged viral suppression with anti-HIV-1 antibody therapy. Nature 2022;606(7913):368–74.

45. Lynch RM, Bar KJ. Development of screening assays for use of broadly neutralizing antibodies in people with HIV. Curr Opin HIV AIDS 2023;18(4):171–7.

46. Sharma VK, Misra B, McManus KT, et al. Characterization of co-formulated high-concentration broadly neutralizing anti-HIV-1 monoclonal antibodies for subcutaneous administration. Antibodies 2020;9(3).

47. Gautam R, Nishimura Y, Gaughan N, et al. A single injection of crystallizable fragment domain-modified antibodies elicits durable protection from SHIV infection. Nat Med 2018;24(5):610–6.
48. Eron JJ, Little SJ, Crofoot G, et al. Safety of teropavimab and zinlirvimab with lenacapavir once every 6 months for HIV treatment: a phase 1b, randomised, proof-of-concept study. Lancet HIV 2024. https://doi.org/10.1016/S2352-3018(23)00293-X.
49. Emu B, Fessel J, Schrader S, et al. Phase 3 Study of Ibalizumab for Multidrug-Resistant HIV-1. N Engl J Med 2018;379(7):645–54.
50. Wang CY, Wong WW, Tsai HC, et al. Effect of Anti-CD4 Antibody UB-421 on HIV-1 Rebound after Treatment Interruption. N Engl J Med 2019;380(16):1535–45.
51. Burkly LC, Olson D, Shapiro R, et al. Inhibition of HIV infection by a novel CD4 domain 2-specific monoclonal antibody. Dissecting the basis for its inhibitory effect on HIV-induced cell fusion. J Immunol 1992;149(5):1779–87.
52. Dickter JK, Martin AL, Ho S, et al. Ibalizumab-uiyk as a bridge therapy for a patient with drug-resistant HIV-1 infection receiving chemotherapy: A case report. J Clin Pharm Therapeut 2021;46(4):1185–7.
53. Chang XL, Reed JS, Webb GM, et al. Suppression of human and simian immunodeficiency virus replication with the CCR5-specific antibody Leronlimab in two species. PLoS Pathog 2022;18(3):e1010396.
54. Jacobson JM, Lalezari JP, Thompson MA, et al. Phase 2a study of the CCR5 monoclonal antibody PRO 140 administered intravenously to HIV-infected adults. Antimicrob Agents Chemother 2010;54(10):4137–42.
55. Dhody K, Kazempour K, Pourhassan N, et al. Pro 140 SC: long-acting, single-agent maintenance therapy for HIV-1 infection. Seattle, WA: Paper presented at: Conference on Retroviruses and Opportunistic Infections (CROI); 2019.
56. A Multicenter, Randomized, Double-blind, Placebo-controlled Trial, Followed by Single-arm Treatment of PRO 140 in Combination With Optimized Background Therapy in Treatment-Experienced HIV-1 Subjects. [Clinical trial registration], Available at: https://clinicaltrials.gov/study/NCT02483078 (Accessed 11 February 2024), 2022.

Switching Human Immunodeficiency Virus Therapy
Basic Principles and Options

Danilo Bacic Lima, MD[a,b], Daniel A. Solomon, MD[b,c],*

KEYWORDS

- HIV • ART • Switch • Antiretroviral

KEY POINTS

- Although contemporary first-line antiretroviral therapy (ART) is highly effective and well tolerated, there remain many scenarios in which clinicians and/or patients may choose to switch medications.
- Consideration of comorbidities, including renal function, bone health, cardiometabolic risk, as well as the prior ART and resistance history, is important to navigate ART switches safely and effectively.
- Simplification of medication regimens is associated with better adherence.
- Long-acting injectable ART is a novel option for human immunodeficiency virus treatment and offers a switch strategy for patients with virologic suppression who prefer to avoid daily oral medications.

INTRODUCTION

The number of options for antiretroviral therapies (ARTs) has expanded significantly over the years, providing patients with human immunodeficiency virus (HIV) with many treatment options. Including both stand-alone agents and combination pills, the current list exceeds 45 available Food and Drug Administration (FDA)–approved antiretrovirals (ARVs).[1] Navigating ART switches in treatment-experienced individuals can be complex, reflecting both the progress in the ART pipeline and unique considerations for individual patients. In this article, we review reasons to pursue ART switch and offer a guiding framework for selecting a new regimen. We then discuss specific recommendations and considerations, first focusing on patients with active viremia

^a Massachusetts General Hospital and Brigham & Women's Hospital; ^b Infectious Diseases Division, Brigham and Women's Hospital, 75 Francis Street, PBB-A4, Boston, MA 02115, USA; ^c Harvard Medical School
* Corresponding author. Infectious Diseases Division, Brigham and Women's Hospital, 75 Francis Street, PBB-A4, Boston, MA 02115.
E-mail address: dasolomon@bwh.harvard.edu
Twitter: @danbacic (D.B.L.)

Infect Dis Clin N Am 38 (2024) 409–422
https://doi.org/10.1016/j.idc.2024.04.002
0891-5520/24/© 2024 Elsevier Inc. All rights reserved.

id.theclinics.com

and then turning attention to optimizing treatment regimens in patients with viral suppression.

REASONS TO CONSIDER ANTIRETROVIRAL THERAPY SWITCH

In the United States, most patients who are engaged in care are virologically suppressed.[2] Treatment failure is typically associated with lapses in adherence, but can also stem from unrecognized drug resistance, suboptimal pharmacokinetics, inadequate absorption, or drug-drug interactions.[3] ART switch should always be considered for patients experiencing treatment failure, with a focus on identification of the underlying cause of virologic failure and the selection of an active regimen that patients can consistently tolerate, absorb, and adhere to.

For patients who are virologically suppressed, ART switch may be considered to simplify a regimen, enhance tolerability, prevent or mitigate drug-drug interactions, eliminate food requirements, switch to a long-acting (LA) injectable regimen, or reduce costs (**Box 1**).

While older regimens may achieve the goal of virologic suppression, newer options may offer advantages in safety, tolerability, and convenience. **Table 1** summarizes older medications clinicians may consider targeting for a switch.

PRACTICAL APPROACH TO ANTIRETROVIRAL THERAPY SWITCH

Once the decision to switch is made, the following framework can help guide the approach to ART switch: (1) compile a cumulative ART history and resistance assessment; (2) optimize efficacy and genetic barrier to resistance; (3) mitigate cumulative drug toxicity, exacerbation of comorbidities and drug-drug interactions; (4) incorporate patient preferences; and (5) follow-up and assess tolerability after the switch.

Box 1
List of common reasons to consider a switch in antiretroviral therapy[4]

Reasons for considering human immunodeficiency virus antiretroviral therapy switch

- Patient preferences
  - Regimen simplification to reduce pill burden and/or dosing frequency
  - Reduce pill size
  - Eliminate food requirements
  - Desire to use injectable long-acting medication
  - Desire to be on the same regimen as partner
  - Upcoming prolonged international travel

- Adverse events, risk for long-term complications, & comorbidities
  - Poor tolerability
  - Comorbid osteoporosis and osteopenia
  - Cardiometabolic risk, weight, and lipids
  - Change in renal function
  - Hepatitis B virus (HBV) coinfection
  - Drug-drug interactions

- Other safety considerations
  - Pregnancy and potential for pregnancy
  - Transition to a regimen with higher genetic barrier to resistance

- Reduce cost & consider insurance coverage of medications

Source: Optimizing Antiretroviral Therapy in the Setting of Virologic Suppression | NIH. Published May 26, 2023. Accessed March 24, 2024. https://clinicalinfo.hiv.gov/en/guidelines/hiv-clinical-guidelines-adult-and-adolescent-arv/optimizing-antiretroviral-therapy

Table 1
Summary of specific antiretroviral therapy agents that are either consistently targeted for switch or that may be targeted for switch

Medication Class	Reasons for Switch	Consistently Target for Switch	May Target for Switch
NRTIs	ABC: Potential increased cardiovascular risk. AZT: Bone marrow and mitochondrial toxicity.	Zidovudine (ZDV/AZT)	Abacavir (ABC)
NNRTIs	EFV: neuropsychiatric side effects, switch if depression. ETR: drug-drug interactions. NVP: Risk of life-threatening allergic reactions upon re-initiation.	-	Efavirenz (EFV) Etravirine (ETR) Nevirapine (NVP)
Older INSTIs	Higher barrier to resistance with DTG or BIC.	-	Raltegravir (RAL) Boosted Elvitegravir (EVG/c)
PIs	Increased cardiovascular risk (exception: ATV/r). Older PIs associated with numerous toxicities. Specific cases on boosted DRV (eg, due to resistance) may benefit from switching to DOR, FTR, or LEN.	Fosamprenavir Lopinavir-ritonavir (LPV/r) Tipranavir	Boosted atazanavir (ATV/r) Boosted darunavir (DRV/c or DRV/r)
Pk boosters	Risk for dangerous drug-drug interactions, for example, with corticosteroids. Cobicistat: pregnancy.	-	Cobicistat Ritonavir

Abbreviations: BIC, bictegravir; DOR, doravirine; DTG, dolutegravir; FTR, fostemsavir; INSTI, integrase strand transfer inhibitor; LEN, lenacapavir; NNRTI, non-nucleoside reverse transcriptase inhibitor; NRTI, nucleoside reverse transcriptase inhibitor; PI, protease inhibitor; Pk, pharmacokinetic.

Compile a Cumulative Antiretroviral Therapy History and Resistance Assessment

The first step in switching ART is a careful review of the patient's prior ART history and developing a cumulative genotype that includes all historical resistance mutations. During periods of ART interruption, there is often a reversion to wild-type virus dominance. Therefore, genotypes obtained greater than several weeks after treatment interruption may not capture certain mutations, especially those that have a discernible impact on viral fitness.[5,6] This underscores the importance of considering all available genotypes and entire treatment history, including any episodes of past ART changes that were prompted by virologic failure. For patients with virologic suppression, a standard genotype cannot be performed, therefore switch is guided by the ART history and cumulative genotypes. In situations when a patient's preceding ART history, genotypic information, and the occurrence of viral failure are uncertain, a proviral "archived" HIV DNA genotype may identify mutations in the viral reservoir. While helpful when a mutation is identified, the detection of proviral "archived" DNA mutations may not align perfectly with traditional RNA genotype mutations, and certain mutations may still go undetected. In addition, there is less clinical information about how proviral genotypes inform care, though some studies have shown its potential usefulness.[7] The selected switch regimen should maintain a comparable or higher relative barrier to resistance, especially when substantial uncertainty persists regarding the presence of prior mutations.

Maximize Efficacy and Genetic Barrier to Resistance

The genetic barrier to resistance roughly corresponds to the approximate number of mutations needed to render a specific ARV agent ineffective. Switching from a higher to a lower barrier to resistance regimen can increase the chance for treatment failure due to resistance patterns that may have been overlooked or are not available for review. Agents with high genetic barrier to resistance include second-generation integrase strand transfer inhibitors (INSTIs), bictegravir (BIC) and dolutegravir (DTG), or the protease inhibitor (PI) boosted darunavir (DRV). **Fig. 1** visually outlines the genetic barrier to resistance of commonly used ART drugs.[8]

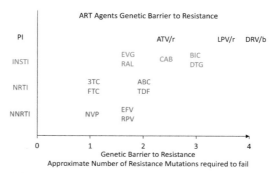

Fig. 1. Antiretroviral therapy (ART) class versus genetic barrier to resistance. ARTs in black font are protease inhibitors (PIs), those in red font are integrase strand transfer inhibitors (INSTIs), those in blue font are nucleotide reverse transcriptase inhibitors (NRTIs), those in green font are non-nucleotide reverse transcriptase inhibitors (NNRTIs). ABC, abacavir; ATV/r, ritonavir-boosted atazanavir; CAB, cabotegravir; DRV/b, ritonavir-boosted darunavir; DTG, dolutegravir; EFV, efavirenz; EVG, elvitegravir; FTC, emtricitabine; LPV/r, ritonavir-boosted lopinavir; NVP, nevirapine; RAL, raltegravir; RPV, rilpivirine; TDF, tenofovir; 3TC, lamivudine. (*Adapted from* Clutter DS et al.[8])

Consider Comorbid Conditions, Drug-Drug Interactions, and Cumulative Drug Toxicities

Considerations for ART switches should incorporate a review of underlying comorbidities with a focus on cardiometabolic disease, chronic kidney disease, and osteoporosis. ARVs that could exacerbate comorbid conditions should be avoided. For example, tenofovir disoproxil fumarate (TDF) should be avoided in patients with kidney disease or bone disease; tenofovir alafenamide (TAF) has less renal and bone toxicity and is preferred.[9] Similarly, abacavir and DRV have both been associated with increased risk of cardiac events in patients with underlying cardiovascular disease, and alternative agents should strongly be considered.[10,11] When switching ART in a person with hepatitis B virus (HBV) coinfection, the new regimen should contain tenofovir to reduce the risk for HBV reactivation and/or resistance.[12] In addition to review of medical comorbidities, it is important to consider both the introduction and the elimination of drug-drug interactions. In particular, discontinuation of pharmacokinetic boosters (ritonavir [RTV] or cobicistat) may require dose adjustments of many concomitant medications. These include statins, antihypertensives, warfarin, psychiatric medications, and numerous others.

Incorporate Patient Preferences

Discussing patient preferences, barriers to adherence, food requirements, pill burden and size, insurance coverage, cost, pregnancy, or potential for pregnancy is crucial to optimizing adherence and efficacy.

Pill burden and size

Pill burden and size are potential barriers to adherence for some patients and the simplification of medication regimens has been associated with improved adherence in clinical trials.[13,14] Fixed-dose combinations have the advantage of decreasing pill burden, preventing patients from taking partial regimens and reducing prescription errors.[14] **Table 2** offers a guide for considering pill size in the context of ART switches.[15,16] In the case of significant pill aversion, candidacy for long-acting (LA) injectable cabotegravir and rilpivirine (LA CAB/RPV) can be explored.

Food requirements

Certain ART agents have a food requirement for improved absorption, while others are best tolerated on an empty stomach (**Table 3**). An example of an important food requirement is RPV which requires a full meal for optimal absorption. Since RPV has a low barrier to resistance, optimizing systemic exposures is critical for avoiding virologic failure.

Pregnancy or the potential for pregnancy

For pregnant patients or those considering pregnancy, a regimen containing DTG, with either TDF or TAF, and either emtricitabine (FTC) or lamivudine (3TC) is preferred.[17] The continuation of regimens for which there are limited safety data such as LA CAB/RPV should be individualized, weighing risks and benefits. The use of cobicistat-boosted regimens is not recommended during pregnancy due to the larger volume of distribution yielding low serum drug levels with the risk for virologic failure.[18–20]

Follow-up and Tolerability Assessment

After modifying a patient's ART regimen, a follow-up at 4 to 8 weeks is recommended to assess tolerability, safety, and efficacy of the new regimen. HIV RNA viral load should be obtained to assess for viral response in patients who were viremic, and for viral rebound in patients who were previously virologically suppressed. This is also an opportunity for targeted laboratory testing if there were pre-existing

Table 2
Rank of commonly used fixed-dose combination pills by size of pill

Commonly Used Fixed-dose Combination Pills Ranked by Size of Pill	Pill Size (mm x mm) or Largest Dimension
DRV 800 mg/COBI 150 mg	23 mm
DRV 800 mg/COBI 150 mg/FTC 200 mg/TAF 10 mg	22 mm
ABC 600 mg/DTG 50 mg/3 TC 300 mg	22 x 11 mm
EFV 600 mg/FTC 200 mg/TDF 300 mg	20 mm
EVG 150 mg/COBI 150 mg/FTC 200 mg/TAF 10 mg	19 x 8.5 mm
TDF 300 mg/FTC 200 mg	19 x 8.5 mm
DTG 50 mg/3 TC 30 mg	19 mm
DOR 100 mg/3TC 300 mg/TDF 300 mg	19 mm
BIC 50 mg/FTC 200 mg/TAF 25 mg	15 x 8 mm
FTC 200 mg/RPV 25 mg/TAF 25 mg	15 mm
DTG 50 mg/RPV 25 mg	14 mm
FTC 200 mg/TAF 25 mg	12.5 x 6.4 mm

Abbreviations: ABC, abacavir; BIC, bictegravir; COBI, cobicistat; DOR, doravirine; DRV, darunavir; EFV, efavirenz; EVG, elvitegravir; FTC, emtricitabine; 3 TC, lamivudine; RPV, rilpivirine; TAF, tenofovir alafenamide; TDF, tenofovir disoproxil fumarate.[15]

Source Antiretroviral fixed-dose combination tablets: minimum body weights and considerations for use in children and adolescents | NIH, Available at: Accessed November 27, 2023. https://clinicalinfo.hiv.gov/en/guidelines/pediatric-arv/appendix-a-table-2-antiretroviral-fixed-dose-combination-tablets-and-copackaged-formulations.

abnormalities that prompted the switch. For example, if the switch was initiated by new renal dysfunction or lipid abnormality, re-assessment of comorbid conditions should be performed after the switch.

SELECTING A NEW REGIMEN

Turning now to specific regimens, we start by reviewing ART switch in the setting of treatment failure then discuss switching for treatment optimization in patients with viral suppression.

Table 3
Food requirement of commonly used antiretroviral therapy agents[15]

Antiretroviral Therapy Agents with a Food Requirement	Antiretroviral Therapy Agents that are Best Tolerated on an Empty Stomach	Antiretroviral Therapy Agents without Food Requirements
• Atazanavir	• Efavirenz	• Abacavir
• Cobicistat		• Bictegravir
• Darunavir		• Doravirine
• Etravirine		• Dolutegravir
• Rilpivirine		• Emtricitabine
• Ritonavir		• Lamivudine
		• Raltegravir
		• Tenofovir
		• Zidovudine

Source FDA-Approved HIV Medicines | NIH. Accessed December 1, 2023. https://hivinfo.nih.gov/understanding-hiv/fact-sheets/fda-approved-hiv-medicines

Switching in the Setting of Virologic Failure

The primary goal of treatment for ART-experienced individuals experiencing treatment failure is to establish virologic suppression. The selection of a new regimen can include 2 fully active ARVs if at least 1 drug has a high barrier to resistance[3] (**Fig. 1**). If no fully active drug with a high resistance barrier is available, then 3 fully active drugs should be included. Selected ARVs may include drugs from the same class with different resistance mechanism pathways, or drugs from classes to which the patient is naïve and the virus is susceptible. Some partially active drugs may be included especially when the drug may select for a virus with lower fitness. We review common scenarios in the following sections.

Virologic failure without resistance

Patients with no confirmed or suspected resistance mutations have all options available to them. Since virologic failure likely occurred secondary to poor adherence, the focus should be on overcoming barriers to taking ART regularly. Regimen selection can focus on similar attributes of initial therapy, aiming for treatments that are tolerable and convenient. Change in regimen must be paired with adherence support both before and after ART switch. Selection of a regimen with a high barrier to resistance is critical to minimize the risk of developing drug resistance in the future.

Long-acting injectable CAB/RPV is an emerging treatment option for patients who struggle to achieve viral suppression due to structural or social barriers to adherence to oral medications. One study demonstrated that after achieving virologic suppression with oral medications, injectable ART was superior to oral medications in maintaining HIV control.[21] There are limited data for the combination of LA CAB/RPV in people with active viremia. One study of patients with HIV in San Francisco with high rates of housing insecurity, mental illness, and substance use disorder showed a high efficacy of CAB/RPV even in patients with viremia[22] demonstrating proof of concept that this treatment strategy may be effective in select patient populations. In March 2024, the International Antiviral Society-USA panel updated guidelines to include consideration of LA CAB/RPV in people at high risk of HIV progression (CD4 < 200 or prior HIV-related opportunistic infection), consistently unable to take oral ART, and with virus susceptible to both CAB and RPV when supported by intensive follow-up and case management services.[23]

Virologic failure with nucleotide reverse transcriptase inhibitor resistance

Several studies have investigated optimal switch strategies for patients who have failed non-nucleotide reverse transcriptase inhibitor (NNRTI)–containing regimens and hence have nucleotide reverse transcriptase inhibitor (NRTI) mutations such as M184V, thymidine-associated mutations, or K65R.[24–26] Since the NRTIs retain some antiviral activity even in the presence of multiple resistance mutations, the use of "recycled" NRTIs (preferably tenofovir with either 3TC or FTC) plus a fully active high-resistance barrier drug (a boosted PI, DTG, or BIC) achieves virologic suppression in over 90% of persons with HIV.[27–29] The DAWNING trial assessed the efficacy of 2 NRTIs plus either lopinavir/ritonavir (LPV/r) or DTG in patients with virologic failure on a first-line NNRTI-based regimen. DTG was superior to LPV/r with 84% achieving suppression at week 48, though a small subset of patients in the INSTI arm developed DTG resistance.[25] In the NADIA (Nucleosides And Darunavir/Dolutegravir In Africa) trial of patients with virologic failure on a first-line regimen of 2 NRTIs and 1 NNRTI, a switch to DTG or DRV/r plus 2 NRTIs resulted in viral suppression in greater than 85% of participants in both arms at week 48.[24] In the setting of M184V, clinicians may continue 3TC or FTC alongside tenofovir as a strategy to preferentially select for M184V viral subpopulations, which imparts both a viral replication fitness cost and augments susceptibility to tenofovir.[30,31] Importantly, while active NNRTIs may be included in the new regimen, they should be avoided as the sole fully active agent given their relatively lower barrier to resistance.

For patients with isolated NRTI resistance, an alternative to continuing background NRTIs is a regimen with fully active boosted PI plus INSTI. In multiple trials of first-line treatment failure, LPV/r plus raltegravir (RAL) has proved as effective as LPV/r plus 2 NRTIs.[32] Since LPV/r and RAL are no longer recommended, the current preferred approach is boosted DRV (either with RTV or cobicistat) plus DTG. The high efficacy of this regimen was demonstrated in the D^2EFT (Dolutegravir and Darunavir Evaluation in Adults Failing Therapy) study, which showed it was superior to DRV/r plus recycled NRTIs.[33]

Virologic failure with integrase strand transfer inhibitor and nucleotide reverse transcriptase inhibitor resistance

Virologic failure in patients on a regimen that included first-generation INSTIs such as RAL or elvitegravir plus 2 NRTIs can occur with resistance to NRTIs, INSTIs, or both.[34] In contrast, in the few patients who have viral failure on regimens with second-generation INSTIs (DTG, BIC) plus 2 NRTIs, resistance to DTG or BIC remains uncommon, underscoring the higher barrier to resistance of these medications.[35,36] Viruses with resistance to first-generation INSTIs sometimes retain susceptibility to DTG and BIC, but in this setting DTG should be dosed twice daily to prevent emergence of additional resistance mutations.[37]

For patients with high-level INSTI resistance, regimens should include at least 2 and ideally 3 medications which are fully active. Available options may include drugs from classes not previously used or drugs from a recycled class with known activity against virus if deemed susceptible on resistance testing. Boosted darunavir may be an option if the virus is susceptible and may require twice-daily dosing if major darunavir mutations are present. Doravirine is an NNRTI with a unique pathway of resistance that often retains activity even in the presence of some NNRTI mutations.[38] Maraviroc can be considered for R5-tropic virus. Several medications with novel mechanisms of action have been approved which specifically target heavily treatment-experienced patients with multiclass resistance. These new agents include ibalizumab, fostemsavir, and lenacapavir. They may be particularly useful for patients who are resistant to boosted darunavir, experience drug-drug interactions due to pharmacokinetic boosting, or have significant cardiovascular risk. Drugs with partial activity such as recycled NRTIs (tenofovir/3TC or FTC) may be added to the regimen but should not replace fully active agents. In this issue, there is a comprehensive review of medications in the HIV pipeline that hold promise to expand treatment options for patients with highly resistant virus.

Optimizing Antiretroviral Therapy in the Setting of Viral Suppression

The goal of switching therapy in patients with viral suppression is to select a new regimen that maintains viral suppression while optimizing effectiveness, safety, convenience, and cost. Maintaining virologic suppression is easier than achieving it in patients with active viremia for several reasons. First, patients who are suppressed are generally adherent to their medications; second, there is no active viral replication; and finally, the virus is less likely to harbor resistance mutations. These factors allow for ART switch without introducing the risk for emergent resistance. This is most relevant for patients switching from a boosted-PI regimen to a second-generation INSTI. In contrast to the cases of emergent DTG resistance in the NADIA and DAWNING trials as discussed earlier, in the 2SD (Second-line Switch to Dolutegravir Study) trial of virologically suppressed patients on a regimen of 2 NRTIs plus RTV-boosted PI, there was no emergent resistance in individuals who were switched from the boosted-PI to DTG.[39] As a result, patients with virologic suppression with no confirmed or suspected history of resistance mutations or virologic failure have all options available to them and can transition to a new regimen without the need for further testing.[3] In addition to standard 3-drug regimens, patients with viral suppression are also eligible for a switch to select 2-drug oral regimens and LA injectable medication. These strategies are discussed in more detail in the following sections.

Switching to 2-drug oral regimens

Several 2-drug regimens have proved safe and effective for select patients and can decrease cumulative drug exposure. Combination DTG/RPV, approved in November 2017, was the first complete single-tablet regimen consisting of only 2 drugs. In 2 identical phase 3, open-label trials, SWORD-1 and SWORD-2 treatment-experienced participants without NNRTI or INSTI resistance, a history of treatment failure, and with good virological control were randomized to switch to DTG plus RPV or remain on their current ART. Participants who were switched to DTG plus RPV maintained virological suppression at 48 weeks, and experienced fewer adverse events with better renal and bone outcomes than participants who remained on their current ART.[40] The renal and bone benefits were accrued from cessation of TDF in the baseline regimen. Multiple observational studies have confirmed that patients maintain durable virological suppression after switching to DTG plus RPV.[41,42] Co-formulated DTG/RPV is an NRTI-sparing regimen for patients with contraindications to or intolerance of NRTIs, or patients with renal impairment as exposure to DTG and RPV is not affected by decreased renal function.

DTG/3TC is another 2-drug regimen that has proven highly effective at maintaining virologic suppression in patients without NRTI or INSTI resistance. Multiple switch studies have demonstrated maintenance of viral suppression when patients are transitioned to DTG plus 3TC, including 2 large phase 3 switch studies, TANGO and SALSA , which both showed that DTG plus 3TC was non-inferior in maintaining virologic suppression when compared with continuing current ARV regimens.[43,44] There are also observational studies showing that DTG/3TC is effective even in patients with complex past treatment histories, but this regimen should not be used in patients with a history of 3TC resistance.[45]

Tenofovir-sparing 2-drug regimens may be of particular benefit for patients with chronic kidney disease or osteoporosis. However, these regimens should not be used in patients with HIV/HBV coinfection unless another antiviral such as entecavir is added to treat HBV.

Switching to long-acting injectable cabotegravir-rilpivirine

In 2021, the FDA approved the first long-acting (LA) injectable treatment, LA CAB/RPV. The ATLAS (Antiretroviral Therapy as Long-Acting Suppression) trial compared LA CAB/RPV versus continuation of current oral therapy in treatment-experienced patients with virologic control and no baseline NNRTI or INSTI resistance. The LA injectable arm was non-inferior at week 48 with 1.6% of participants found to have HIV-1 RNA $\geq$ 50 copies/mL compared to 1.0% in the oral arm.[46] In the follow-up ATLAS-2M study, the efficacy of CAB/RPV injections administered every 8 weeks was non-inferior to every 4 weeks with 2% and 1% virologic failure, respectively.[46] Risk factors for virologic failure on injectable CAB/RPV include any resistance to rilpivirine, subtype A6/A1 virus, and body mass index above 30.[47]

This treatment regimen is currently approved as a monthly or bimonthly intramuscular injection for patients who are virally suppressed, and do not have HBV coinfection, without INSTI or NNRTI resistance. Although patients with the K103N resistance mutation were included in the original studies, LA CAB/RPV in these patients should be approached with caution due to the risk of unrecognized additional NNRTI mutations. Injectable ART is an appealing option for patients who have pill aversion, have a desire for increased convenience, or have concerns about confidentiality. Patients must be able to reliably present to their monthly or bimonthly injection appointments but can temporarily transition back to oral therapy if needed, for example, in the case of travel or missed appointments. The switch to injectable ART can create cumbersome clinical operations with increased number of visits, prior authorizations, and staff required for safe administration of the medications.

SUMMARY

The guiding principles for safely navigating ART switches highlight the importance of a careful review of the patient's ART history and genotypes, optimizing for efficacy and genetic barrier to resistance, while also considering cumulative drug toxicities, comorbidities, and patient preferences. For patients who are viremic, focus should be on selection a fully active regimen paired with adherence support. LA injectable medication may be a salvage option for patients with viremia with barriers to adherence to oral regimens. For patients who are virologically suppressed, 2-drug regimens and LA injectable regimens offer potential advantages in tolerability, safety, cumulative drug exposure, and convenience. The ART pipeline holds promise for newer options for patients with multiclass resistance as well as additional options for LA alternatives to daily medications.

CLINICS CARE POINTS

- When contemplating an ART switch, thoroughly review the complete HIV treatment history and compile a comprehensive aggregate of all prior genotypes to inform the choice of the new regimen.
- Patients with no resistance and no history of virologic failure can be safely switched to regimens generally recommended for first-line therapy.
- Preferentially opt for regimens with a high genetic barrier to resistance to minimize the risk of virologic failure.
- In patients with renal disease or bone disease, consider tenofovir-sparing 2-drug regimens such as DTG/3TC or DTG/RPV.
- LA injectable ART offers a unique treatment modality for patients who prefer to avoid daily oral medications.

DISCLOSURE

The authors have nothing to disclose.

REFERENCES

1. Appendix A. Table 2. Antiretroviral fixed-dose combination tablets: minimum body weights and considerations for use in children and adolescents | NIH. Available at: https://clinicalinfo.hiv.gov/en/guidelines/pediatric-arv/appendix-a-table-

2-antiretroviral-fixed-dose-combination-tablets-and-copackaged-formulations. [Accessed 27 November 2023].

2. HIV Surveillance | Reports| Resource Library | HIV/AIDS | CDC. 2024. Available at: https://www.cdc.gov/hiv/library/reports/hiv-surveillance.html. [Accessed 24 March 2024].

3. Virologic Failure | Clinicalinfo.HIV.gov. 2023. Available at: https://clinicalinfo.hiv.gov/en/guidelines/hiv-clinical-guidelines-adult-and-adolescent-arv/virologic-failure. [Accessed 24 March 2024].

4. Optimizing Antiretroviral Therapy in the Setting of Virologic Suppression | NIH 2023. Available at: https://clinicalinfo.hiv.gov/en/guidelines/hiv-clinical-guidelines-adult-and-adolescent-arv/optimizing-antiretroviral-therapy. [Accessed 24 March 2024].

5. Miller V, Sabin C, Hertogs K, et al. Virological and immunological effects of treatment interruptions in HIV-1 infected patients with treatment failure. AIDS Lond Engl 2000;14(18):2857–67.

6. Verhofstede C, Wanzeele FV, Van Der Gucht B, et al. Interruption of reverse transcriptase inhibitors or a switch from reverse transcriptase to protease inhibitors resulted in a fast reappearance of virus strains with a reverse transcriptase inhibitor-sensitive genotype. AIDS Lond Engl 1999;13(18):2541–6.

7. Ellis KE, Nawas GT, Chan C, et al. Clinical Outcomes Following the Use of Archived Proviral HIV-1 DNA Genotype to Guide Antiretroviral Therapy Adjustment. Open Forum Infect Dis 2020;7(1):ofz533.

8. Clutter DS, Jordan MR, Bertagnolio S, et al. HIV-1 Drug Resistance and Resistance Testing. Infect Genet Evol J Mol Epidemiol Evol Genet Infect Dis 2016; 46:292–307.

9. Sax PE, Wohl D, Yin MT, et al. Tenofovir alafenamide versus tenofovir disoproxil fumarate, coformulated with elvitegravir, cobicistat, and emtricitabine, for initial treatment of HIV-1 infection: two randomised, double-blind, phase 3, non-inferiority trials. Lancet Lond Engl 2015;385(9987):2606–15.

10. Triant VA, Siedner MJ. Darunavir and cardiovascular risk: evaluating the data to inform clinical care. J Infect Dis 2020;221(4):498–500.

11. Cruciani M, Zanichelli V, Serpelloni G, et al. Abacavir use and cardiovascular disease events: a meta-analysis of published and unpublished data. AIDS Lond Engl 2011;25(16):1993–2004.

12. Benhamou Y, Bochet M, Thibault V, et al. Long-term incidence of hepatitis B virus resistance to lamivudine in human immunodeficiency virus-infected patients. Hepatol Baltim Md 1999;30(5):1302–6.

13. Langebeek N, Gisolf EH, Reiss P, et al. Predictors and correlates of adherence to combination antiretroviral therapy (ART) for chronic HIV infection: a meta-analysis. BMC Med 2014;12:142.

14. Nachega JB, Mugavero MJ, Zeier M, et al. Treatment simplification in HIV-infected adults as a strategy to prevent toxicity, improve adherence, quality of life and decrease healthcare costs. Patient Prefer Adherence 2011;5:357–67.

15. FDA-Approved HIV Medicines | NIH. Available at: https://hivinfo.nih.gov/understanding-hiv/fact-sheets/fda-approved-hiv-medicines. [Accessed 1 December 2023].

16. Table 7. Antiretroviral regimen considerations for initial therapy based on specific clinical scenarios | NIH. 2022. Available at: https://clinicalinfo.hiv.gov/en/guidelines/hiv-clinical-guidelines-adult-and-adolescent-arv/table-7-antiretroviral-regimen. [Accessed 24 March 2024].

17. Overview | NIH. 2023. Available at: https://clinicalinfo.hiv.gov/en/guidelines/perinatal/recommendations-arv-drugs-pregnancy-overview. [Accessed 1 December 2023].

18. Cobicistat (Tybost, COBI) | NIH. Available at: https://clinicalinfo.hiv.gov/en/guidelines/perinatal/safety-toxicity-arv-agents-pharmacoenhancers-cobicistat-tybost. [Accessed 1 December 2023].

19. Crauwels HM, Osiyemi O, Zorrilla C, et al. Reduced exposure to darunavir and cobicistat in HIV-1-infected pregnant women receiving a darunavir/cobicistat-based regimen. HIV Med 2019;20(5):337–43.

20. Momper JD, Wang J, Stek A, et al. Pharmacokinetics of Atazanavir Boosted With Cobicistat in Pregnant and Postpartum Women With HIV. J Acquir Immune Defic Syndr 1999 2022;89(3):303–9.

21. Rana AI, Bao Y, et al. Long-acting injectable CAB/RPV is superior to oral ART in PWH with adherence Challenges: ACTG A5359. Abstract #212. Denver, Colorado: Presented at Conference on Retroviruses and Opportunistic Infections; 2024.

22. Gandhi M, Hickey M, Imbert E, et al. Demonstration project of long-acting antiretroviral therapy in a diverse population of people with HIV. Ann Intern Med 2023; 176(7):969–74.

23. Sax PE, Thompson MA, Saag MS, IAS-USA Treatment Guidelines Panel. Updated treatment recommendation on use of cabotegravir and rilpivirine for people with HIV from the IAS-USA guidelines panel. JAMA 2024. https://doi.org/10.1001/jama.2024.2985.

24. Paton NI, Musaazi J, Kityo C, et al. Dolutegravir or Darunavir in Combination with Zidovudine or Tenofovir to Treat HIV. N Engl J Med 2021;385(4):330–41.

25. Aboud M, Kaplan R, Lombaard J, et al. Dolutegravir versus ritonavir-boosted lopinavir both with dual nucleoside reverse transcriptase inhibitor therapy in adults with HIV-1 infection in whom first-line therapy has failed (DAWNING): an open-label, non-inferiority, phase 3b trial. Lancet Infect Dis 2019;19(3):253–64.

26. Acosta RK, Willkom M, Andreatta K, et al. Switching to Bictegravir/Emtricitabine/Tenofovir Alafenamide (B/F/TAF) From Dolutegravir (DTG)+F/TAF or DTG+F/Tenofovir Disoproxil Fumarate (TDF) in the Presence of Pre-existing NRTI Resistance. J Acquir Immune Defic Syndr 1999 2020;85(3):363–71.

27. Campbell TB, Shulman NS, Johnson SC, et al. Antiviral activity of lamivudine in salvage therapy for multidrug-resistant HIV-1 infection. Clin Infect Dis 2005; 41(2):236–42.

28. Ciaffi L, Koulla-Shiro S, Sawadogo AB, et al. Boosted protease inhibitor monotherapy versus boosted protease inhibitor plus lamivudine dual therapy as second-line maintenance treatment for HIV-1-infected patients in sub-Saharan Africa (ANRS12 286/MOBIDIP): a multicentre, randomised, parallel, open-label, superiority trial. Lancet HIV 2017;4(9):e384–92.

29. Deeks SG, Hoh R, Neilands TB, et al. Interruption of treatment with individual therapeutic drug classes in adults with multidrug-resistant HIV-1 infection. J Infect Dis 2005;192(9):1537–44.

30. Turner D, Brenner B, Wainberg MA. Multiple effects of the M184V resistance mutation in the reverse transcriptase of human immunodeficiency virus type 1. Clin Diagn Lab Immunol 2003;10(6):979–81.

31. Whitcomb JM, Parkin NT, Chappey C, et al. Broad nucleoside reverse-transcriptase inhibitor cross-resistance in human immunodeficiency virus type 1 clinical isolates. J Infect Dis 2003;188(7):992–1000.

32. SECOND-LINE Study Group, Boyd MA, Kumarasamy N, et al. Ritonavir-boosted lopinavir plus nucleoside or nucleotide reverse transcriptase inhibitors versus ritonavir-boosted lopinavir plus raltegravir for treatment of HIV-1 infection in adults with virological failure of a standard first-line ART regimen (SECOND-LINE): a randomised, open-label, non-inferiority study. Lancet Lond Engl 2013; 381(9883):2091–9.

33. D2EFT: Dolutegravir and Darunavir evaluation in adults failing first-line NNRTI therapy. Abstract #12. Presented at Conference on Retroviruses and Opportunistic Infections (CROI). 2023. Available at: https://www.natap.org/2023/CROI/croi_34.htm. [Accessed 24 March 2024].

34. White KL, Raffi F, Miller MD. Resistance analyses of integrase strand transfer inhibitors within phase 3 clinical trials of treatment-naive patients. Viruses 2014; 6(7):2858–79.

35. Sax PE, Pozniak A, Montes ML, et al. Coformulated bictegravir, emtricitabine, and tenofovir alafenamide versus dolutegravir with emtricitabine and tenofovir alafenamide, for initial treatment of HIV-1 infection (GS-US-380-1490): a randomised, double-blind, multicentre, phase 3, non-inferiority trial. Lancet Lond Engl 2017; 390(10107):2073–82.

36. Gallant J, Lazzarin A, Mills A, et al. Bictegravir, emtricitabine, and tenofovir alafenamide versus dolutegravir, abacavir, and lamivudine for initial treatment of HIV-1 infection (GS-US-380-1489): a double-blind, multicentre, phase 3, randomised controlled non-inferiority trial. Lancet Lond Engl 2017;390(10107):2063–72.

37. Saladini F, Giannini A, Boccuto A, et al. Comparable in vitro activities of second-generation HIV-1 integrase strand transfer inhibitors (INSTIs) on HIV-1 clinical isolates with INSTI resistance mutations. Antimicrob Agents Chemother 2019;64(1): e01717–9.

38. Martin EA, Lai MT, Ngo W, et al. Review of doravirine resistance patterns identified in participants during clinical development. J Acquir Immune Defic Syndr 1999 2020;85(5):635–42.

39. Ombajo LA, Penner J, Nkuranga J, et al. Second-line switch to dolutegravir for treatment of HIV infection. N Engl J Med 2023;388(25):2349–59.

40. Aboud M, Orkin C, Podzamczer D, et al. Efficacy and safety of dolutegravir–rilpivirine for maintenance of virological suppression in adults with HIV-1: 100-week data from the randomised, open-label, phase 3 SWORD-1 and SWORD-2 studies. Lancet HIV 2019;6(9):e576–87.

41. Palacios R, Mayorga M, González-Domenech CM, et al. Safety and efficacy of dolutegravir plus rilpivirine in treatment-experienced HIV-infected patients: the DORIVIR study. J Int Assoc Provid AIDS Care 2018;17. 2325958218760847.

42. Capetti AF, Cossu MV, Sterrantino G, et al. Dolutegravir plus rilpivirine as a switch option in cART-experienced patients: 96-week data. Ann Pharmacother 2018; 52(8):740–6.

43. Van Wyk J, Ajana F, Bisshop F, et al. Efficacy and safety of switching to dolutegravir/lamivudine fixed-dose 2-drug regimen vs continuing a tenofovir alafenamide–based 3- or 4-drug regimen for maintenance of virologic suppression in adults living with human immunodeficiency virus type 1: phase 3, randomized, noninferiority TANGO study. Clin Infect Dis 2020;71(8):1920–9.

44. Llibre JM, Brites C, Cheng CY, et al. Efficacy and safety of switching to the 2-drug regimen dolutegravir/lamivudine versus continuing a 3- or 4-drug regimen for maintaining virologic suppression in adults living with human immunodeficiency virus 1 (HIV-1): week 48 results from the phase 3, noninferiority SALSA Randomized Trial. Clin Infect Dis 2023;76(4):720–9.

45. Suárez-García I, Alejos B, Hernando V, et al. Effectiveness and tolerability of do-lutegravir/lamivudine for the treatment of HIV-1 infection in clinical practice. J Antimicrob Chemother 2023;78(6):1423–32.

46. Overton ET, Richmond G, Rizzardini G, et al. Long-acting cabotegravir and rilpi-virine dosed every 2 months in adults with HIV-1 infection (ATLAS-2M), 48-week results: a randomised, multicentre, open-label, phase 3b, non-inferiority study. Lancet 2020;396(10267):1994–2005.

47. Orkin C, Schapiro JM, Perno CF, et al. Expanded multivariable models to assist patient selection for long-acting cabotegravir + rilpivirine treatment: clinical utility of a combination of patient, drug concentration, and viral factors associated with virologic failure. Clin Infect Dis Off Publ Infect Dis Soc Am 2023;77(10):1423–31.

Advances in HIV Management During Pregnancy and Infant Feeding

Mariana Espinal, MD, Lynn M. Yee, MD, MPH*,
Stephanie A. Fisher, MD, MPH

KEYWORDS

- HIV • Antiretroviral therapy • Integrase inhibitors • Pregnancy • Infant feeding
- Breastfeeding • Lactation

KEY POINTS

- HIV testing should be performed for all pregnant individuals at initiation of prenatal care, with repeat third trimester testing indicated for individuals at high risk of HIV infection based on risk factors and/or residence in areas with high HIV incidence. Universal repeat third trimester testing is employed in some regions and should be considered given the limitations of risk-based screening.
- Dolutegravir is a *preferred* drug of choice in pregnancy and breastfeeding people with HIV, and bictegravir is now considered an *alternative* drug for this population.
- Previously excluded from clinical trials evaluating novel antiretroviral regimens, pregnant and breastfeeding people with HIV should be included in drug trials from the time of study inception to provide timely safety and pharmacokinetic data in this population.
- Shared decision-making regarding method of infant feeding with a multidisciplinary health care team should be employed early and often throughout pregnancy, at delivery, and postpartum, with avoidance of breastfeeding and use of replacement feeding methods (eg, formula or donor human milk) considered the only way to assure 0 risk of postnatal HIV transmission. If breastfeeding is chosen, expert consultation regarding risk-reducing measures is necessary.

INTRODUCTION

Prevention of perinatal human immunodeficiency virus (HIV) transmission represents a significant triumph in contemporary medical practice. Perinatal HIV transmission occurs during pregnancy (ie, transplacental) or labor and delivery, while postnatal HIV transmission occurs through breastfeeding. Perinatal HIV transmission has previously

Division of Maternal-Fetal Medicine, Department of Obstetrics and Gynecology, Northwestern University Feinberg School of Medicine, 250 East Superior Street, Suite 05-2303, Chicago, IL, USA
* Corresponding author.
E-mail address: lynn.yee@northwestern.edu

Infect Dis Clin N Am 38 (2024) 423–452
https://doi.org/10.1016/j.idc.2024.06.005   **id.theclinics.com**
0891-5520/24/© 2024 Elsevier Inc. All rights reserved, including those for text and data mining, AI training, and similar technologies.

been referred to as vertical or mother-to-child transmission, although the latter term is not recommended. Since the 1990s, perinatal transmission has decreased substantially, largely due to the use of combination antiretroviral therapy (ART). Rates of perinatally acquired HIV infections in the United States decreased from 74 in 2010 to 32 in 2019, representing a decline in annual perinatal HIV diagnosis rates from 1.9 to 0.9 per 100,000 live births, and perinatal HIV transmission rates from 1.6% to 0.9%.[1] Data on safety, virologic efficacy, and pharmacokinetics (PK) support ART use in pregnancy. In addition, universal HIV screening of pregnant people has improved detection of HIV, facilitating implementation of several strategies to prevent perinatal and postnatal transmission, including early initiation of ART to achieve virologic suppression and special considerations regarding mode of delivery, infant post-exposure prophylaxis (PEP), and feeding.[2] Substantial progress has been achieved on a global scale with the advancements in perinatal HIV care over the past 2 decades; nevertheless, much work remains to be done.

The authors will review the latest advancements in HIV management that are revolutionizing pregnancy and postpartum care in pursuit of elimination of perinatal HIV transmission.

HUMAN IMMUNODEFICIENCY VIRUS TESTING DURING PREGNANCY AND POSTPARTUM

Pregnancy and the peripartum period are times of heightened risk of HIV acquisition due to both behavioral factors, such as engagement in unprotected sex and increased risk of sexual violence, and physiologic changes, including alterations in innate and adaptive immunity. Detection of HIV infection should ideally occur prior to conception or as early as possible during pregnancy to facilitate early virologic control and effectively eliminate perinatal transmission. For this reason, universal, voluntary opt-out HIV testing in the United States has been recommended for all pregnant people since 1999 by the Institute of Medicine, including those who present in labor or at delivery with unknown HIV status, based on clear evidence that antepartum, intrapartum, and postpartum interventions are associated with marked reduction in risk of perinatal transmission.[3]

To facilitate early HIV diagnosis and ART initiation in pregnancy, HIV testing should be completed as early as the pregnant person seeks care, including during emergency department and prenatal visits. Furthermore, HIV testing should be incorporated in preconception counseling in non-pregnant people considering pregnancy. Similar to the care of non-pregnant individuals, the preferred screening test is a fourth-generation or fifth-generation HIV antigen/antibody immunoassay, followed by an HIV-1/HIV-2 antibody differentiation assay.[4] Individuals with a reactive antigen/antibody immunoassay and a nonreactive antibody differentiation assay or with negative screening test but clinical symptoms that could be consistent with acute HIV should undergo viral load testing with a plasma HIV RNA assay to assess for acute HIV infection during the window period before the HIV-1 or HIV-2 antibody can be detected.[5]

Despite universal HIV testing in early pregnancy, perinatal transmissions can occur when maternal HIV is acquired after initial testing. Most (80%) perinatal HIV transmissions occur between 36 weeks' gestation and delivery, highlighting that even late detection of maternal HIV represents an opportunity for implementation of prevention measures. Thus, repeat third trimester HIV testing is recommended for people who are at increased risk of acquiring HIV (eg, individuals who engage in injection drug use, exchange sex for money or drugs, have a partner with HIV, have multiple new sex partners during pregnancy, have suspected or diagnosed sexually transmitted or other genitourinary tract infections, incarceration, or recent immigration from high-burden HIV areas), live in areas of high HIV incidence, or exhibit signs or symptoms of acute HIV infection.[6–8] Studies have affirmed that repeat third trimester screening is cost-effective, and at least 15 states (Arizona, Connecticut, Delaware, Florida, Georgia, Illinois, Louisiana, Maryland, Nevada, New Jersey, North Carolina, Tennessee, Texas, Virginia, and West Virginia) have statutes that mandate universal third trimester HIV testing, with testing performed for neonates if maternal testing is missed or declined.[9–12] At the local level, some institutions have further instituted universal testing intrapartum on their labor and delivery units, including in individuals who previously had negative first and third trimester testing, to further prevent missed cases of late sero-conversion prior to delivery.

Given available intrapartum and postpartum interventions to minimize perinatal transmission, and the limitations of risk-based screening that may contribute to missed diagnoses, HIV testing should be completed in pregnant people with unknown or undocumented HIV status who present to care in labor before delivery or during the immediate postpartum period.[8,11,13] Moreover, assessing the risk of HIV exposure should not be limited to the pregnancy and should be extended to the postpartum period; all breastfeeding individuals need to know their HIV status, and individuals who are at elevated risk of HIV acquisition should be counseled about their increased risk in the postpartum period related to hormonal, immune, and other physiologic changes postpartum.[14] Therefore, postpartum individuals who have signs or symptoms of acute HIV infection should also undergo HIV testing, and the results should guide recommendations on infant feeding.[15]

CLINICS CARE POINTS

- HIV infection should be identified before pregnancy or as early as possible during pregnancy through universal testing.
- Repeat third trimester HIV testing is recommended for people who are at increased risk of acquiring HIV or who are living in areas of high HIV incidence. The authors recommend universal repeat third trimester, which is already mandated by state public health laws or guidelines in some regions of the country.
- Pregnant people with unknown or undocumented HIV status who present to care in labor should be tested before delivery or as soon as possible after delivery.
- HIV testing should be performed any time there is concern for acute HIV infection, including during the postpartum period.
- When the birthing parent's HIV testing is unavailable, the infant should undergo HIV testing.

ANTIRETROVIRAL THERAPY IN PREGNANCY
Preferred and Alternative Regimens

Achieving virologic suppression during pregnancy is essential for the health of pregnant PWH and their offspring. Rapid reduction of the birthing parent's viral load to undetectable as early as possible in pregnancy reduces the risk of antenatal and intrapartum HIV transmission. Based on pharmacokinetic, efficacy, and safety considerations during pregnancy, the US Department of Health and Human Services (DHHS) Perinatal HIV Clinical Guidelines categorize antiretroviral drugs into 5 groups for their utilization during pregnancy: preferred, alternative, lacking sufficient data for recommendation, not recommended except under specific conditions, and not recommended.[8]

Since 2014, after observing the rapid virologic suppression achieved with integrase strand-transfer inhibitor (INSTI)-based regimens, the US Panel on Antiretroviral Guidelines for Adults and Adolescents identified dolutegravir (DTG) as a recommended agent for nonpregnant PWH.[16,17] One study of nonpregnant adults demonstrated INSTI-based regimens achieved initial virologic suppression in 21.4 days compared to 58.6 days for non-INSTI regimens.[18] INSTI-based ART also results in more rapid virologic suppression in pregnancy, and faster first-phase HIV RNA half-life decay, compared to that achieved with other frequently used first-line regimens.[19,20]

Preliminary findings from a prospective study in Botswana regarding a potential association of periconceptional DTG exposure and neural tube defects led the World Health Organization and DHHS Guidelines to initially issue guidance in 2018 against DTG's use as a first-line agent in pregnancy; however, these findings were not confirmed in larger follow-up studies, effectively absolving this earlier concern.[21–23] INSTI-based regimens are preferred in pregnancy, and dolutegravir (DTG) is currently considered the first-line INSTI of choice.[8] The endorsement of DTG-based ART in pregnancy is backed by safety and effectiveness data from the Dolutegravir in Pregnant HIV Mothers and Their Neonates (DolPHIN-1 and DolPHIN-2) and International Maternal Pediatric Adolescent AIDS Clinical Trials Network (IMPAACT) 2010/Virologic Efficacy and Safety of ART Combinations with Tenofovir, Efavirenz [EFV], and DTG (VESTED) trials.[24]

The DolPHIN-1 and DolPHIN-2 trials randomized pregnant, treatment-naïve PWH to either DTG-containing or EFV-containing ART and found that both regimens were well-tolerated with no significant differences in frequency of adverse events or congenital anomalies; however, DTG achieved significantly faster viral suppression.[25,26] The IMPAACT 2010/VESTED trial completed a multicenter, open-label, randomized controlled, phase 3 trial in 9 countries in pregnant, treatment-naïve PWH randomized to either DTG/emtricitabine (FTC)/tenofovir alafenamide fumarate (TAF), DTG/FTC/tenofovir disoproxil fumarate (TDF), or EFV/FTC/TDF. DTG-containing ART, compared to EFV/FTC/TDF, had superior virological efficacy at delivery and postpartum, and lower frequency of adverse pregnancy and neonatal outcomes.[27,28] Additionally, Patel and colleagues on behalf of the Pediatric HIV/AIDS Cohort Study compared the effectiveness of DTG-based ART regimens with non-DTG-based regimens in 1257 pregnant individuals, and found that DTG-based ART was superior to several non-DTG-based regimens in achieving viral suppression at delivery without increasing adverse birth outcomes.[29] As a result, the DHHS Guidelines now advocate for DTG as the preferred medication when selecting initial INSTI-based regimens for pregnant PWH, in combination with a dual-nucleoside reverse transcriptase inhibitors (NRTI) backbone (eg, abacavir (ABC)/lamivudine (3TC), TAF/FTC, TAF/3TC, TDF/FTC, or TDF/3TC). An exception to this consideration is for pregnant PWH with a history of cabotegravir (CAB) exposure for pre-exposure prophylaxis (PrEP), where initiating a protease inhibitor (PI)-based ART regimen is recommended due to concerns regarding INSTI resistance mutations.[8,24]

Previously indexed under the category of insufficient data for use as initial ART regimen in pregnancy, bictegravir (BIC) was upgraded in 2024 to an *alternative* drug when selecting an INSTI-based regimen in pregnant PWH after several prospective studies demonstrated it was a safe, efficacious option for the treatment of HIV in women.[8,30,31] Several case reports and clinical trials designed to monitor both PK parameters and virologic response to BIC have disproven initial concerns regarding the attainment of adequate plasma concentrations for therapeutic efficacy of BIC during pregnancy, stemming from its metabolism by CYP3A4 and UGT1A1 and physiologic alterations in pregnancy such as enzyme induction.[32,33] Prospective BIC PK monitoring trials by the IMPAACT Network are ongoing, yet preliminary data show adequate drug levels and virologic efficacy during pregnancy and at delivery, and no adverse events attributable to BIC.[34] As BIC is a *preferred* agent for non-pregnant adult PWH, it is expected that BIC use will continue to rise among reproductive-age females, including those who become pregnant; future studies of pregnancies among PWH who conceive while taking BIC will be the key to potentially further expanding its classification from *alternative* to *preferred*.

Experience with Injectable Regimens

Approval of novel long-acting injectable ART formulations represents a significant advancement in the treatment of PWH. These formulations are designed to sustain virologic suppression in PWH facing challenges related to daily oral ART adherence, such as stigma, apprehension regarding disclosure of their HIV status, anxiety about adherence, and pill aversion.[35] However, both the CAB/rilpivirine (RPV) and lenacapavir (LEN) injectable formulations are categorized as *not recommended* during pregnancy due to limited PK, toxicity, and efficacy data during pregnancy.[8]

Long-acting CAB/RPV is not recommended for pregnant, treatment-naïve PWH. Nevertheless, in shared decision-making between patients and providers understanding that the data are insufficient for pregnancy, those who become pregnant while taking this regimen may continue CAB/RPV in pregnancy provided HIV viral load remains fully suppressed and the injection is well-tolerated without side effects.[8] The limited safety data in pregnancy originate from participants who conceived while receiving CAB/RPV as part of clinical trials, although this regimen was discontinued upon confirmation of pregnancy. These limited data suggest that plasma concentrations were within the range of observed concentrations of nonpregnant participants and detectable plasma concentrations persisted for up to 12 months after the last dose.[36,37] The HPTN 084 trial, which demonstrated the superiority of long-acting CAB over TDF/FTC for PrEP in individuals assigned female at birth who engage in receptive vaginal intercourse, reported 29 unintended pregnancies exposed to CAB; most pregnancies resulted in a livebirth and no congenital anomalies were observed.[36] Likewise, outcomes of 25 pregnancies exposed to CAB/RPV during Phase 2 b/3/3b clinical trials have been described and included 8 induced abortions, 6 spontaneous abortions (5 occurring in the first trimester), 1 ectopic pregnancy, and 10 live births, among which 1 infant displayed congenital ptosis, which spontaneously resolved without intervention.[37]

Currently, recommendations for CAB/RPV pregnancy dosing are limited as no antenatal PK studies currently exist. Two physiologically-based pharmacokinetic models have been described to assess the impact of pregnancy on the PK of long-acting injectable CAB/RPV. The first model suggested minimal influence of pregnancy on PK, with no need for dose adjustments.[38] The second model, focusing on pregnant individuals initiating CAB and RPV in the early second trimester, predicted reductions in plasma concentrations after each injection, attributed to induced enzymatic activity during pregnancy.[39] A case report describing the use of bimonthly CAB/RPV during pregnancy showed that CAB concentrations were comparable to non-pregnant individuals, yet RPV concentrations were 70% to 75% lower.[40] Future data regarding long-acting CAB/RPV pharmacokinetics and pregnancy outcomes are required to understand appropriate use for pregnant or pregnancy-capable individuals.

Long-acting LEN, an HIV-1 capsid inhibitor, is another emerging injectable drug currently undergoing evaluation for first-line treatment in treatment-naïve PWH and for PrEP.[41] The reported data to date do not include information from pregnant participants, leading to extremely limited data regarding its pharmacokinetics, toxicity, and efficacy in pregnancy. The DHHS Guidelines do not currently recommend initiation of long-acting LEN in treatment-naïve PWH; however, it can be considered in special circumstances, such as heavily treatment-experienced adults with multidrug-resistant HIV-1.[8] Expectantly, the dearth of pregnancy data should improve, as an ongoing study is assessing the effectiveness of LEN and TAF/FTC for PrEP in adolescent and young individuals assigned female at birth at risk of HIV infection in Uganda and South Africa. If participants become pregnant after randomization, they have the option to continue in the study and still receive the study drug, allowing for the evaluation of pregnancy and breastfeeding outcomes.[42,43]

Studying Novel Antiretroviral Drugs in Pregnancy

Pregnant individuals are frequently excluded from clinical trials involving new medications due to the unique circumstance where the safety of both the pregnant person and fetus must be considered. Furthermore, studies evaluating perinatal HIV transmission preventive measures have largely emphasized protecting the health of the fetus, with lesser consideration for the health of the pregnant individual.[44] This practice extends to trials focusing on ART, thereby limiting the data on PK, safety, and efficacy of new ART agents during pregnancy and breastfeeding.

The gaps in PK and safety data of novel ART have resulted in inadequate access and considerable delays in accessing potentially beneficial therapies. For instance, although BIC was first approved by the US Food and Drug Administration for use in nonpregnant adults in 2018, not until 2024 did the DHHS Guidelines first recommend use of BIC in pregnancy, given limited pregnancy data available; even now, BIC is relegated to an *alternative,* not *preferred,* regimen for pregnancy.[8] Similarly, until additional data become available, CAB/RPV and LEN remain not recommended for pregnancy. Given the importance of maintaining viral suppression throughout pregnancy, pregnant PWH are among those who could benefit the most from these formulations, as an injectable route could help alleviate pregnancy-specific challenges to oral ART adherence such as pregnancy-related nausea and vomiting or hyperemesis gravidarum.[45]

In 2016, the National Institute of Child Health and Human Development established the Task Force on Research Specific to Pregnant Women and Lactating Women aiming to identify and address gaps in knowledge and research regarding safe and effective therapies for pregnant and lactating people.[46,47] Taking a proactive stance, the Task Force suggests that investigators and sponsors must provide justifications for excluding pregnant and lactating women from their study designs, and they should develop studies aimed at capturing the physiologic changes that occur in these populations over time.[48] The notion that excluding pregnant and lactating individuals from clinical studies serves as a means of protecting both the pregnant person and their offspring is outdated. Rather, this practice proves detrimental by withholding and postponing therapeutic approaches that could enhance their disease management and, in the case of pregnant PWH and their offspring, prevent perinatal HIV transmission. Instead, involving pregnant individuals in clinical research should be viewed as a safeguarding measure, amplifying safety monitoring of new medications within this population.

Perinatal HIV clinicians have advocated for expediting investigation of new ART during pregnancy. Initially, the efficacy of antiretroviral drugs in pregnant individuals can be inferred from established efficacy in non-pregnant populations, provided that drug levels remain consistent during pregnancy. However, the initial development process for all new ART should incorporate examination of short-term safety and PK in pregnant and lactating people. This approach ensures that relevant data specific to pregnancy are available at the time of approval. Additionally, assessing teratogenic risks prior to attaining drug licensure is not practically feasible, as it requires robust post-marketing surveillance systems, including reporting to the Antiretroviral Pregnancy Registry (APR).[42,49,50] Health care providers managing pregnant PWH and their new-borns are strongly advised to report events of prenatal exposure to antiretroviral (ARV) drugs, whether administered alone or in combination, to the APR to strengthen information available about safety and toxicity associated with ARV.

CLINICS CARE POINTS

- DTG is the *preferred* drug of choice when selecting INSTI-based regimens in pregnancy, in combination with a *preferred* dual-NRTI backbone.
- Based on recent PK and safety data in pregnancy, ART regimens containing BIC are now considered *alternative* ART regimens in pregnancy.
- Additional data on long-acting CAB/RPV and LEN during pregnancy are needed.
- Pregnant and lactating PWH should be included in clinical trials for new ART reg-imens since their inception to provide timely safety and PK data specific to pregnancy.

INFANT FEEDING

Breast milk-associated HIV transmission remains a major route of pediatric HIV infec-tion globally, accounting for up to half of new pediatric infections, with a baseline transmission risk of 14% to 29% in the first 2 years postpartum without the use of ART.[51–53] This risk is substantially reduced to 0.3% to 1.1%, yet not completely elim-inated, by the use of maternal ART to maintain viral suppression while breastfeeding in conjunction with neonatal post-exposure prophylaxis (PEP).[8,52,54–57] The term "breastfeeding" herein encompasses the act of feeding one's own milk to one's child with expressed milk or via direct breast-feeding, chest-feeding, or body-feeding, by women, transgender men, or gender-diverse individuals.[8]

Decisions about infant feeding in the context of maternal HIV involve nuanced balancing of risks and benefits. In low-income and middle-income countries, lack of access to clean water, cost of formula, and other resource limitations often prohibit the avoidance of breastfeeding in birthing PWH.[58] Comparatively, balancing breast milk-associated HIV transmission risk with the availability of safe, feasible, and afford-able replacement feeding options in resource-rich settings (ie, infant formula or donor human milk), guidelines for birthing PWH in the United States and other high-income countries had previously recommended against routine breastfeeding.[51,59,60] In the era of contemporary ART regimens, neonatal PEP, and emerging evidence that the risk of HIV transmission is lower than previously believed with risk-reducing measures while breastfeeding, breastfeeding uptake by birthing PWH in high-income countries is increasing.[58,59,61,62]

Mechanisms of Breast Milk-Associated Human Immunodeficiency Virus Transmission

Despite viral suppression in maternal plasma with effective ART, the HIV virus can still be present in breast milk and contribute to viral transmission. Cell-free (RNA) and cell-associated (DNA) HIV viral shedding in breastmilk contribute to residual risk of breast milk-associated HIV transmission.[63] Breast milk-associated transmission can occur early in the postnatal period, throughout the duration of breastfeeding, and during weaning off breast milk.[51,64] CD4 + T-lymphocytes in breast milk are an inducible reservoir for HIV proviral DNA, and are up to 17 times more effective than those in blood in producing viral antigens.[53,65] Routine viral load tests cannot detect HIV viral particles dormant within immune cells in breast milk, and ART cannot attack these viral particles hiding within immune cells.[53] Considering these viral reservoirs for HIV and the uncertain pharmacodynamics of ART in breast milk, the principle "undetectable equals untransmittable" (ie, U = U), referring to evidence that an undetectable plasma viral load in PWH taking ART indicates they cannot sexually transmit the virus, cannot be applied to breastmilk.[66]

Certain circumstances heighten the risk of HIV transmission through breast milk. Upregulation of proinflammatory cytokines during breast infection or inflammation (eg, a breast abscess, mastitis, or breast engorgement with milk stasis) activates these CD4 + T-lymphocytes in breast milk to replicate viral antigens, augmenting the risk of HIV transmission to the infant.[52,53] High maternal HIV viral load and ART drug resistance are also associated with viral replication and breast milk-associated HIV transmission.[54,55,63]

HIV virus in breast milk can then be transmitted to the infant via transcytosis through the infant gut mucosa.[52,53] Disruption of the infant gut mucosa (eg, via mixed feeding with formula or abrupt cessation of breastfeeding) promotes a proinflammatory milieu and enhanced gut permeability that can facilitate mucosal transmission of the virus.[53] As such, in those who choose to breastfeed, the World Health Organization recommends exclusive breastfeeding for the first 6 months postnatally, at which point solid foods are introduced, and breastfeeding should be continued thereafter, unless environmental and social circumstances are safe for, and supportive of, replacement feeding.[51,52] In high-income countries, weaning off breastfeeding after 6 months may be encouraged in favor of replacement feeding as longer duration of breastfeeding contributes to compounded risk of HIV exposure through breast milk.[63]

Perinatal HIV Transmission in the Era of Antenatal Antiretroviral Therapy and Postnatal Infant Prophylaxis

Studies of breastfeeding PWH from low-income and middle-income countries provide the most abundant evidence regarding breast milk-associated HIV transmission risk, including in PWH with viral suppression on ART.[54–57,67,68] In most studies, maternal ART was initiated in the second or third trimester of pregnancy or postpartum; data are limited on breast milk-associated HIV transmission risk when ART is initiated earlier and maintained for the duration of pregnancy and breastfeeding.

The most recent evidence comes from the previously described DolPHIN-2 trial in 2018 that randomized 268 PWH to DTG-versus EFV-based ART beginning in the third trimester of pregnancy and continued postpartum up to 72 weeks.[57] In this trial, a case of transmission during breastfeeding occurred despite maternal viral load less than 50 copies/mL.[57] Prior to DolPHIN-2, the postpartum component of the Promoting Maternal and Infant Survival Everywhere (PROMISE) trial from 2011 to 2014 was the largest randomized trial of 2431 breastfeeding PWH that evaluated treatment with maternal ART versus extended nevirapine (NVP) infant prophylaxis through 18 months postnatally.[55] Two infants in the maternal ART arm of PROMISE acquired HIV despite maternal undetectable viral load or viral load less than 40 copies/mL.[55] Two cases of breastfeeding-associated HIV transmission also occurred in the Mma Bana interventional cohort study from 2006 to 2008 that evaluated different maternal ART regimens postpartum, even though maternal plasma and breast milk HIV RNA levels were less than 50 copies/mL at the time that each neonatal infection was identified at 1 and 3 months postpartum, respectively. Additional randomized trials, observational cohort studies, and a systematic review and meta-analysis of additional cohort studies that

Table 1
Studies evaluating breastfeeding-associated human immunodeficiency virus transmission in low-income and middle-income countries

Study	Setting	Years of Study	Study Design	Sample Size	Intervention/ Treatment	Timing of Assessment of Transmission	Human Immunodeficiency Virus Transmission During Breastfeeding	Additional Comments
Dolutegravir in Pregnant HIV Mothers and Their Neonates (DolPHIN-2)[57]	South Africa, Uganda	2018	RCT	268 PWH	DTG- (n = 135) vs. EFV- (n = 130) based maternal ART started in the third trimester	72 wk (16 mo)	1 of 268 (0.37%)	Maternal viral load was <50 copies/mL at 12 wk, 24 wk, 48 wk, and 72 wk postpartum
Promoting Maternal and Infant Survival Everywhere (PROMISE)[54,55]	14 sites in Sub-Saharan Africa and India	2011–14	RCT	2431 PWH	Maternal ART (ZDV/3TC/LPVr or TDF/FTC/LPV; n = 1219) vs. extended infant NVP prophylaxis (n = 1211), until 18 mo postpartum (or cessation of breastfeeding) in both arms _All infants:_ single-dose NVP intrapartum with TDF/FTC tail until the postpartum wk 1 visit and daily NVP for 6 wk	6 mo 12 mo 18 mo 24 mo	0.3% 0.6% cumulative infections Maternal ART: 7/1219 (0.57%) Infant NVP: 7/1211 (0.58%) Maternal ART: 8 cumulative infections Infant NVP: 10 cumulative infections (0.8%)	2 infants in the maternal ART arm acquired HIV despite maternal undetectable viral load or viral load <40 copies/mL on the date that the infants' first samples tested positive for HIV RNA

(continued on next page)

Table 1
(continued)

Study	Setting	Years of Study	Study Design	Sample Size	Intervention/ Treatment	Timing of Assessment of Transmission	Human Immunodeficiency Virus Transmission During Breastfeeding	Additional Comments
Kilombero and Ulanga Antiretroviral Cohort (KIULARCO)[75]	Tanzania	2013–2016	Prospective cohort	214 PWH, 228 infants; 186 infants with known final HIV serostatus	Maternal ART initiated before delivery + postnatal daily infant NVP 4–6 wk Mothers had a negative viral load in the first trimester and exclusively breastfed for ≥6 mo	11 mo	2 of 186 infants (1%, 95% CI 0.3%–4%) in mothers with detectable viral load or interrupted ART 0 infants in mothers with nondetectable viral load	1 infant born to a mother with high viral load (144,111 copies/mL) 5 wk postpartum; 1 infant born to a mother who had undetectable viral load at 6 wk postpartum, but shortly after interrupted ART during breastfeeding

Mma Bana[56]	Botswana	2006–08	Interventional cohort	Interventional: 560 PWH, CD4+ >200; Observational: 170 PWH, CD4+ ≤200; 709 liveborn infants	Interventional, PWH with CD4+ count >200: Maternal ART ZDV/3TC/Abacavir (n = 283 infants) vs. ZDV/3TC/LPVr (n = 270 infants) from 26-34 wga to 6 mo postpartum. Observational: Maternal ART ZDV/3TC/NVP (n = 156 infants) from 18-34wga, continued indefinitely All Infants: Single-dose NVP and 4 wk of postnatal ZDV	6 and 18 mo	2 of 703 (0.28%) at-risk infants (excluding 6 transmissions in utero)	In both cases of transmission, maternal plasma and breast milk HIV RNA levels were <50 copies/mL at 1 mo and 3 mo postpartum.
Breastfeeding, Antiretrovirals, and Nutrition (BAN)[67,76]	Malawi	2004–10	RCT	2369 PWH	Maternal ART, initiated ≤30 wga (n = 849) vs. Postnatal extended daily infant NVP (n = 852) vs. Control (intrapartum single dose NVP + 7 d ZDV/3TC, n = 668), each through 28 wk postpartum	11 mo (48 wk)	Maternal ART: 4% (95% CI 3%–6%) Infant NVP: 4% (95% CI 2%–5%) Control: 7% (95% CI 5%–9%)	

(continued on next page)

Table 1
(continued)

Study	Setting	Years of Study	Study Design	Sample Size	Intervention/Treatment	Timing of Assessment of Transmission	Human Immunodeficiency Virus Transmission During Breastfeeding	Additional Comments
Safe Milk for African Children (SMAC)[77]	Malawi	2008–2009	Observational	288 infants	Maternal ART (ZDV/3TC/NVP) from 25 wga-6 mo postpartum vs. infant single dose NVP	6 mo 12 mo	2 infants (0.7%) Additional 4 infants (1.4%)	1 at 3 mo, 1 at 6 mo All 4 infants had negative HIV-testing at 6 mo. Risk of late postnatal transmission (>6 mo) was higher ($P = .013$), in PWH who breastfed >6 mo
Kesho Bora[78]	5 study sites in Burkina Faso, Kenya, and South Africa	2005–2008	RCT	824 PWH	Maternal triple ART (n = 412) vs. maternal ZDV (n = 412) and single-dose NVP intrapartum; study ART started at 28–36 wk' gestation. *All infants:* single dose NVP and ZDV for 1 wk postnatally	6 wk 6 wk-6 mo 12 mo	Triple ART: cumulative rate: 3.3% (95% CI 1.9%–5.6%) ZDV + NVP: 5.0% (3.3%–7.7%) 6wk-6 mo: Triple ART: 6 cases ZDV + NVP: 13 cases Triple ART: 5.4% (3.6%–8.1%) ZDV + NVP: 9.5% (70%–12.9%)	

| Pregnant Women and Infants (PROMOTE)[79] | Uganda | 2009–2013 | Secondary analysis of RCT | 389 PWH | Maternal ART: ZDV/3TC/EFV (n = 195) vs. ZDV/3TC/LPVr (n = 194) | 6 mo 12 mo | No cases of transmission 1 infant in the LPVr arm – The infant received extended nevirapine prophylaxis beyond 6 wk and was exclusively breastfed for 28 wk and partially breastfed until 1 y of age. Infant HIV-1 DNA polymerase chain reaction (PCR) testing was negative at birth and 24 wk of life, then positive at 58 & 61 wk. | mother's HIV-1 RNA: *During pregnancy:* 23 wga: 253,000 copies/mL 8wk after ART initiation: ≤400 copies/mL *Delivery:* 30, 800 copies/mL *Postpartum: 4270– 24,400 copies/mL* |

(continued on next page)

Table 1
(continued)

Study	Setting	Years of Study	Study Design	Sample Size	Intervention/Treatment	Timing of Assessment of Transmission	Human Immunodeficiency Virus Transmission During Breastfeeding	Additional Comments
Tshilo Dikotla Study[80]	Botswana	2016–22	Secondary analysis of RCT	247 PWH	Infants randomized to 4 wk of prophylactic ZDV (n = 120) vs. NVP (n = 127) Maternal ART (TDF/FTC +/DTG (n = 139) or EFV (n = 110)) since 16–36 wga	6 mo	No cases of transmission to infants	19 PWH had detectable viral loads during breastfeeding. 12 stopped breastfeeding, 7 continued to breastfeed with ongoing counseling and frequent viral load checks
ANRS 12174[81]	Burkina Faso, South Africa, Uganda, and Zambia	2009–2012	RCT	1236 infants	Postnatal extended infant LPVr (n = 615) vs. 3TC (n = 621) up to 1 wk after complete cessation of breastfeeding or at the final visit at wk 50 Mothers were not eligible for ART (CD4 count >350 cells/mL) prior to 2013	12 mo (50 wk)	LPVr: 8 infants, cumulative infection rate 1.4% (95% CI 0.4–2.5) 3TC: 9 infants, cumulative infection rate 1.5% (95% CI 0.7–2.5)	

Study	Location	Years	Design	N	Intervention	Timing	Results
HPTN 046[82]	South Africa, Tanzania, Uganda, Zimbabwe	2008–2010	RCT	1527 infants	Postnatal extended infant NVP (n = 762) from 6 wk to 6 mo vs. placebo (n = 765), both after initial infant NVP for 6 wk after birth. Mothers received the local standard of care for ART	6 mo	Extended NVP: 1.1% (95% CI 0·3–1.8) Placebo: 2.4% (95% CI 1.3–3.6)
Bispo et al,[68] 2017	11 studies (7 observational, 4 nested cohorts within RCTs throughout Africa)	2005–2015	Systematic review and meta-analysis (includes SMAC, BAN, HPTN046)		Maternal ART initiated 15–34 wk' gestation and continued through 6 mo postpartum	4–6 wk to 6 mo 4–6 wk to 12 mo	1.08% (95% CI 0.32%–1.85%) 2.93% (95% CI 0.68–5.18)

Abbreviation: 3TC, lamivudine; ART, antiretroviral therapy; DTG, dolutegravir; EFV, efavirenz; FTC, emtricitabine: LPVr, lopivarine boosted with ritonavir; NVP, nevirapine; PWH, people with HIV; RCT, randomized controlled trial; RNA, ribonucleic acid; TDF, tenofovir disoproxil difumarate: wga, weeks gestational age; ZDV, zidovudine.

Table 2
Studies evaluating breastfeeding-associated human immunodeficiency virus transmission in high-income countries

Study/Author	Setting	Years of Study	Study Design	Sample Size	Intervention/Treatment	Breastfeeding Duration and Type	Follow-up Duration	Human Immunodeficiency Virus Transmission During Breastfeeding	Additional Comments
Levison et al,[69] 2023	US (8 sites), Canada (3 sites)	2014–22	Retrospective cohort	72 PWH and infants (US: 44; Canada: 28)	Maternal ART during pregnancy: 38 integrase strand-transfer inhibitor (INSTI)–based, 21 NNRTI-based, 7 protease inhibitor (PI)-based, 6 unknown regimen Variable infant prophylaxis protocols, ranging from ZDV or NVP monotherapy 4–6 wk postnatally to triple therapy until cessation of breastfeeding	Median 24 wk (range 1 day–72 weeks); 16 cases with mixed feeding, 54 with exclusive breastfeeding, (2 unknown)	12 mo	No neonatal transmissions among 68 infants for whom results were available ≥6 wk after weaning	62 PWH were on ART prior to pregnancy, at least 65 had undetectable viral load (<40 copies/mL) at delivery

Study	Location	Years	Study type	Sample	ART/Intervention	Feeding	Follow-up	Transmission	Notes
Weiss et al,[70] 2022; Haberl et al,[62] 2021	Germany	2016–2020	Retrospective cohort	30 PWH and infants	Maternal ART (37% NNRTI-based, 33% INSTI-based, 17% PI-based, 13% other) throughout pregnancy and postpartum during breastfeeding ZDV infant prophylaxis between 2–8 wk postnatally (declined from 5 breastfeeding virally suppressed PWH)	<2 weeks–12 months (mostly exclusive)	18 mo	No cases of transmission	25 PWH had HIV RNA <50 copies/mL during pregnancy and postpartum, 4 PWH had HIV RNA 50–70 copies/mL at some point postpartum, 2 PWH had a detectable viral load early in pregnancy
Nashid et al,[61] 2020	Toronto, Canada	Published 2020	Case series	2 PWH, 3 infants	Case 1: maternal ART (FTC/TDF/RAL) + infant ZDV/3TC/NVP for duration of exclusive breastfeeding (6 wk) Case 2 & 3: Maternal ART (FTC/TDF/RPV) + infant ZDV/3TC/NVP for duration of mixed feeding (12 wk)	Case 1: 6 wk, exclusive Cases 2–3: 12 wk, mixed feeding	20 wk	No cases of transmission Both PWH with undetectable viral load in pregnancy and postpartum	Case 1: proviral DNA in breastmilk detected by PCR, reflecting latent virus within the CD4+ T cells or macrophages Cases 2–3: insufficient sample to measure breastmilk proviral DNA

(continued on next page)

Table 2
(continued)

Study/ Author	Setting	Years of Study	Study Design	Sample Size	Intervention/ Treatment	Breastfeeding Duration and Type	Follow-up Duration	Human Immunodeficiency Virus Transmission During Breastfeeding	Additional Comments
Yusuf et al,[72] 2022	Baltimore, Maryland, US	Published 2021	Case series	9 PWH, 10 infants	All PWH on maternal ART pre-pregnancy, throughout pregnancy, and postpartum during breastfeeding All infants on AZT/3TC/NVP for 4-6 wk postnatally, then NVP monotherapy through 6 wk after discontinuation of breastfeeding	Mean 4.4 (1.0–8.6) mo, exclusive	Median 16 mo	No cases of transmission	70% of PWH were virally suppressed at initial prenatal visit. All 9 PWH had HIV RNA <30 copies/mL at delivery.
Koay et al,[71] 2022	Washington, DC, US	2018–2021	Case series	6 PWH, 7 infants	All PWH on maternal ART pre-pregnancy, throughout pregnancy, and postpartum during breastfeeding	2 wk–6 ms, exclusive	6 mo	No cases of transmission	4 PWH were virally suppressed (<20 copies/mL), 2 had low levels of viremia (30–40 copies/mL) at delivery

| Prestileo et al,[73] 2022 | Italy | 2017–2021 | Case series | 13 PWH | All PWH on maternal ART (TDF/FTC/RAL or LPV/r) pre-pregnancy, throughout pregnancy, and postpartum during breastfeeding All infants on ZDV for 4 wk postnatally. All infants on ZDV and/or NVP for 4–6 wk postnatally (ZDV × 4 weeks [n = 1], ZDV × 6 weeks [n = 3], ZDV/NVP × 6 weeks[n = 2] ZDV/3TC/NVP × 2 weeks then 4 wk ZDV [n = 1]) | 5.4 mo | 6 mo after cessation of breastfeeding | No cases of transmission | All 13 PWH were virally suppressed during pregnancy and postpartum. |

Abbreviation: 3TC, lamivudine; ART, antiretroviral therapy; DTG, dolutegravir; EFV, efavirenz; FTC, emtricitabine; LPVr, lopivarine boosted with ritonavir; NNRTI, nonnucleoside reverse transcriptase inhibitor; NVP, nevirapine; PWH, people with HIV; RAL, raltegravir; RNA, ribonucleic acid; TDF, tenofovir disoproxil difumarate; ZDV, zidovudine.

Table 3 Multidisciplinary approach and key discussion points for development of an infant feeding plan[8,59,66,74]	
Multidisciplinary team members and Staff education	• *Clinician team:* maternal-fetal medicine specialist or general obstetrician, adult HIV specialist, pediatric HIV specialist, neonatologist • *Nursing team:* labor and delivery, postpartum, newborn nursery staff • *Additional consultants:* lactation consultant, social worker, case manager, peer and/or community support • Hospital Staff should receive education in caring for PWH who choose to breastfeed and promote stigma reduction. • Devising a written copy of the infant feeding plan for PWH to have at their delivery hospitalization may improve communication, promote transparency, and avoid confusion among other health care providers at delivery.
Discussion points	• Assessment of feeding intentions with clear and informed discussion about risks and benefits of breastfeeding vs alternative feeding methods • Emphasis on the importance of sustained viral suppression throughout pregnancy and postpartum and anticipation of challenges to ongoing ART adherence postpartum. • Establishment of a plan for maternal and neonatal ART and laboratory monitoring for the duration of breastfeeding • Setting a realistic yet optimized plan for exclusive breastfeeding in their day-to-day life postpartum, including avoidance of mixed feeding, promotion of breast care, development of a plan for harm reduction measures should lactation delays, infant illness, or other challenges arise postnatally, and slow weaning plan • Assessment of psychosocial support and facilitation of HIV status disclosure to family members assisting with infant feeding • Provision of additional resources to support their choice of feeding (ie, referral to a lactation consultant or breastfeeding support groups vs referral to a donor milk bank or governmental assistance programs for infant formula; linkage to mental health or substance use treatment programs, etc.)

Expanded details regarding these discussion points for development of the infant feeding plan are included in **Tables 4** and **5**

identified cases of transmission while taking maternal ART and/or extended infant PEP in low-income and middle-income countries over the past 2 decades are highlighted in **Table 1**.

As interest in breastfeeding has increased in high-income countries, at least 6 additional small retrospective cohort studies and case series from the United States, Canada, Germany, and Italy have collectively reported on 135 infants with breastmilk-associated HIV exposure.[61,62,69–73] No cases of HIV transmission occurred in these studies. All PWH were on ART preconceptionally, throughout pregnancy, and postpartum while breastfeeding; most were virally suppressed since early pregnancy through delivery and postpartum, and breastfeeding continued from less than 2 weeks up to 72 weeks postpartum. Infant PEP regimens ranged from ZDV or NVP monotherapy for 2 to 8 weeks postnatally to triple ART for the duration of breastfeeding. Additional details regarding these reports on breastfeeding among PWH in high-income settings are outlined in **Table 2**.

Table 4
Key components of virologic control and surveillance in people with human immunodeficiency virus who opt to breastfeed

Key component	Additional notes and discussion points
Virologic control and surveillance	
100% maternal ART adherence and maintenance of sustained viral suppression throughout pregnancy, at delivery, and throughout infant feeding	• With optimal ART adherence and maintenance of viral suppression throughout pregnancy, at delivery, and throughout breastfeeding, HIV transmission risk through breast milk is <1%, but U = U cannot be applied to breastmilk. • Active viremia, suboptimal maternal ART use, or nonadherence to infant PEP raises HIV transmission risk. • Choice of ART regimen should be consistent with recommended agents per the DHHS Perinatal HIV Clinical Guidelines, and acceptable and well-tolerated to the individual with minimal side effects and without evidence of drug resistance. • Consider simplifying regimen postpartum (eg, single pill regimen, once daily dosing) to facilitate adherence.
Maternal and infant virologic surveillance postnatally	• Monitor maternal plasma viral load every 1–2 mo throughout breastfeeding to ensure maintenance of viral suppression and inform HIV transmission risk. • PWH should be counseled on the increased frequency of clinic visits and laboratory testing postpartum. Clarify which clinician is responsible for monitoring viral load postpartum (obstetrician, primary care provider, or HIV specialist). • Consult with an infectious disease expert immediately if viremia is detected during breastfeeding, and recommend temporarily or permanently discontinuing breastfeeding. • Infant virologic HIV testing should occur at birth then at 14–21 d, 1–2 mo, and 4–6 mo postnatally, with an additional test between the 1–2 mo and 4–6 mo time points if the gap between tests exceeds 3 mo. Then, testing should occur every 3 mo for the duration of breastfeeding, followed by monitoring at 4–6 wk, 3 mo, and 6 mo after cessation of breastfeeding.
Appropriate infant PEP	• The optimal regimen for infant PEP remains unclear. • Infant PEP options include postnatal ZDV for 2 wk (if meet the lowest risk criteria), ZDV for 4–6 k, NVP for 6 wk, NVP continued for the duration of breastfeeding, or a 3-drug presumptive regimen with continuation until 4 wk following cessation of breastfeeding. • Expert opinion suggests continuation of infant PEP with extended NVP throughout breastfeeding until 4 wk following breastfeeding cessation.

ART, antiretroviral therapy; ARV, antiretroviral; DHHS, US Department of Health and Human Services; NVP, nevirapine; PEP, post-exposure prophylaxis; PWH, people with HIV; ZDV, zidovudine.
Table adapted from the DHHS Guidelines and subsequent reviews by Pollock et al. and Powell et al.[8,66,74].

Table 5
Best practices for counseling and management of safer breastfeeding in people with human immunodeficiency virus

Key component	Additional notes and discussion points
Exclusive breastfeeding for the infant's first 6 mo	• In individuals who opt to breastfeed, exclusive breastfeeding for the infant's first 6 mo with avoidance of mixed feeding (ie, breast milk plus other liquid or solid foods, including formula) is recommended, followed by the introduction of solid foods, but not before. • With maternal ART, infant ARV prophylaxis, and viral suppression, it is unclear to what degree formula supplementation increases risk of HIV transmission; however, mixed feeding can increase intestinal inflammation and permeability that can increase this risk. If formula substitution is required and the infant initially refuses formula, mix a bottle with half breast milk and half formula and slowly increase the volume of formula overtime. Avoid frequent switching of formula type as this can cause gastrointestinal irritation. • When approaching 6 mo postpartum, the birthing person together with the health care team should reassess whether to continue breastfeeding vs initiate weaning. • Stop breastfeeding as early as possible to reduce duration of HIV exposure. Some PWH may choose to breastfeed <6 mo, and some experts discourage breastfeeding beyond 6 mo given the higher risk of HIV transmission with longer duration of breastfeeding. • If the birthing person develops a detectable viral load postpartum, breastfeeding should be stopped and replacement feeding initiated until viral load testing is repeated and confirmed to be nondetectable again; however, once the infant starts formula feeding, a return to breastfeeding is not recommended given the higher risk of HIV transmission with mixed feeding.
Slow weaning plan	• Abrupt cessation of breastfeeding and rapid weaning can increase HIV viral shedding into breast milk and raise HIV transmission risk. Weaning over 2–4 wk as the infant approaches 6 mo of age is safer, with attention to healthy breast care to avoid engorgement or mastitis. • If not already, start feeding the infant expressed breast milk, and progressively drop a pumping or breastfeeding session every 3–4 d, substituting solid foods (or formula) for one of the infant's feedings, until no longer breastfeeding. Over time the body will respond to the signal to reduce breast milk production. • If engorgement occurs, expression of a small volume of milk can reduce breast pressure and discomfort, as can applying cold compresses to the breast. Consider use of cabergoline for lactation inhibition.
Healthy breast care	• Regular breastfeeding or expression of breast milk every few hours can help avoid breast engorgement and milk stasis, and prevent mastitis or breast abscesses, all of which can raise HIV viral load in the affected breast.

(continued on next page)

Table 5
(continued)

Key component	Additional notes and discussion points
	• Proactive counseling by a lactation consultant to avoid latching/feeding problems and reduce these risks. If the birthing person develops mastitis, bleeding or cracked nipples, or nipple thrush, defer feeding breastmilk from the affected breast (instead, pump and discard breastmilk) until healed. • These conditions should be promptly identified, disclosed to the health care team, and treated, and the health care team should provide an interim, alternative safe feeding plan until resolved.
Healthy infant	• Avoid direct breastfeeding or feeding expressed breast milk to an infant with gastrointestinal upset (ie, diarrhea, vomiting) given increased risk of HIV transmission via microbial translocation and transcytosis across the intestine in the setting of intestinal inflammation, in addition to lower prophylactic ARV absorption. • Avoid feeding the infant breast milk if oral thrush is present.
Open communication and engagement with health care team throughout pregnancy and infant feeding	• Encourage transparency regarding feeding plans, including reporting challenges with infant feeding. • Only formula feeding completely eliminates the risk of postnatal HIV transmission, but the health care team can help mitigate this risk with guidance on harm reduction measures and referrals to case management, social work, and lactation consultant with perinatal support experience for PWH. • Early cessation of breastfeeding may be necessary for a variety of reasons. Should this occur, having a supply of stored breast milk or other rescue strategy for replacement feeding developed in collaboration with the health care team can help. • Routine screening and treatment of postpartum depression and other mental health conditions that may affect ART adherence is encouraged.

Abbreviation: ART, antiretroviral therapy; ARV, antiretroviral; DHHS, US Department of Health and Human Services; NVP, nevirapine; PEP, post-exposure prophylaxis; PWH, people with HIV; ZDV, zidovudine.

Table adapted from the DHHS Guidelines and subsequent reviews by Pollock and colleagues and Powell and colleagues[8,66,74]

Updates to the Department of Health and Human Services Guidelines on Infant Feeding in the United States

Incorporating this body of evidence, and in response to community desires, cultural norms, and health equity concerns, the 2023 DHHS Guidelines emphasized a major shift in recommendations regarding infant feeding.[8,74] Previously, the DHHS Guidelines had recommended avoidance of breastfeeding in favor of replacement feeding methods as standard of care in birthing PWH in the United States, highlighting replacement feeding as the only manner to completely eliminate the risk of postnatal HIV transmission.[74] The updated DHHS Guidelines still emphasize that replacement feeding is the only manner to eliminate postnatal HIV transmission risk, that PWH who choose to formula feed should be supported in this decision, and any potential barriers to formula feeding should be addressed. However, with respect to patient autonomy, the revised DHHS Guidelines have shifted toward a more inclusive, shared-decision making approach to infant feeding including endorsement that PWH with sustained viral suppression throughout pregnancy, at delivery, and postpartum who receive informed, evidence-based counseling and choose to breastfeed should be supported in this decision.[8] The British, Canadian, Swiss, European, and Australian perinatal guidelines endorse a similar approach.[66] Best practices for implementing a multidisciplinary shared decision-making approach, longitudinal patient counseling across the perinatal period, risk-reducing counseling, and other considerations for management of safer breastfeeding are summarized in **Table 3** and **Tables 4** and **5**, with further details in the DHHS guidelines and expert reviews by Powell and Pollock and colleagues[8,66,74]

CLINICS CARE POINTS

- Although adherence to ART and sustained viral suppression during pregnancy and breastfeeding reduce breast milk-associated HIV transmission to less than 1%, HIV viral reservoirs can remain present in present breast milk despite an undetectable plasma viral load. Formula or pasteurized donor human milk are the only infant feeding options that completely eliminate the risk of postnatal HIV transmission.

- Additional studies are needed evaluating breast milk-associated HIV transmission risk in high-resource settings among individuals who demonstrate ART adherence on current first-line regimens and achieve sustained viral suppression beginning before or early in pregnancy. Further studies to determine optimal infant PEP and frequency of postnatal maternal and infant viral load monitoring are also required.

- When individuals opt to breastfeed, exclusive breastfeeding for 6 months is recommended over mixed feeding until solid foods can be introduced, with slow weaning thereafter.

- Open communication regarding infant feeding plans and engagement with a multidisciplinary care team throughout pregnancy and postpartum are essential for PWH who choose to breastfeed.

SUMMARY

Recent advances in the management of HIV during pregnancy and infant feeding include improved diagnosis of HIV through expanded HIV testing and the use of newer INSTI-based ART regimens, supported by emerging safety, efficacy, and PK data. Furthermore, the inclusion of pregnant PWH participants in clinical trials is the key to eliminating delays in accessing novel ART among this population. Finally, a shared decision-making approach to infant feeding among PWH, and engagement in risk-reducing measures in individuals who choose to breastfeed, is now endorsed by US national guidelines.

DISCLOSURE

The authors report no financial or non-financial competing interests that are relevant to the content of this article, or other conflict of interest to disclose. All authors consent to publication of this manuscript. All authors contributed to conception and design of this review article. M. Espinal and S.A. Fisher drafted the initial manuscript. L.M. Yee provided critical content expertise for the manuscript. All authors critically revised the manuscript for important intellectual context. All authors have read and approved the final manuscript to be published and agree to be accountable for the accuracy and integrity of this work.

REFERENCES

1. Lampe MA, Nesheim SR, Oladapo KL, et al. Achieving elimination of perinatal HIV in the United States. Pediatrics 2023;151(5).
2. Sibiude J, Le Chenadec J, Mandelbrot L, et al. Update of perinatal human immunodeficiency virus type 1 transmission in france: zero transmission for 5482 mothers on continuous antiretroviral therapy from conception and with undetectable viral load at delivery. Clin Infect Dis 2023;76(3):e590–8.
3. Branson BM, Handsfield HH, Lampe MA, et al. Revised recommendations for HIV testing of adults, adolescents, and pregnant women in health-care settings. MMWR Recomm Rep (Morb Mortal Wkly Rep) 2006;55(RR-14):1–17 [quiz CE1-4].
4. Alexander Thomas S. Human immunodeficiency virus diagnostic testing: 30 years of evolution. Clin Vaccine Immunol 2016;23(4):249–53.
5. National Center for HIV/AIDS, Viral Hepatitis, and TB Prevention (U.S.). Division of HIV/AIDS Prevention. Association of Public Health Laboratories. 2018 Quick reference guide: Recommended laboratory HIV testing algorithm for serum or plasma specimens. 2018. Available at: https://stacks.cdc.gov/view/cdc/50872.
6. Kourtis AP, Bulterys M, Nesheim SR, et al. Understanding the timing of HIV transmission from mother to infant. JAMA 2001;285(6):709–12.
7. Singh ALM, Surendera Babu A, Rao S, et al. HIV seroconversion during prgnancy and mother-to-child HIV transmission: data from the Enhanced Perinatal Surveillance Project, United States, 2005–2010. Washington, District of Columbia, US: Abstract presented at: 19th International AIDS Conference; 2012.
8. Panel on Treatment of HIV During Pregnancy and Prevention of Perinatal Transmission. Recommendations for the Use of Antiretroviral Drugs During Pregnancy and Interventions to Reduce Perinatal HIV Transmission in the United States. Department of Health and Human Services. 2024. Available at: https://clinicalinfo.hiv.gov/en/guidelines/perinatal. Accessed April 15, 2024.
9. Ishikawa N, Dalal S, Johnson C, et al. Should HIV testing for all pregnant women continue? Cost-effectiveness of universal antenatal testing compared to focused approaches across high to very low HIV prevalence settings. J Int AIDS Soc 2016;19(1).
10. Scott RK, Crochet S, Huang CC. Universal rapid human immunodeficiency virus screening at delivery: a cost-effectiveness analysis. Infect Dis Obstet Gynecol 2018;2018:6024698.
11. Cassimatis IR, Ayala LD, Miller ES, et al. Third-trimester repeat HIV testing: it is time we make it universal. Am J Obstet Gynecol 2021;225(5):494–9.
12. Salvant Valentine S, Caldwell J, Tailor A. Effect of CDC 2006 Revised HIV testing recommendations for adults, adolescents, pregnant women, and newborns on state laws, 2018. Publ Health Rep 2020;135(1_suppl):189S–96S.
13. Liao C, Golden WC, Anderson JR, et al. Missed opportunities for repeat HIV testing in pregnancy: implications for elimination of mother-to-child transmission in the United States. AIDS Patient Care STDS 2017;31(1):20–6.
14. Thomson KA, Hughes J, Baeten JM, et al. Increased risk of HIV acquisition among women throughout pregnancy and during the postpartum period: a prospective per-coital-act analysis among women with HIV-Infected Partners. J Infect Dis 2018;218(1):16–25.
15. Graybill LA, Kasaro M, Freeborn K, et al. Incident HIV among pregnant and breast-feeding women in sub-Saharan Africa: a systematic review and meta-analysis. AIDS 2020;34(5):761–76.

16. Panel on Antiretroviral Guidelines for Adults and Adolescents: Guidelines for the use of antiretroviral agents in HIV-1-infected adults and adolescents. 2014. Department of Health and Human Services. Available at: https://clinicalinfo.hiv. gov/sites/default/files/guidelines/archive/AdultandAdolescentGL003392.pdf. Accessed May 11, 2024.

17. Walmsley SL, Antela A, Clumeck N, et al. Dolutegravir plus abacavir-lamivudine for the treatment of HIV-1 infection. N Engl J Med 2013;369(19):1807–18.

18. Zhu J, Rozada I, David J, et al. The potential impact of initiating antiretroviral therapy with integrase inhibitors on HIV transmission risk in British Columbia, Canada. EClinicalMedicine 2019;13:101–11.

19. Smith C, Silveira L, Crotteau M, et al. Modern antiretroviral regimens in pregnant women: virologic outcomes and durability. AIDS 2024;38(1):21–9.

20. Alagaratnam J, Peters H, Francis K, et al. An observational study of initial HIV RNA decay following initiation of combination antiretroviral treatment during pregnancy. AIDS Res Ther 2020;17(1):41.

21. Zash R, Makhema J, Shapiro RL. Neural-tube defects with dolutegravir treatment from the time of conception. N Engl J Med 2018;379(10):979–81.

22. Zash R, Holmes LB, Diseko M, et al. Update on neural tube defects with antiretroviral exposure in the Tsepamo Study, Botswana. Montreal, Canada: Abstract presented at: The 24th International AIDS Conference; 2022.

23. Kourtis AP, Zhu W, Lampe MA, et al. Dolutegravir and pregnancy outcomes including neural tube defects in the USA during 2008-20: a national cohort study. Lancet HIV 2023;10(9):e588–96.

24. Fisher SA, Madden N, Espinal M, et al. Clinical trials that have changed clinical practice and care of pregnant people with HIV. Clin Obstet Gynecol 2024. https://doi.org/10.1097/grf.0000000000000860.

25. Waitt C, Orrell C, Walimbwa S, et al. Safety and pharmacokinetics of dolutegravir in pregnant mothers with HIV infection and their neonates: A randomised trial (DolPHIN-1 study). PLoS Med 2019;16(9):e1002895.

26. Kintu K, Malaba TR, Nakibuka J, et al. Dolutegravir versus efavirenz in women starting HIV therapy in late pregnancy (DolPHIN-2): an open-label, randomised controlled trial. Lancet HIV 2020;7(5):e332–9.

27. Lockman S, Brummel SS, Ziemba L, et al. Efficacy and safety of dolutegravir with emtricitabine and tenofovir alafenamide fumarate or tenofovir disoproxil fumarate, and efavirenz, emtricitabine, and tenofovir disoproxil fumarate HIV antiretroviral therapy regimens started in pregnancy (IMPAACT 2010/VESTED): a multicentre, open-label, randomised, controlled, phase 3 trial. Lancet 2021;397(10281):1276–92.

28. Chinula L, Ziemba L, Brummel S, et al. Efficacy and safety of three antiretroviral therapy regimens started in pregnancy up to 50 weeks post partum: a multicentre, open-label, randomised, controlled, phase 3 trial. Lancet HIV 2023;10(6):e363–74.

29. Patel K, Huo Y, Jao J, et al. Dolutegravir in pregnancy as compared with current HIV Regimens in the United States. N Engl J Med 2022;387(9):799–809.

30. Kityo C, Hagins D, Koenig E, et al. Switching to fixed-dose bictegravir, emtricitabine, and tenofovir alafenamide (B/F/TAF) in Virologically Suppressed HIV-1 Infected Women: A Randomized, Open-Label, Multicenter, Active-Controlled, Phase 3, Noninferiority Trial. J Acquir Immune Defic Syndr 2019;82(3):321–8.

31. Orkin C, DeJesus E, Sax PE, et al. Fixed-dose combination bictegravir, emtricitabine, and tenofovir alafenamide versus dolutegravir-containing regimens for initial treatment of HIV-1 infection: week 144 results from two randomised, double-blind, multicentre, phase 3, non-inferiority trials. Lancet HIV 2020;7(6):e389–400.

32. Bukkems VE, Hidalgo-Tenorio C, Garcia C, et al. First pharmacokinetic data of bictegravir in pregnant women living with HIV. AIDS 2021;35(14):2405–6.

33. Zhang H, Hindman JT, Lin L, et al. A study of the pharmacokinetics, safety, and efficacy of bictegravir/emtricitabine/tenofovir alafenamide in virologically suppressed pregnant women with HIV. AIDS 2024;38(1):F1–9.

34. Powis K.M., Pinilla M., Bergam L., et al., Pharmacokinetics and Virologic Outcomes of Bictegravir in Pregnancy and Postpartum. Abstract presented at: Conference on Retroviruses and Opportunistic Infections; 2023; Seattle, WA, Available at: https://www.croiconference.org/wp-content/uploads/sites/2/posters/2023/IMPAACT_PHARMACOKINETICS_AND_VIROLOGIC_15Feb23-133209845782009090.pdf. Accessed April 13, 2024.

35. Overton ET, Richmond G, Rizzardini G, et al. Long-acting cabotegravir and rilpivirine dosed every 2 months in adults with HIV-1 infection (ATLAS-2M), 48-week results: a randomised, multicentre, open-label, phase 3b, non-inferiority study. Lancet 2021;396(10267):1994–2005.

36. Delany-Moretlwe S, Hughes JP, Bock P, et al. Cabotegravir for the prevention of HIV-1 in women: results from HPTN 084, a phase 3, randomised clinical trial. Lancet 2022;399(10337):1779–89.

37. Patel P, Ford SL, Baker M, et al. Pregnancy outcomes and pharmacokinetics in pregnant women living with HIV exposed to long-acting cabotegravir and rilpivirine in clinical trials. HIV Med 2023;24(5):568–79.

38. Atoyebi S.A., Bunglawala F.S., Cottura N., et al., PBPK modeling of long-acting injectable cabotegravir in pregnancy. Abstract presented at: Conference on Retroviruses and Opportunistic Infections 2022; Virtual, Available at: https://www.croiconference.org/abstract/pbpk-modeling-of-long-acting-injectable-cabotegravir-in-pregnancy/. Accessed April 16, 2024.

39. Yu Y., Bekker A., Li X., et al., PBPK model prediction of long-acting cab and RPV concentrations in pregnancy. Abstract Seattle, WA, Available at: https://www.croiconference.org/abstract/pbpk-model-prediction-of-long-acting-cab-and-rpv-concentrations-in-pregnancy/, Accessed April 16, 2024. 2023.

40. van der Wekken-Pas L, Weiss F, Simon-Zuber C, et al. Cabotegravir and rilpivirine long acting injectables in a pregnant woman living with HIV. Clin Infect Dis 2024. https://doi.org/10.1093/cid/ciae242.

41. Ogbuagu O, Segal-Maurer S, Ratanasuwan W, et al. Efficacy and safety of the novel capsid inhibitor lenacapavir to treat multidrug-resistant HIV: week 52 results of a phase 2/3 trial. Lancet HIV 2023;10(8):e497–505.

42. Joseph Davey DL, Bekker LG, Bukusi EA, et al. Where are the pregnant and breastfeeding women in new pre-exposure prophylaxis trials? The imperative to overcome the evidence gap. Lancet HIV 2022;9(3):e214–22.

43. Pregnant and Lactating People in the Lenacapavir for HIV PrEP PURPOSE Program. Available at: https://www.purposestudies.com. Accessed April 17, 2024.

44. Wickremsinhe MN, Little MO, Carter AS, et al. Beyond "vessels and vectors": a global review of registered HIV-related clinical trials with pregnant women. J Womens Health (Larchmt) 2019;28(1):93–9.

45. Brooks KM, Scarsi KK, Mirochnick M. Antiretrovirals for human immunodeficiency virus treatment and prevention in pregnancy. Obstet Gynecol Clin N Am 2023; 50(1):205–18.

46. Byrne JJ, Saucedo AM, Spong CY. Task force on research specific to pregnant and lactating women. Semin Perinatol 2020;44(3):151226.

47. Thiele L, Thompson J, Pruszynski J, et al. Gaps in evidence-based medicine: underrepresented populations still excluded from research trials following 2018

recommendations from the Health and Human Services Task Force on Research Specific to Pregnant Women and Lactating Women. Am J Obstet Gynecol 2022; 227(6):908–9.

48. PRGLAC. Task force on research specific to pregnant women and lactating women. Available at: https://www.nichd.nih.gov/sites/default/files/2018-09/PRGLAC_Report.pdf. Accessed May 11, 2024.

49. Penazzato M, Lockman S, Colbers A, et al. Accelerating investigation of new HIV drugs in pregnancy: advancing the research agenda from theory to action. J Int AIDS Soc 2022;25(Suppl 2):e25912.

50. Abrams EJ, Calmy A, Fairlie L, et al. Approaches to accelerating the study of new antiretrovirals in pregnancy. J Int AIDS Soc 2022;25(Suppl 2):e25916.

51. World Health Organization. HIV Transmission through breastfeeding: a review of available evidence; 2007 update. Available at: http://apps.who.int/iris/bitstream/10665/43879/1/9789241596596_eng.pdf. [Accessed 18 April 2024].

52. Njom Nlend AE. Mother-to-child transmission of HIV through breastfeeding improving awareness and education: a short narrative review. Int J Womens Health 2022;14:697–703.

53. Van de Perre P, Rubbo PA, Viljoen J, et al. HIV-1 reservoirs in breast milk and challenges to elimination of breast-feeding transmission of HIV-1. Sci Transl Med 2012;4(143):143sr3.

54. Flynn PM, Taha TE, Cababasay M, et al. Association of maternal viral load and CD4 count with perinatal HIV-1 transmission risk during breastfeeding in the PROMISE postpartum component. J Acquir Immune Defic Syndr 2021;88(2):206–13.

55. Flynn PM, Taha TE, Cababasay M, et al. Prevention of HIV-1 transmission through breastfeeding: efficacy and safety of maternal antiretroviral therapy versus infant nevirapine prophylaxis for duration of breastfeeding in HIV-1-infected women with high CD4 cell count (IMPAACT PROMISE): a randomized, open-label, clinical trial. J Acquir Immune Defic Syndr 2018;77(4):383–92.

56. Shapiro RL, Hughes MD, Ogwu A, et al. Antiretroviral regimens in pregnancy and breast-feeding in Botswana. N Engl J Med 2010;362(24):2282–94.

57. Malaba TR, Nakatudde I, Kintu K, et al. 72 weeks post-partum follow-up of dolutegravir versus efavirenz initiated in late pregnancy (DolPHIN-2): an open-label, randomised controlled study. Lancet HIV 2022;9(8):e534–43.

58. Freeman-Romilly N, Nyatsanza F, Namiba A, et al. Moving closer to what women want? A review of breastfeeding and women living with HIV in the UK and high-income countries. HIV Med 2020;21(1):1–8.

59. Levison J, Weber S, Cohan D. Breastfeeding and HIV-Infected Women in the United States: Harm Reduction Counseling Strategies. Clin Infect Dis 2014; 59(2):304–9.

60. Powell A, Agwu A. In support of breast/chest feeding by people with HIV in high-income settings. Clin Infect Dis 2024. https://doi.org/10.1093/cid/ciae027.

61. Nashid N, Khan S, Loutfy M, et al. Breastfeeding by women living with human immunodeficiency virus in a resource-rich setting: a case series of maternal and infant management and outcomes. J Pediatric Infect Dis Soc 2020;9(2):228–31.

62. Haberl L, Audebert F, Feiterna-Sperling C, et al. Not recommended, but done: breastfeeding with HIV in Germany. AIDS Patient Care STDS 2021;35(2):33–8.

63. Ndirangu J, Viljoen J, Bland RM, et al. Cell-free (RNA) and cell-associated (DNA) HIV-1 and postnatal transmission through breastfeeding. PLoS One 2012;7(12): e51493.

64. Kuhn L, Kim HY, Walter J, et al. HIV-1 concentrations in human breast milk before and after weaning. Sci Transl Med 2013;5(181):181ra51.

65. Waitt C, Low N, Van de Perre P, et al. Does U=U for breastfeeding mothers and infants? Breastfeeding by mothers on effective treatment for HIV infection in high-income settings. Lancet HIV 2018;5(9):e531–6.

66. Powell AM, Knott-Grasso MA, Anderson J, et al. Infant feeding for people living with HIV in high resource settings: a multi-disciplinary approach with best practices to maximise risk reduction. Lancet Reg Health Am 2023;22:100509.

67. Jamieson DJ, Chasela CS, Hudgens MG, et al. Maternal and infant antiretroviral regimens to prevent postnatal HIV-1 transmission: 48-week follow-up of the BAN randomised controlled trial. Lancet 2012;379(9835):2449–58.

68. Bispo S, Chikhungu L, Rollins N, et al. Postnatal HIV transmission in breastfed infants of HIV-infected women on ART: a systematic review and meta-analysis. J Int AIDS Soc 2017;20(1):21251.

69. Levison J, McKinney J, Duque A, et al. Breastfeeding among people with human immunodeficiency virus in North America: a multisite study. Clin Infect Dis 2023; 77(10):1416–22.

70. Weiss F, von Both U, Rack-Hoch A, et al. Brief report: HIV-positive and breastfeeding in high-income settings: 5-year experience from a perinatal center in Germany. J Acquir Immune Defic Syndr 2022;91(4):364–7.

71. Koay WLA, Rakhmanina NY. Supporting Mothers Living With HIV in the United States Who Choose to Breastfeed. Journal of the Pediatric Infectious Diseases Society 2022;11(5):239.

72. Yusuf HE, Knott-Grasso MA, Anderson J, et al. experience and outcomes of breastfed infants of women living with HIV in the United States: findings from a single-center breastfeeding support initiative. Journal of the Pediatric Infectious Diseases Society 2022;11(1):24–7.

73. Prestileo T, Adriana S, Lorenza DM, et al. From undetectable equals untransmittable (U=U) to breastfeeding: is the jump short? Infect Dis Rep 2022;14(2): 220–7.

74. Pollock L, Levison J. 2023 Updated guidelines on infant feeding and HIV in the United States: what are they and why have recommendations changed. Top Antivir Med 2023;31(5):576–86.

75. Luoga E, Vanobberghen F, Bircher R, et al. Brief report: No HIV transmission from virally suppressed mothers during breastfeeding in rural tanzania. J Acquir Immune Defic Syndr 2018;79(1):e17–20.

76. Davis NL, Miller WC, Hudgens MG, et al. Maternal and breastmilk viral load: impacts of adherence on peripartum HIV infections averted-the breastfeeding, antiretrovirals, and nutrition study. J Acquir Immune Defic Syndr 2016;73(5):572–80.

77. Giuliano M, Andreotti M, Liotta G, et al. Maternal antiretroviral therapy for the prevention of mother-to-child transmission of HIV in Malawi: maternal and infant outcomes two years after delivery. PLoS One 2013;8(7):e68950.

78. de Vincenzi I. Triple antiretroviral compared with zidovudine and single-dose nevirapine prophylaxis during pregnancy and breastfeeding for prevention of mother-to-child transmission of HIV-1 (Kesho Bora study): a randomised controlled trial. Lancet Infect Dis 2011;11(3):171–80.

79. Cohan D, Natureeba P, Koss CA, et al. Efficacy and safety of lopinavir/ritonavir versus efavirenz-based antiretroviral therapy in HIV-infected pregnant Ugandan women. AIDS 2015;29(2):183–91.

80. Volpe LJ, Powis KM, Legbedze J, et al. A counseling and monitoring approach for supporting breastfeeding women living with HIV in Botswana. J Acquir Immune Defic Syndr 2022;89(2):e16.
81. Nagot N, Kankasa C, Tumwine JK, et al. Extended pre-exposure prophylaxis with lopinavir-ritonavir versus lamivudine to prevent HIV-1 transmission through breastfeeding up to 50 weeks in infants in Africa (ANRS 12174): a randomised controlled trial. Lancet 2016;387(10018):566–73.
82. Coovadia HM, Brown ER, Fowler MG, et al. Efficacy and safety of an extended nevirapine regimen in infant children of breastfeeding mothers with HIV-1 infection for prevention of postnatal HIV-1 transmission (HPTN 046): a randomised, double-blind, placebo-controlled trial. Lancet 2012;379(9812):221–8.

HIV Pre-Exposure Prophylaxis

Geoffroy Liegeon, MD, PhD[a],*,
Constance Delaugerre, PharmD, PhD[b,c,d],
Jean-Michel Molina, MD, PhD[c,d,e]

KEYWORDS

- Human immunodeficiency virus • Prevention • Pre-exposure prophylaxis • Tenofovir
- Cabotegravir • Men • Women • Transgender

KEY POINTS

- Pre-exposure prophylaxis (PrEP) consists of using antiretroviral therapy among human immunodeficiency virus (HIV)-uninfected individuals to prevent HIV infection.
- This strategy effectively prevents HIV in all individuals, providing high adherence.
- Daily oral tenofovir disoproxil–emtricitabine or long-acting injectable cabotegravir can be used among all individuals.
- Large PrEP roll-out, as part of a combination prevention approach, has the potential to significantly reduce the number of new HIV infections at the population level.
- Long-acting PrEP formulations are being developed to address the gaps in uptake, adherence, and persistence to oral PrEP.

INTRODUCTION

Pre-exposure prophylaxis (PrEP) has revolutionized the human immunodeficiency virus (HIV) prevention strategy during the past 15 years. Despite of the fact that people living with HIV (PLWH) on antiretroviral therapy (ART) do not transmit the virus (Undetectable = Untransmittable), the impact of the test-and-treat approach to preventing HIV transmission has been limited at the population level, notably because of delays in HIV diagnosis and persistence on ART.[1] With one-third of the global PLWH population still untreated, additional HIV prevention measures are required to control the global HIV epidemic.[2] PrEP, which consists of using ART among HIV-uninfected individuals

[a] Department of Infectious Diseases and Global Health, University of Chicago Medicine, Office L043 5841 South Maryland Avenue, Chicago 60637, IL, USA; [b] Virology Department, Assistance Publique - Hôpitaux de Paris, Hôpital Saint Louis, Paris, France; [c] Paris Cité University, Paris, France; [d] INSERM UMR 944, Paris, France; [e] Department of Infectious Diseases, Assistance Publique - Hôpitaux de Paris, Hôpitaux Saint Louis et Lariboisière, Paris, France
* Corresponding author.
E-mail address: geoffroy.liegeon@bsd.uchicago.edu

Infect Dis Clin N Am 38 (2024) 453–474
https://doi.org/10.1016/j.idc.2024.04.003
0891-5520/24/© 2024 Elsevier Inc. All rights reserved.

to prevent HIV infection, emerged as a game changer in the HIV prevention field, pending the development of an effective HIV vaccine. From 2016 to 2023, nearly 5 million individuals have initiated PrEP worldwide, while the range of PrEP options has progressively expanded.[3] Research in the PrEP field has shown that adherence and pharmacokinetics considerations, which varied widely across population groups, were the key drivers of PrEP effectiveness. To highlight the importance of those factors, the authors review the evidence supporting PrEP use across different population groups before addressing the issue of breakthrough HIV infections, the challenges in implementation, and the advances in the development of next-generation PrEP formulations.

GAY, BISEXUAL, AND OTHER MEN WHO HAVE SEX WITH MEN

Historically, cisgender gay, bisexual, and other men who have sex with men (GBMSM) were the first group for whom the efficacy and safety of oral PrEP were demonstrated in clinical trials.[4] Over a decade after the Food and Drug Administration (FDA) approved the daily combination of tenofovir (TFV) disoproxil–emtricitabine (TDF/FTC) for HIV PrEP, the landscape of PrEP options has expanded significantly among GBMSM. These alternatives include a daily TAF/FTC combination, an event-driven TDF-based regimen, and long-acting injectable cabotegravir (CAB-LA). **Table 1** summarizes the results of clinical trials of PrEP by agents and **Table 2** presents the grade of evidence supporting PrEP effectiveness categorized by transmission risk behavior.

Daily Tenofovir-emtricitabine Based Pre-exposure Prophylaxis

Extensive research has focused on the daily combination of TDF/FTC for HIV PrEP among GBMSM. These 2 nucleoside reverse transcriptase inhibitors have generated significant interest because of their complementary pharmacokinetic profiles. Emtricitabine triphosphate, the active form of FTC, rapidly accumulates in rectal tissue, preventing early-stage of HIV infection at the mucosal level.[5] In contrast, TFV-diphosphate (TFV-DP), the active form of TFV, progressively concentrates in peripheral blood mononuclear cells (PBMCs) avoiding early HIV trapping in lymph nodes and systemic diffusion of HIV. Studies in non-human primate models of Simian HIV (SHIV) (a Simian immunodeficiency virus [SIV]/HIV chimera) infection demonstrated the effectiveness of this combination after rectal exposure to SHIV, paving the way for further clinical investigations in human.[6]

The iPrEx study was the first clinical trial to demonstrate that daily TDF/FTC was effective in preventing HIV infection in GBMSM.[4] In this multicenter, randomized, double-blinded, and placebo-controlled clinical trial including 2499 HIV-seronegative men and transgender women (TGW) having sex with men, daily TDF/FTC led to a 44% HIV relative risk reduction (95% confidence interval [CI] [15–63]). Insights from the study's open-label extension revealed a strong correlation between TFV-DP concentration in dried blood spot (DBS) and the reduction in HIV risk. Notably, participants with TFV-DP levels more than 700 fmol/punch (equivalent to more than 4 TDF/FTC pills per week) achieved over 95% HIV risk reduction, underscoring the critical role of adherence in PrEP effectiveness.[7] These findings were further corroborated in the PROUD clinical trial in England in which 544 GBMSM were randomly assigned to either immediate or deferred PrEP initiation using daily TDF/FTC.[8] Immediate PrEP initiation led to 86% relative risk reduction in HIV transmission.

These studies, and others on daily TDF-based PrEP across diverse populations, also underscore the excellent safety profile of this combination. Meta-analyses of PrEP clinical trials showed that daily TDF/FTC did not result in a higher risk of serious

Table 1
Main randomized efficacy clinical trials in human immunodeficiency virus pre-exposure prophylaxis

Study	Location	Study Population	Number of Participants	Intervention	Controlled Arm	PrEP Effectiveness (95%CI)[a]
Oral PrEP with a TDF based regimen						
iPrEx	Peru, Ecuador, South Africa, Brazil, Thailand, US	GBMSM and transgender women	2499	Daily TDF/FTC	Placebo	44% (15% to 63%)
PROUD	England	GBMSM and transgender women	544	Daily TDF/FTC	No PrEP	86% (64% to 96%)
IPERGAY	France, Canada	GBMSM and transgender women	400	On-demand TDF/FTC	Placebo	86% (40% to 99%)
Bangkok Tenofovir Study	Thailand	People who inject drugs	2413	Daily TDF	Placebo	48.9% (9.6% to 72.2%)
Partners PrEP	Kenya, Uganda	Sero-discordant couples	4747 couples	Daily TDF or Daily TDF/FTC	Placebo	TDF/FTC: 75% (55% to 87%) TDF: 67% (44% to 81%)
TDF-2	Botswana	Heterosexual men and cisgender women	1219	Daily TDF/FTC	Placebo	61.7% (15.9% to 82.6%)
FEM-PrEP	Tanzania, South Africa, Kenya	Cisgender women	2056	Daily TDF/FTC	Placebo	6% (−52% to −41%)
VOICE	South Africa, Uganda, Zimbabwe	Cisgender women	4969	Daily TDF or Daily TDF/FTC	Placebo	TDF/FTC: −4.4% (−50% to 27%) TDF: −49% (−130% to 3%)
Oral PrEP with TAF/FTC						
DISCOVER	Europe and North America	GBMSM and transgender women	5857	Daily TAF/FTC	Daily TDF/FTC	53% (−15% to 81%) relative risk reduction of TAF/FTC vs TDF/FTC
PURPOSE 1 NCT 04994509	South Africa	Cisgender women	5010	Daily TAF/FTC	Counterfactual HIV incidence	On-going

(continued on next page)

Table 1
(continued)

Study	Location	Study Population	Number of Participants	Intervention	Controlled Arm	PrEP Effectiveness (95%CI)[a]
Once Monthly Oral Islatravir						
IMPOWER-022 NCT 04644029	Unites States, South Africa, Uganda	Cisgender women	4500	Once monthly oral Islatravir	Counterfactual HIV incidence	Halted for a significant decrease in CD4 count
IMPOWER-024 NCT 04652700	US, France, Japan, Peru, South Africa, Thailand	GBMSM and transgender women	1500	Once monthly oral Islatravir	Counterfactual HIV incidence	
Cabotegravir Long-Acting						
HPTN 083	US, Latin America, Asia, and Africa	GBMSM and transgender women	4566	Cabotegravir Long Acting	Daily TDF/FTC	66% (38%–82%) relative risk reduction on CAB
HPTN 084	Sub-Saharan Africa	Cisgender women	3224	Cabotegravir Long Acting	Daily TDF/FTC	89% (69%–99%) relative risk reduction on CAB
Lenacapavir Long-Acting						
PURPOSE 1 NCT 04994509	South Africa	Cisgender women	5010	Lenacapavir	Counterfactual HIV incidence	On-going
PURPOSE 2 NCT 04925752	US	GBMSM and transgender women	3000	Lenacapavir	Counterfactual HIV incidence	On-going
Broadly Neutralizing Antibody						
HPTN 081	Sub-Saharan Africa	Cisgender women	1924	VRCO1	Placebo	8.8% (−45.1%–42.6%)
HPTN 085	Americas and Europe	GBMSM and transgender women	2699	VRCO1	Placebo	26.6% (−11.7%–51.8%)
Dapivirine vaginal ring						
ASPIRE	Malawi, South Africa, Uganda, and Zimbabwe	Cisgender women	2629	Dapivirine vaginal ring	Placebo	27% (1%–46%)
RING	South Africa and Uganda.	Cisgender women	1959	Dapivirine vaginal ring	Placebo	31% (1%–51%)

Abbreviations: FTC, emtricitabine. GBMSM, gay, bisexual, and other men who have sex with men; TAF, tenofovir alafenamide; TDF, tenofovir disoproxil fumarate.
[a] Intention to treat analysis.

Table 2
Grade of evidence supporting PrEP effectiveness by transmission risk behavior

	Daily TDF/FTC	Daily TAF/FTC	Event-Driven TDF/FTC	CAB-LA	LEN
Insertive sex (vaginal or anal)	Grade AIa	Grade AIa	Grade BIa[b]	Grade AIa	Under Evaluation
Receptive vaginal sex	Grade AIa	Under Evaluation	Insufficient Data	Grade AIa	Under Evaluation
Receptive neo-vaginal sex	Grade BIII	Insufficient Data	Insufficient Data	Grade BIII	Under Evaluation
Receptive anal sex	Grade AIa	Grade AIa	Grade AIa[b]	Grade AIa	Under Evaluation
Injection drug use[a]	Grade AIa	Insufficient Data	Insufficient Data	Insufficient Data	Under Evaluation

Abbreviations: CAB-LA, long-acting injectable cabotegravir; DPV-VR, dapivirine vaginal ring; Grade AIa, Evidence from 1 or more randomized clinical trials with strong panel expert support for recommendations; Grade BIa, Evidence from 1 or more randomized clinical trials with moderate panel expert support for the recommendations; Grade BIII, Recommendation based on the expert panel's analysis of the accumulated available evidence with moderate panel expert support for the recommendations. LEN, lenacapavir; TAF/FTC, tenofovir alafenamide–emtricitabine; TDF/FTC, tenofovir disoproxil–emtricitabine.

[a] Refer to the other categories for people who inject drugs who are also at-risk of sexual exposure to HIV.

[b] Grade CIII, if patients using gender affirming hormone therapy (Recommendation based on the expert panel's analysis of the accumulated available evidence with limited panel or weak panel support for the recommendations).

Adapted from Gandhi, Antiretroviral Drugs for Treatment and Prevention of HIV Infection in Adults: 2022 Recommendations of the International Antiviral Society-USA Panel, JAMA, 2023[70] adverse events compared with placebo or no intervention.[9] While gastrointestinal issues remain the most common side effects among users, these symptoms are typically transient and resolve within a few weeks. Additionally, TDF-based PrEP results in a slight but non-clinically relevant decline in estimated glomerular filtration rate (eGFR) and bone mineral density over time, which tends to normalize upon PrEP discontinuation.[10]

As an alternative to TDF-based PrEP, a daily combination of tenofovir alafenamide (TAF) – FTC has also been studied for HIV prevention. As compared with TDF, oral TAF administration results in significantly higher and sustained concentrations of TFV-DP in PBMCs, a critical driver of PrEP effectiveness.[11] The efficacy of TAF/FTC in HIV PrEP was evaluated in the double-blinded, non-inferiority DISCOVER clinical trial.[12] In this study, 5,387 HIV-uninfected men and TGW who have sex with men were randomized to receive daily PrEP with either TAF/FTC or TDF/FTC. Over 8,756 person-years of follow-up, 7 infections occurred in the TAF/FTC group compared with 15 in the TDF/FTC group, resulting in an incidence rate ratio of 0.47 (95% CI: 0.19–1.15). These findings demonstrate that TAF/FTC was non-inferior to daily TDF/FTC for HIV PrEP. While TAF-based PrEP exhibited a more favorable renal and bone safety profile based on biomarkers, no significant differences in meaningful clinical outcomes were observed between the 2 groups. Nevertheless, TAF/FTC remains the exclusive oral PrEP option for GBMSM with an eGFR ranging from 30 to 60 mL/min. A recent post-marketing study in the United States (US) suggests a potential association between TAF/FTC and a higher incidence of hypertension and statin initiation, particularly among users aged 40 years or older.[13] Despite its FDA approval in 2019, daily TAF/FTC remains largely unavailable in most countries because of cost-effectiveness considerations when compared with low-cost TDF/FTC generics.

Event-driven Tenofovir Disoproxil–Emtricitabine Based PrEP

To offer a non-daily oral PrEP option that could improve adherence, an intermittent PrEP regimen with TDF/FTC was developed. Based on data derived from macaque models of SHIV infection, the 2-1-1 regimen (also called event-driven [ED], intermittent, or on-demand PrEP) consists of a loading dose of 2 tablets of TDF/FTC 2 to 24 hours before sexual intercourse, a third tablet 24 hours after the first drug intake and a fourth tablet 24 hours later.[14] The efficacy of this regimen was evaluated in the ANRS Ipergay trial in France and Canada.[15,16] In this randomized, controlled, double-blinded clinical trial, and 400 HIV-uninfected GBMSM were randomized to follow a "2-1-1" regimen with either TDF/FTC or a placebo. After 9.3 months, the trial was halted because of the high efficacy of ED TDF/FTC: only 2 infections occurred in the TDF/FTC group (incidence of 0.91 per 100 person-years) compared with 14 in the placebo group (incidence of 6.60 per 100 person-years). This resulted in an 86% (95% CI: 40% to 98%) HIV-related risk reduction. This finding was further confirmed in the open-label extension study with a 97% HIV relative reduction compared with the placebo arm of the trial.[16] Real-world evidence from the ANRS PREVENIR cohort study, which enrolled 3,057 PrEP users in the Paris region, further validated the effectiveness of ED-PrEP in GBMSM.[17] Over 5623 person-years of follow-up, only 6 infections occurred for a 1.1 (95% CI: 0.4–2.3) per 1000 person-years HIV-1 incidence. Although not a randomized comparison, the incidence did not differ between participants using daily and ED-PrEP. Beyond its remarkable efficacy, the '2-1-1' regimen remains the most cost-effective approach for HIV PrEP and offers potential renal safety benefits for users at risk of kidney dysfunction who cannot access other PrEP alternatives.[18,19] The '2-1-1' regimen for GBMSM has been endorsed by World Health Organisation (WHO) guidelines since 2018 and has been incorporated into the 2021 Centers for Disease Control and Prevention (CDC) PrEP guidelines.[20,21] Pending the results of specific studies, TAF/FTC is not recommended for ED-PrEP, but a clinical trial is on-going to evaluate a simplified "1-1" regimen based on this combination (NCT 05813964).

Long-acting Injectable Cabotegravir

CAB, an integrase transfer inhibitor (INSTI) structurally related to dolutegravir, is available in both short-acting oral and long-acting injectable forms. The extended half-life of the injectable suspension has prompted extensive research into its use as the first injectable PrEP agent. Although CAB penetration remains limited in rectal and vaginal tissue, studies in non-human primate models have demonstrated its effectiveness in preventing SIV/SHIV infection after repeated rectal, vaginal, penile, and intravenous challenges.[22] Achieving a plasma concentration of CAB more than 4-fold the protein-adjusted IC90 (PA-IC90 = 166 ng/mL) after vaginal exposure and more than 3-fold, the PA-IC90 after rectal challenge predicts a 90% probability of in vivo protection against SHIV acquisition. In humans, this protective threshold is achieved through a single 600-mg intramuscular CAB injection given at 2-month intervals after an initial 2 injections 1 month apart.[23] This regimen ensures long-term CAB persistence in the body. The tail phase, defined as the median time from the last injection to the time when CAB concentration is undetectable, reach 44 weeks for men and 67 weeks for women.[24]

The randomized, double-blinded, and placebo-controlled HIV Prevention Trails Network (HPTN) 083 clinical trial evaluated the CAB-LA efficacy in 3999 HIV-uninfected men and 567 trans-women having sex with men.[25] Participants were randomized to receive CAB-LA plus TDF/FTC placebo or active TDF/FTC plus CAB-LA placebo after a 5-week oral lead-in period at 43 sites across Africa, Asia, Latin America, and the US. After a median follow-up time of 1.4 years, HIV incidence was 0.41% in the CAB-LA arm (13 infections) and 1.22% in the daily TDF/FTC arm (31 infections). CAB-LA was significantly superior to daily TDF/FTC in preventing HIV infection with a 66% HIV relative risk reduction. The superiority of CAB-LA was primarily driven by low adherence to oral TDF/FTC. In a randomly selected sub-group of 390 participants, 28% of the DBS showed a TFV-DP concentration indicating the use of fewer than 4 TDF–FTC doses per week over the previous 1 to 2 months.[25] In the first 1-year unblinded period, CAB-LA effectiveness remained unchanged, with 12 additional HIV infections in the CAB-LA group (incidence 0.82 per 100 persons-year [PY]) versus 32 in the TDF/FTC group (2.27 per 100 PY) (HR 0.31; 95% CI: 0.17–0.58) for a similar reduction in HIV incidence.[26] Injection site reactions (ISRs) were the most common adverse events, occurring in 81.4% of CAB-LA participants and 31.3% of those receiving TDF/FTC. These ISRs led to study discontinuation in 50 participants (2.4%) who received CAB-LA. Additionally, the mean annualized increase in body weight was higher in the CAB-LA group (1.23 kg per year) compared with TDF/FTC (0.37 kg). Importantly, CAB-LA did not result in a higher risk of serious grade greater than or equal to 2 adverse events when compared with TDF/FTC.

The HPTN 083 clinical trial provided the initial proof of concept that a single long-acting agent could effectively serve as HIV PrEP, positioning CAB-LA as a potential game-changer in HIV prevention field. However, several factors may hinder its integration into clinical practice.[27] Among the 12 breakthrough HIV infections observed with CAB-LA in HPTN 083, 4 occurred despite continuous and timely injections with appropriate plasma CAB concentration, suggesting that CAB-LA may not consistently prevent HIV infection among all individuals. Additionally, CAB-LA significantly alters the timing and patterns of HIV seroconversion, which may warrant more complex testing algorithms based on nucleic acid test that are not widely available in low- and middle-income countries.[28] The long and variable tail phase after CAB-LA injection may favor the emergence of HIV drug resistance in case of HIV infection during this period, resulting in challenges for safely discontinuing PrEP.[29] However, so far in clinical trials, such emergence of resistance did not occur. Challenges related to the inherent medicalization because of intramuscular injections, the health care infrastructure's additional burden, and the cost-effectiveness compared with TDF/FTC generics also pose barriers to CAB-LA adoption. The licensing agreement between ViiV Healthcare and the Medicines Patent Pool will improve access to CAB-LA in low- and middle-income countries in the coming years.[30]

In 2021, both CDC and WHO endorsed CAB-LA as part of their PrEP guidelines following the positive results from the HPTN 083 and 084 clinical trials.[20,31] Despite the US FDA approved CAB-LA for HIV prevention, the utilization of CAB-LA in the US remains limited, with only 1 out of 200 PrEP prescriptions being for CAB-LA. This underscores the significant barriers faced by health care providers and PrEP users in accessing this prophylaxis. Addressing these challenges will require a concerted effort from all stakeholders and policymakers to position CAB-LA as a game-changer in the global HIV response.

TRANSGENDER PEOPLE

In the US, approximately 1 million individuals identify as transgender. Of the new HIV diagnoses in the country, 2% occurs among transgender individuals, with TGW accounting for 90% of these new infections.[32] Transgender individuals often face stigma, socioeconomic disadvantages, and psychologic challenges, which not only increase their risk of HIV infection but also limit their access to HIV prevention services. PrEP serves as a powerful instrument to address these HIV-related disparities within the transgender community.

The iPrEx trial, which enrolled 399 TGW, provided evidence for the effectiveness of daily PrEP with TDF/FTC among TGW. In this trial, 11 HIV infections were reported in the daily TDF/FTC group and 10 in the placebo group (hazard ratio 1.1, 0.5–2.7).[4] The infections in the daily TDF/FTC group were generally associated with lower plasma drug concentrations. This finding was corroborated in the open-label extension study involving 151 TGW taking daily TDF/FTC.[7] No infections were reported among TGW with TFV-DP concentrations in DBS indicating intake of at least 2 to 3 tablets per week, a pattern similar to that observed in GBMSM. Three seroconversions were reported in TGW with drug levels below this threshold. Data on the efficacy of TAF/FTC among TGW are more limited, as only 74 TGW (1.4% of study participants) were included in the DISCOVER trial; 29 were randomized to TDF/FTC; and 45 to TAF/FTC. No HIV infections occurred among these participants. As per FDA approval, daily PrEP with TAF/FTC can be used among transgender people who do not engage in receptive vaginal sex.[20]

Gender-affirming therapy with feminizing (eg, estradiol) or masculinizing (eg, testosterone) hormones concur to the physical and psychologic well-being of transgender people and are widely used in this population. The potential for drug-drug interactions that could impact the effectiveness of either PrEP or gender-affirming hormone therapy (GAHT) poses an additional barrier to PrEP uptake among transgender individuals. Several pharmacologic studies have evaluated the interaction between TDF-based PrEP and feminizing hormone therapy (FHT). Those studies showed that FHT slightly decreases the plasma concentration of TFV and the ratio of TFV active metabolites to competing deoxynucleotides in rectal tissues, which could theoretically affect PrEP effectiveness.[33,34] However, the plasma TVF-DP concentration, a critical driver of

PrEP efficacy, seems not significantly affected. The iBrEATHEe study evaluated the TFV-DP in DBS and sex hormone concentration at 2 and 4 weeks among 24 trans gender men (TGM) and 24 TGW on stable sex hormone therapy for at least 6 months who received directly observed dosing of daily oral TDF/FTC for 4 weeks.[35] After 4 weeks of PrEP use, testosterone (total and free), and estradiol concentrations remained stable and did not result in changes in hormone dosing. Moreover, the TFV-DP concentration in DBS at 4 weeks in TGW was comparable to that observed in a historical control group of cisgender men (mean difference, −12%, 95% CI: −27% to 7%). Importantly, all individuals achieved a TFV-DP concentration of greater than 700 fmol per punch, a level associated with high protection from HIV. This study demonstrates that GAHT and daily TDF/FTC can be co-administered safely without compromising HIV prevention or gender-affirming care. Data on potential interactions with TAF/FTC are more limited. In the DISCOVER trial, which included 32 TGW who received TAF/FTC and GAHT, the TFV-DP concentration was similar to that observed among GBMSM in the study, suggesting no adverse drug-drug interactions of GAHT with TAF/FTC.[36] Regarding event-driven PrEP, no studies to date have evaluated the impact of GHAT on the efficacy of this dosing regimen. The lower ratio of TFV active metabolites with FHT in the rectal tissue may increase the risk of PrEP failure when the "2-1-1" regimen is initiated or resumed after a prolonged break.[33] Furthermore, the ef-ficacy of event-driven PrEP has not been evaluated for receptive vaginal intercourse among cisgender women or transgender individuals who have undergone vagino-plasty. As a result, most guidelines do not recommend event-driven PrEP for trans-gender individuals.[20,37]

Regarding long-acting agents, the HPTN083 clinical trial, which included 570 TGW, provided efficacy and safety data for long-acting cabotegravir. Of these, 266 (47%) received CAB-LA injections and 330 (58%) used GAHT. The HIV incidence among TGW on TDF/FTC (1.8 per 100 PY) and CAB-LA (0.54 per 100 PY) was similar to that observed in GBMSM.[38] This resulted in a similar relative reduction in HIV inci-dence among TGW, suggesting that the efficacy of CAB-LA was maintained in this population. The frequency of adverse events was also similar between the treatment groups, and GAHT had no impact on CAB-LA concentration. These results suggest that CAB-LA is also a safe and effective PrEP option for TGW.

While there is a lack of specific efficacy data about PrEP in TGM, evidence from other demographic groups suggests that a daily TDF/FTC regimen or CAB-LA could offer protection for both insertive and receptive vaginal and anal sex within this pop-ulation. A recent US study found that a quarter of the TGM surveyed, fulfilled the eligi-bility requirements for PrEP, underscoring the need of specific PrEP studies in this group.[39]

CISGENDER WOMEN

The initial evidence that ART could prevent HIV infection in HIV-negative individuals was first demonstrated in 2010 among heterosexual women through the CAPRISA 004 study.[40] This randomized, double-blind, placebo-controlled clinical trial conduct-ed in South Africa, found that the daily application of a 1% TFV vaginal gel formulation reduced the relative risk of HIV infection by 39%. Although this formulation did not achieve regulatory approval, this study paved the way for further PrEP research with oral and topical ART agents in cisgender women. Main PrEP clinical trials results among cisgender women are summarized by PrEP agents in **Table 1**.

Daily oral PrEP with TDF/FTC has been extensively studied among cisgender women in Sub-Saharan Africa.[41] These studies have shown that maintaining PrEP efficacy over time in women requires a high level of adherence and that some women poorly accept a daily dosing regimen. Consequently, 2 large, randomized, placebo-controlled clinical trials in Sub-Saharan Africa failed to demonstrate the efficacy of daily TDF/FTC for HIV PrEP among heterosexual women. The FEM-PrEP study randomized 2,120 heterosexual women in Sub-Saharan Africa to receive either a placebo or daily oral TDF/FTC but found no evidence for the clinical efficacy of this regimen (hazard ratio 0.94, 0.59–1.52).[42] Similar results were reported in the VOICE trial, where a daily TDF-based regimen did not outperform a placebo in protecting heterosexual women from HIV infection among the 5,029 women enrolled in the trial (Daily TDF/FTC: HR 1.04 [0.73–1.49] & daily TDF: 1.49 [0.97–2.29]).[43] Despite high self-reported adherence, the study drug was detected in less than 40% of women taking daily TDF-based PrEP in both studies. The most compelling evidence of daily TDF/FTC effectiveness in heterosexual women comes from studies in serodiscordant heterosexual couples. In the Partners PrEP clinical trial, 4,747 couples were randomized to receive a single (TDF alone) or dual agent (TDF/FTC) PrEP or a placebo. In the 1,785 women included in the study, TDF and TDF/FTC taken daily resulted in a relative HIV risk reduction of 71% (95% CI: 0.13–0.63) and 66% (95% CI: 0.16–0.72), respectively.[44] These findings were confirmed in the randomized placebo-controlled clinical trial TDF2, which randomized 1,219 heterosexual couples. Daily TDF/FTC led to a 49% HIV relative risk reduction among the 557 women enrolled in the study.[45]

A pooled analysis of pharmacologic data from the FEM-PrEP, VOICE, and Partners PrEP clinical trials demonstrated a significant correlation between PrEP adherence and HIV risk reduction in cisgender women.[46] The incidence of HIV was reduced by 59% (95% credible interval: 30%–96%), 84% (95% CI: 52–100), and 96% (95% CI: 73%–100%) with the administration of 2, 4, and 7 pills of TDF/FTC per week, respectively. These results are aligned with modeling study and observational meta-analysis including 11 demonstration project of TDF/FTC in cisgender women.[47,48] Compared with GBMSM, cisgender women may need to adhere more strictly to daily TDF/FTC to achieve a similar level of protection. Data from the TDF/FTC arm of the HPTN 083 and 084 clinical trials, which assessed CAB-LA for HIV PrEP, showed that approximately 99% efficacy was achieved with daily dosages among cisgender women, compared with greater than or equal to 2 doses per week for GBMSM.[49] Since the concentration of FTC-TP is 10 times higher in vaginal tissue compared with rectal tissue, and that TFV-DP achieves similar concentrations in PBMCs regardless of sex, this difference in pharmacologic forgiveness profiles may be driven by the lower concentrations of TFV-DP in the vaginal tissue reported in pharmacokinetic studies.[50] This lower TFV-DP concentration in the women genital tract and the longer time required to achieve mucosal level protection have raised concerns about the potential efficacy of the on-demand '2–1–1' PrEP regimen in cisgender women. Pending the results of clinical trials, this dosing regimen is not recommended for women.[20] In cisgender women, the use of TAF results in a lower concentration of TFV-DP in vaginal tissue compared with TDF.[51] However, TAF leads to a higher concentration of TFV-DP in PBMCs. The efficacy of daily TAF/FTC is currently under investigation in a phase 3 clinical trial (NCT04994509). To date, daily TDF/FTC remains the only oral PrEP option for cisgender women. This regimen can be safely used during pregnancy and breastfeeding and in association with hormonal contraception.[52] Given the challenges associated with adherence to a daily regimen and the less forgiving pharmacologic profile in the event of sub-optimal adherence, long-acting PrEP options are eagerly awaited in this population.

The efficacy of CAB-LA in cisgender women was assessed in the HPTN084 clinical trial.[53] This double-blind, double-dummy, active-controlled, superiority trial involved

3224 women aged 18 to 45 years at risk of HIV infection in 7 sub-Saharan African countries. Participants were randomized to receive either CAB-LA plus TDF/FTC placebo or active TDF/FTC plus CAB-LA placebo following a 5-week oral lead-in period. After a median follow-up of 1.24 years, the HIV incidence was 0.2 per 100 PY in the CAB-LA arm compared with 1.85 per 100 PY in the TDF/FTC arm. This corresponds to an 89% relative risk reduction in HIV (HR 0.12; 95%CI: 0.05–0.31), demonstrating the superiority of CAB-LA over daily TDF/FTC for HIV prevention in cisgender women. No additional HIV infections occurred during the unblinded phase of the trial among women receiving CAB-LA, and 78% of study participants opted for CAB LA during the open-label extension phase.[54,55] The safety profile of CAB-LA was similar to that observed among GBMSM in the HPTN083 trial, but ISRs were less frequent (38%) and did not lead to PrEP discontinuation.[53] Forty-nine pregnancies occurred during the HPTN 084 trial, none of which resulted in congenital abnormalities.[56] Additional data on pregnancy outcomes and pharmacokinetic parameters are being collected through the open-label extension study. Preliminary data also suggested no clinically significant drug-drug interactions between CAB-LA and hormonal contraception in women of reproductive age.[57] Interestingly, the HIV incidence among women receiving CAB-LA was lower than that reported in GBMSM, and more importantly, no breakthrough HIV infections occurred among women receiving timely injections.[53] The reasons for this difference between men and women remain unclear but may be because of a shorter follow-up period in women, a higher number of HIV exposures among GBMSM, or differences in the pharmacokinetic profile, as women have slower CAB-LA absorption, resulting in a longer terminal-phase half-life.[24] CAB-LA is anticipated to mitigate the challenges associated with the uptake, adherence, and retention of oral PrEP in cisgender women. However, large implementation challenges remain among cisgender women, requiring pilot studies to facilitate CAB-LA uptake in clinical practice and support its large-scale rollout.

Drawing from experiences in contraception, a monthly vaginal ring containing 25 mg of the non-NRTI dapivirine (DPV) has been developed as an additional PrEP option for cisgender women. This silicone ring, which is easy to bend and insert into the vagina, slowly releases DPV over a 28-day period, after which it should be replaced with a new one. The efficacy of this long-acting formulation was evaluated in 2 double-blind, placebo-controlled randomized trials in Sub-Saharan Africa.[58,59] The DPV vaginal ring (DPV-VR) resulted in a 35% and 27% relative risk reduction of HIV among Sub-Saharan African women in the Ring and ASPIRE studies, respectively. The ring was well-tolerated in both studies. Results from the open-label extension studies of these trials showed improved adherence and efficacy, with a greater than 50% relative risk reduction of HIV compared with the estimated HIV incidence in the study population.[60,61] The DELIVER and B-PROTECTED studies also confirmed that DPV-VG could be safely used in the third trimester of pregnancy and during breastfeeding.[62,63] Based on these positive outcomes, WHO has recommended in 2021 that the DPV-VR may be offered as an additional prevention choice for women at substantial risk of HIV infection. A randomized open-label crossover clinical trial among African adolescent girls and young women recently evaluated the adherence, safety, and choice of oral PrEP compared with the DPV-VR.[64] In this study, 247 adolescent girls and young women were randomized to receive DPV-VR for 6 months followed by 6 months of oral PrEP or vice versa. During the 6-month randomized periods, the adherence level was similar for both groups, with 57% of women having pharmacologic evidence of high adherence to the DPV-VR and oral PrEP. Safety and tolerability of both products were high. Interestingly, after 6 months of use of oral PrEP and the DPV-VR, two-thirds of study participants chose the DPV-VR. Those data support the DPV-VR as an additional HIV prevention option for women who do not want or cannot properly follow a daily oral tablet or CAB-LA injection. Longer-duration rings (3 months or more) containing DPV or tenofovir, as well as multi-purpose technology rings that contain an antiretroviral drug and a hormonal contraceptive, are also being explored to expand the HIV prevention menu in women. However, the efficacy of the DPV-VR has never been directly compared with daily TDF/FTC or CAB-LA in women, leading to the withdrawal of this product from consideration for FDA regulatory approval in the US.

PEOPLE WHO INJECT DRUGS

In 2021, people who inject drugs (PWID) accounted for 7% (2,512) of the 36,136 new HIV diagnoses in the US.[65] Substance use disorders (SUD) increase the risk of HIV infection by sharing drug injection equipment and condomless sexual intercourse. SUD fuels additional barriers to uptake and retention in HIV prevention programs. Insurance issue, housing instability, poverty, criminalization of drug use, associated mental illness, racism, or stigma should be evaluated and addressed as part of a comprehensive reduction risk strategy. Reducing or eliminating injection risk practices can be achieved by offering social support, drug treatment plus relapse prevention services, access to clean injection material, and replacement opioid therapy. PrEP should be integrated and offered to all PWID as part of harm reduction program.

The Bangkok Tenofovir Study is the only randomized, double-blinded, and placebo-controlled clinical trial that evaluated the efficacy of daily TDF among 2413 PWID in Thailand. Daily TDF led to 49% (10% to 72%; $P = .01$) HIV relative risk reduction.[66] PrEP efficacy was strongly correlated to adherence to daily TDF.[67] Factors independently associated with poor adherence included being men, being aged under 40 years, injecting methamphetamine, and incarceration.[68] Several of the study participants reported risk factors for sexual HIV acquisition, suggesting that the efficacy of TDF in the study may not be solely attributable to its action in preventing HIV infection following intravenous exposure. Furthermore, the trial sites did not provide access to clean injection equipment, which limits the extrapolation of the study outcomes to settings that provide such access as part of standard care.

Currently, there are no clinical trial data that support the use of event-driven TDF/FTC or daily TAF/FTC for the prevention of HIV infection following intravenous exposure. However, as PWID may also acquire HIV via condomless sexual intercourse, those PrEP options remain relevant to prevent HIV infection as part of harm reduction programs especially for people who practice transactional sex. CAB-LA has been shown effective in protecting macaques after intravenous challenges with SHIV and pilot projects generating data with CAB-LA are expected in the coming years.[69] This option may be particularly suitable for many PWID drugs facing adherence or persistence issues with oral regimen.

HETEROSEXUAL MEN

The efficacy of daily TDF/FTC among heterosexual men has been specifically evaluated in the TDF-2 and Partner PrEP trials, which enrolled HIV-1 serodiscordant couples in Sub-saharan Africa.[44,45] These studies demonstrated that daily TDF/FTC was safe and highly effective in protecting heterosexual men from HIV-1 infection when adherence was high. Additional data on PrEP efficacy after insertive sex are derived from PrEP clinical trials among GBMSM.[4,8] Although these studies did not provide efficacy data after vaginal insertive sex, daily TAF/FTC and CAB-LA have been recommended as additional prevention option among heterosexual men. Similarly, the WHO and the International Antivirus Society-USA Panel guidelines also consider the event-driven "2-1-1" regimen among heterosexual men.[70,71] This regimen has not yet been approved by CDC guidelines pending the results of specific data in heterosexual men.[20]

BREAKTHROUGH HUMAN IMMUNODEFICIENCY VIRUS INFECTION

Despite the high efficacy of pre-exposure prophylaxis, breakthrough HIV infections among PrEP users can occur under various circumstances: (i) undiagnosed HIV infection at the time of PrEP initiation, (ii) sub-optimal adherence to PrEP, and (iii) HIV infection with a virus harboring drug resistance, such as FTC/3 TC resistant virus, TDF-resistant virus, or both.[72] Breakthrough HIV infections with a drug-resistant virus have been rarely reported among oral PrEP users, with fewer than 10 cases worldwide.[73] Most new HIV infection cases occur among users non-adherent to PrEP, with few consequences in terms of HIV resistance and management. The emergence of HIV resistance-associated mutations (RAM) to FTC or TDF predominantly occurs when PrEP is initiated during an undiagnosed acute HIV-1 infection. In this situation, approximately 45% of PrEP users developed RAM to TDF and/or FTC, necessitating the use of ART with a high genetic barrier pending the results of resistance testing. **Table 3** summarizes the prevalence of HIV drug resistance mutations among patients who acquired HIV during the main PrEP clinical trials. Consistent with these data, a pooled analysis of 72 global PrEP studies found that M184V/I mutations, K65R mutations, and both mutations were detected in 23%, 1.3%, and 3.8%, respectively, of the 78 PrEP users who experienced breakthrough HIV infection.[74]

PrEP also significantly alters the timing and patterns of HIV seroconversion. These findings, initially detected among oral PrEP users, have been more frequently reported among users receiving CAB-LA injections and described as the long-acting early viral inhibition (LEVI) syndrome.[75,76] The LEVI syndrome occurs among users with undiagnosed HIV infection starting CAB-LA or in the rare cases of breakthrough HIV infection despite on-time CAB injections. This syndrome is characterized by a smoldering, minimal, asymptomatic HIV viral replication that can persist for several months before being detected through HIV serologic testing.[76] This delay in HIV diagnosis promotes the emergence of RAM to INSTI, leading to potential cross resistance with the WHO-recommended first-line dolutegravir-based regimen. Nucleic acid testing (NAT) can detect HIV infections earlier, often before RAM to INSTIs emerge.[77] Consequently, the US FDA package insert, as well as the US CDC guidelines, recommend using a NAT-based strategy to monitor PrEP users on CAB-LA.[20] Further research is still needed to evaluate the advantages and drawbacks of this approach, especially in low- and middle-income countries, where a NAT-based strategy would be a significant obstacle for CAB-LA rollout. A recent modeling study suggest that large scale CAB-LA implementation along with standard antibody-based rapid testing is likely to reducing HIV incidence and acquired immunodeficiency syndrome (AIDS) deaths despite a significant increase in the prevalence of INSTI resistance.[78] Beyond CAB-LA, the LEVI syndrome represents a new challenge in the development and implementation of next-generation long-acting PrEP agents.

GLOBAL PrEP ROLL-OUT

Following the 2015 WHO guidelines that integrated oral TDF-based PrEP into the combined HIV prevention strategy for all individuals, there has been a global PrEP roll-out. This has resulted in nearly 5 million PrEP initiations worldwide from 2016 to 2023, with 450,000 of these in the US, over 90% of which were men.[3,79] There is a strong evidence suggesting that the large PrEP roll-out, as part of a combination HIV prevention

Table 3
Frequency of human immunodeficiency virus drug resistance mutations in pre-exposure prophylaxis clinical trials

TDF based PrEP	Acute HIV Infection at Study Enrollment				HIV Infection Occurred during the Study			
	HIV cases	HIVDR to TDF and/or XTC	K65 R/K70 E	M184IV	HIV cases	HIVDR to TDF and/or XTC	K65 R/K70 E	M184IV
Bangkok Tenofovir Study	0	–	–	–	17[a]	0	0	–
FEM-PrEP	1	0	0	0	33	4	0	4
iPrEx	2	2	0	2	48	0	0	0
Partners PrEP	12	3	1	2	51	4	1	4
TDF2	1	1	1	1	9	0	0	0
VOICE	14	2	0	2	113	1	0	1
IPERGAY	3[b]	NR	NR	NR	2	0	0	0
PROUD	3	2	0	2	3	0	0	0
iPrEx OLE	0	–	–	–	28	1	0	1
USA DEMO	3	1	0	1	2	0	0	0
HPTN-067	3	2	1	1	9	1	1	1
DISCOVER	5	4	0	4	18	1[c]	0	1
HPTN 083	3	2	0	2	39	4	1	3
Total (%)	50	19 (38)	3 (6)	17 (34)	372	16 (4.3)	3 (0.8)	15 (4.0)

CAB long acting	HIV cases	HIVDR to CAB	Mutations to INSTI		HIV cases	HIVDR to CAB	Mutations to INSTI	
HPTN 084	1	0	None		3	0	None	
HPTN 083	4	1	E138 K + Q148 K		12	4	L74I + Q148 R; E138 A+ Q148 R; R263 K; G140 A+ Q148 R	

Resistance mutation abbreviations reflect standard amino acid nomenclature.

Abbreviations: CAB, cabotegravir; FTC, emtricitabine; HIVDR, HIV drug resistance; INSTI, integrase strand transfer inhibitor; NR, not reported; TDF, tenofovir disoproxil fumarate; XTC, lamivudine or emtricitabine.

[a] Two of the 17 cases were excluded from the total number of HIV cases because HIVDR testing was not successful.

[b] The 3 cases were excluded from the total number of HIV cases because HIVDR were not reported.

[c] After exposure to tenofovir alafenamide.

Adapted from Gibas, Drug Resistance during HIV Prophylaxis. Drugs 2019[72] strategy, has significantly reduced the number of new HIV infections in some communities. For instance, in San Francisco, PrEP uptake as part of the 'Getting to Zero' campaign has contributed to reducing the number of new HIV infections by half between 2012 and 2017.[80] In Australia, the rapid implementation of daily TDF/FTC among 3,700 high risk GBMSM in a network of 21 clinical sites across the state of New South Wales has led to a 31.5% decline in recent HIV infections after 1 year.[81] However, significant disparities in PrEP access continue to exist both globally and within countries. In the US, less than a quarter of eligible black and Hispanic or Latino individuals were prescribed PrEP, compared with three-quarters of eligible White individuals.[79] The effectiveness of oral PrEP in real-world scenarios is significantly hindered by both the high rate of suboptimal PrEP adherence and users' non persistence. Real-world evaluations of PrEP persistence estimated that between 30% and 60% of GBMSM discontinue PrEP by 1 year, despite the persistence of risk factors for HIV acquisition.[82] Early PrEP discontinuation leads to a higher risk of HIV infection and recent studies suggest that 20% to 30% of new HIV diagnosis among GBMSM occur among former PrEP users.[83] Although barriers to adherence and persistence are multidimensional, oral PrEP fatigue related to the burden of oral drug remains a significant issue. CAB-LA represents a first step to offer an alternative to oral PrEP for all populations at risk of HIV infection. Furthermore, next-generation PrEP formulations are being developed to address the gaps in uptake, adherence, and persistence.

NEXT GENERATION PrEP OPTION

To broaden the range of PrEP options, new PrEP agents and extended-release formulations are under development. Lenacapavir is the first long-acting inhibitor of HIV capsid that can be administered subcutaneously every 6 months. Following promising efficacy data in macaque models, lenacapavir has entered its final development stage, with several phase III clinical trials underway to assess its safety and efficacy as a PrEP agent in GBMSM and cis-women (NCT04994509, NCT04925752). A phase 3 clinical trial evaluating an islatravir once-monthly oral tablet for HIV PrEP has been recently halted by the US FDA due to a significant decrease in total lymphocytes and CD4 count. Investigations are ongoing to uncover the underlying mechanism, but a new nucleoside reverse transcriptase translocation inhibitor (MK-8527) is being evaluated in phase 2 trial as a monthly oral pill for PrEP (NCT06045507). Implants that release ART agents also show promise in the PrEP field. A phase 2 clinical trial is presently underway to assess a subdermal implant that provides sustained-release of TAF in cis-women.[84] Additionally, an implant that elutes islatravir has also demonstrated convincing results in a phase 1 trial. As part of CAB development, an injectable, biodegradable, and removable in-situ forming implants demonstrated effectiveness in releasing CAB above protective benchmarks for more than 6 months, offering effective protection to macaques after SHIV rectal challenges.[85] PrEP formulations in the early development phase also include patches, gels, douches, implants, films, vaginal and rectal inserts, and topical agents.[86] Despite limited efficacy data in phase 3 clinical trials, broadly neutralizing antibodies targeting HIV also represent a promising strategy for long-acting PrEP formulation.[87]

SUMMARY

Pre-exposure prophylaxis represents the most significant advancement in HIV prevention over the past decade. The large-scale roll-out of PrEP, as part of a combination prevention approach, is anticipated to address the continuing HIV epidemic and has been established as a cornerstone of global HIV prevention policy. Although the expansion of PrEP options holds potential to address challenges related to uptake, adherence, and persistence in the coming years, this strategy alone will not be sufficient to effectively control the HIV epidemic. A holistic approach involving multilevel interventions is necessary to address individual, structural, social, economic, and political barriers to PrEP use. Particular emphasis must be placed on raising awareness about PrEP and providing education, ensuring easy and free access to all HIV prevention tools, reducing stigma, and involving the community. Along these interventions, a strong commitment from stakeholders and policymakers will be required to fully realize the potential of PrEP in responding to HIV and to achieve the Joint United Nations Programme on HIV and AIDS' goal of ending the AIDS epidemic as a public health threat by 2030.

CLINICS CARE POINTS

- PrEP should be discussed with all individuals who engage in risk behaviors associated with HIV transmission, such as condomless sex or sharing needles or equipment. PrEP is generally not required for individuals who consistently use condoms or are in a mutually monogamous relationship with a partner who has tested negative for HIV or is undetectable on ART.

- There are several PrEP options available in the form of oral, intravaginal ring or injectable regimens. Daily oral TDF/FTC is a safe and effective PrEP option for all individuals at risk of HIV. The use of event-driven TDF/FTC and daily TAF/FTC remains, pending further data, limited to specific populations. Long-acting injectable cabotegravir administered by intramuscular injection every 2 months can be used in all individuals at risk of sexual acquisition of HIV.

- Adherence to PrEP is critical for its effectiveness in preventing HIV acquisition Providers should engage in a comprehensive discussion with all individuals about the available PrEP options to determine the most appropriate PrEP agent based on their individual risk factors, preferences, and lifestyle. The best PrEP regimen is the one the patient can adhere to.

- HIV testing should be performed in all individuals before initiating PrEP to rule out pre-existing HIV infection. In cases of suspected acute HIV NAT can detect HIV should be performed to detect HIV infection early and initiate appropriate treatment.

- PrEP users should have regular follow-up visits with a health care provider to monitor for potential side effects, detect acute HIV infection, and undergo testing for other sexually transmitted infections. Patients should be counseled to take PrEP consistently as prescribed and educated to recognize signs and symptoms of acute HIV infection so that they can promptly seek medical attention.

ACKNOWLEDGMENTS

Dr G. Liegeon was supported by an ANRS, France | Emerging Infectious Diseases grant for this work.

DISCLOSURE

Dr J.M. Molina reports receiving support as an adviser for Gilead Sciences, Merck, and ViiV Healthcare.

REFERENCES

1. Abdool Karim SS. HIV-1 epidemic control - insights from test-and-treat trials. N Engl J Med 2019;381(3):286–8.

2. Joint United Nations Programme on HIV/AIDS. Global HIV and AIDS statistics — 2022 fact sheet. UNAIDS. Available at: https://www.unaids.org/en/resources/fact-sheet.

3. AVAC: The Global PrEP Tracker. Cumulative number of PrEP initiations. Available at: https://data.prepwatch.org/.

4. Grant RM, Lama JR, Anderson PL, et al. Preexposure chemoprophylaxis for HIV prevention in men who have sex with men. N Engl J Med 2010;363(27):2587–99.

5. Chawki S, Goldwirt L, Mouhebb ME, et al. Ex-vivo rectal tissue infection with HIV-1 to assess time to protection following oral preexposure prophylaxis with tenofovir disoproxil/emtricitabine. AIDS 2024;38(4):455–64.

6. García-Lerma JG, McNicholl JM, Heneine W. The predictive value of macaque models of preexposure prophylaxis for HIV prevention. Curr Opin HIV AIDS 2022;17(4):179–85.

7. Grant RM, Anderson PL, McMahan V, et al. Uptake of pre-exposure prophylaxis, sexual practices, and HIV incidence in men and transgender women who have sex with men: a cohort study. Lancet Infect Dis 2014;14(9):820–9.

8. McCormack S, Dunn DT, Desai M, et al. Pre-exposure prophylaxis to prevent the acquisition of HIV-1 infection (PROUD): effectiveness results from the pilot phase of a pragmatic open-label randomised trial. Lancet 2016;387(10013):53–60.

9. Pilkington V, Hill A, Hughes S, et al. How safe is TDF/FTC as PrEP? A systematic review and meta-analysis of the risk of adverse events in 13 randomised trials of PrEP. J Virus Erad 2018;4(4):215–24.

10. Liegeon G. Safety of oral tenofovir disoproxil - emtricitabine for HIV preexposure prophylaxis in adults. Curr Opin HIV AIDS 2022;17(4):199–204.

11. Ruane PJ, DeJesus E, Berger D, et al. Antiviral activity, safety, and pharmacokinetics/pharmacodynamics of tenofovir alafenamide as 10-day monotherapy in HIV-1-positive adults. J Acquir Immune Defic Syndr 2013;63(4):449–55.

12. Mayer KH, Molina JM, Thompson MA, et al. Emtricitabine and tenofovir alafenamide vs emtricitabine and tenofovir disoproxil fumarate for HIV pre-exposure prophylaxis (DISCOVER): primary results from a randomised, double-blind, multicentre, active-controlled, phase 3, non-inferiority trial. Lancet 2020; 396(10246):239–54.

13. Rivera AS, Pak KJ, Mefford MT, et al. Use of tenofovir alafenamide fumarate for HIV pre-exposure prophylaxis and incidence of hypertension and initiation of statins. JAMA Netw Open 2023;6(9):e2332968.

14. García-Lerma JG, Otten RA, Qari SH, et al. Prevention of rectal SHIV transmission in macaques by daily or intermittent prophylaxis with emtricitabine and tenofovir. PLoS Med 2008;5(2):e28.

15. Molina JM, Capitant C, Spire B, et al. On-Demand Preexposure Prophylaxis in Men at High Risk for HIV-1 Infection. N Engl J Med 2015;373(23):2237–46.

16. Molina JM, Charreau I, Spire B, et al. Efficacy, safety, and effect on sexual behaviour of on-demand pre-exposure prophylaxis for HIV in men who have sex with men: an observational cohort study. Lancet HIV 2017;4(9):e402–10.

17. Molina JM, Ghosn J, Assoumou L, et al. Daily and on-demand HIV pre-exposure prophylaxis with emtricitabine and tenofovir disoproxil (ANRS PREVENIR): a prospective observational cohort study. Lancet HIV 2022;S2352-3018(22):00133–43.

18. Liegeon G, Assoumou L, Ghosn J, et al. Impact on renal function of daily and on-demand HIV pre-exposure prophylaxis in the ANRS-PREVENIR study. J Antimicrob Chemother 2022;dkac336.

19. Cambiano V, Miners A, Dunn D, et al. Cost-effectiveness of pre-exposure prophylaxis for HIV prevention in men who have sex with men in the UK: a modelling study and health economic evaluation. Lancet Infect Dis 2018;18(1):85–94.

20. Centers for Disease Control and Prevention. US Public Health Service: Preexposure prophylaxis for the prevention of HIV infection in the United States—2021 Update: a clinical practice guideline. Available at: https://www.cdc.gov/hiv/pdf/risk/prep/cdc-hiv-prep-guidelines-2021.pdf.

21. World Health Organization. What's the 2+1+1? Event-driven oral pre-exposure prophylaxis to prevent HIV for men who have sex with men: Update to WHO's recommendation on oral PrEP. 2019. Available at: https://apps.who.int/iris/bitstream/handle/10665/325955/WHO-CDS-HIV-19.8-eng.pdf?ua=1.

22. Andrews CD, Spreen WR, Mohri H, et al. Long-acting integrase inhibitor protects macaques from intrarectal simian/human immunodeficiency virus. Science 2014;343(6175):1151–4.

23. Markowitz M, Frank I, Grant RM, et al. Safety and tolerability of long-acting cabotegravir injections in HIV-uninfected men (ECLAIR): a multicentre, double-blind, randomised, placebo-controlled, phase 2a trial. Lancet HIV 2017;4(8):e331–40.

24. Landovitz RJ, Li S, Eron JJ, et al. Tail-phase safety, tolerability, and pharmacokinetics of long-acting injectable cabotegravir in HIV-uninfected adults: a secondary analysis of the HPTN 077 trial. Lancet HIV 2020;7(7):e472–81.

25. Landovitz RJ, Donnell D, Clement ME, et al. Cabotegravir for HIV prevention in cisgender men and transgender women. N Engl J Med 2021;385(7):595–608.

26. Landovitz RJ, Hanscom BS, Clement ME, et al. Efficacy and safety of long-acting cabotegravir compared with daily oral tenofovir disoproxil fumarate plus emtricitabine to prevent HIV infection in cisgender men and transgender women who have sex with men 1 year after study unblinding: a secondary analysis of the phase 2b and 3 HPTN 083 randomised controlled trial. Lancet HIV 2023;S2352-3018(23):00261–8.

27. Liegeon G, Ghosn J. Long-acting injectable cabotegravir for PrEP : A game-changer in HIV prevention? HIV Med 2022;hiv:13451.

28. Marzinke MA, Fogel JM, Wang Z, et al. Extended analysis of HIV infection in cisgender men and transgender women who have sex with men receiving injectable cabotegravir for HIV prevention: HPTN 083. Antimicrob Agents Chemother 2023;67(4):e0005323.

29. Meyers K, Nguyen N, Zucker JE, et al. The long-acting cabotegravir tail as an implementation challenge: planning for safe discontinuation. AIDS Behav 2023;27(1):4–9.

30. The Lancet Hiv null. Equitable access to long-acting PrEP on the way? Lancet HIV 2022;9(7):e449.

31. World Health Organization. Guidelines on long-acting injectable cabotegravir for HIV prevention. Geneva. 2022. Available at: https://www.who.int/publications/i/item/9789240054097.

32. Centers for Disease Control and Prevention. HIV and transgender people. Available at: https://www.cdc.gov/hiv/group/gender/transgender/index.html.

33. Cottrell ML, Prince HMA, Schauer AP, et al. Decreased tenofovir diphosphate concentrations in a transgender female cohort: implications for human immunodeficiency virus preexposure prophylaxis. Clin Infect Dis 2019;69(12):2201–4.

34. Hiransuthikul A, Janamnuaysook R, Himmad K, et al. Drug-drug interactions between feminizing hormone therapy and pre-exposure prophylaxis among transgender women: the iFACT study. J Int AIDS Soc 2019;22(7). https://doi.org/10.1002/jia2.25338.

35. Grant RM, Pellegrini M, Defechereux PA, et al. Sex hormone therapy and tenofovir diphosphate concentration in dried blood spots: primary results of the interactions between antiretrovirals and transgender hormones study. Clin Infect Dis 2021;73(7):e2117–23.

36. Cespedes MS, Das M, Yager J, et al. Gender affirming hormones do not affect the exposure and efficacy of F/TDF or F/TAF for HIV preexposure prophylaxis: a subgroup analysis from the DISCOVER trial. Transgender Health 2022;trgh.2022:0048.

37. World Health Organization. Consolidated guidelines on HIV prevention, testing, treatment, service delivery and monitoring: recommendations for a public health approach. 2021. Available at: https://www.who.int/publications/i/item/9789240031593.

38. Marzinke MA, Hanscom B, Wang Z, et al. Efficacy, safety, tolerability, and pharmacokinetics of long-acting injectable cabotegravir for HIV pre-exposure prophylaxis in transgender women: a secondary analysis of the HPTN 083 trial. Lancet HIV 2023;10(11):e703–12.

39. Golub SA, Fikslin RA, Starbuck L, et al. High rates of PrEP eligibility but low rates of PrEP access among a national sample of transmasculine individuals. J Acquir Immune Defic Syndr 2019;82(1):e1–7.

40. Abdool Karim Q, Abdool Karim SS, Frohlich JA, et al. Effectiveness and safety of tenofovir gel, an antiretroviral microbicide, for the prevention of HIV infection in women. Science 2010;329(5996):1168–74.

41. Fonner VA, Dalglish SL, Kennedy CE, et al. Effectiveness and safety of oral HIV preexposure prophylaxis for all populations. AIDS 2016;30(12):1973–83.

42. Van Damme L, Corneli A, Ahmed K, et al. Preexposure prophylaxis for HIV infection among African women. N Engl J Med 2012;367(5):411–22.

43. Marrazzo JM, Ramjee G, Richardson BA, et al. Tenofovir-based preexposure prophylaxis for HIV infection among African women. N Engl J Med 2015;372(6):509–18.

44. Baeten JM, Donnell D, Ndase P, et al. Antiretroviral prophylaxis for HIV prevention in heterosexual men and women. N Engl J Med 2012;367(5):399–410.

45. Thigpen MC, Kebaabetswe PM, Paxton LA, et al. Antiretroviral preexposure prophylaxis for heterosexual HIV transmission in botswana. N Engl J Med 2012;367(5):423–34.

46. Moore M, Stansfield S, Donnell DJ, et al. Efficacy estimates of oral pre-exposure prophylaxis for HIV prevention in cisgender women with partial adherence. Nat Med 2023. https://doi.org/10.1038/s41591-023-02564-5.

47. Zhang L, Iannuzzi S, Chaturvedula A, et al. Model-based predictions of protective HIV pre-exposure prophylaxis adherence levels in cisgender women. Nat Med 2023. https://doi.org/10.1038/s41591-023-02615-x.

48. Marrazzo J, Tao L, Becker M, et al. HIV preexposure prophylaxis with emtricitabine and tenofovir disoproxil fumarate among cisgender women. JAMA 2024;331(11):930–7.

49. Anderson PL, Marzinke MA, Glidden DV. Updating the adherence–response for oral emtricitabine/tenofovir disoproxil fumarate for human immunodeficiency virus pre-exposure prophylaxis among cisgender women. Clin Infect Dis 2023;76(10):1850–3.

50. Cottrell ML, Yang KH, Prince HMA, et al. A translational pharmacology approach to predicting outcomes of preexposure prophylaxis against HIV in men and women using tenofovir disoproxil fumarate with or without emtricitabine. JID (J Infect Dis) 2016;214(1):55–64.

51. Cottrell ML, Garrett KL, Prince HMA, et al. Single-dose pharmacokinetics of tenofovir alafenamide and its active metabolite in the mucosal tissues. J Antimicrob Chemother 2017;72(6):1731–40.
52. Mofenson LM, Baggaley RC, Mameletzis I. Tenofovir disoproxil fumarate safety for women and their infants during pregnancy and breastfeeding. AIDS 2017; 31(2):213–32.
53. Delany-Moretlwe S, Hughes JP, Bock P, et al. Cabotegravir for the prevention of HIV-1 in women: results from HPTN 084, a phase 3, randomised clinical trial. Lancet 2022;S0140-6736(22):00538–44.
54. Delany-Moretlwe S, Hughes JP, Bock P, et al. Long acting injectable cabotegravir: updated efficacy and safety results from HPTN 084. Montreal. Canada: AIDS; 2022. Abstract #OALBX0108. Available at: https://programme.aids2022.org/Abstract/Abstract/?abstractid=13063.
55. Delany-Moretlwe S, Hanscom B, Angira F, et al. Initial PrEP product choice: results from the HPTN 084 open-label extension. Brisbane, Australia: IAS; 2023. Abstract 5998. Available at: https://www.hptn.org/sites/default/files/inline-files/220725%20IAS%202023%20product%20choice%20revised.pdf.
56. Sahloff EG, Hamons N, Baumgartner K, et al. Is long-acting cabotegravir a preexposure prophylaxis option for women of childbearing potential? Open Forum Infect Dis 2022;9(7):ofac230.
57. Blair CS, Li S, Chau G, et al. Brief report: hormonal contraception use and cabotegravir pharmacokinetics in hiv-uninfected women enrolled in HPTN 077. J Acquir Immune Defic Syndr 2020;85(1):93–7.
58. Baeten JM, Palanee-Phillips T, Brown ER, et al. Use of a vaginal ring containing dapivirine for HIV-1 prevention in women. N Engl J Med 2016;375(22):2121–32.
59. Nel A, van Niekerk N, Kapiga S, et al. Safety and efficacy of a dapivirine vaginal ring for HIV prevention in women. N Engl J Med 2016;375(22):2133–43.
60. Nel A, van Niekerk N, Van Baelen B, et al. Safety, adherence, and HIV-1 seroconversion among women using the dapivirine vaginal ring (DREAM): an open-label, extension study. Lancet HIV 2021;8(2):e77–86.
61. Baeten JM, Palanee-Phillips T, Mgodi NM, et al. Safety, uptake, and use of a dapivirine vaginal ring for HIV-1 prevention in African women (HOPE): an open-label, extension study. Lancet HIV 2021;8(2):e87–95.
62. Bunge K, Balkus JE, Fairlie L, et al. DELIVER: a safety study of a dapivirine vaginal ring and oral PrEP for the prevention of HIV during pregnancy. J Acquir Immune Defic Syndr 2023.
63. Owor M, Nogochi L, Horne E, et al. Dapivirine ring safety and drug detection in breastfeeding mother-infant pairs. CROI 2023, February 19-22, Seattle, United States. Abstract 785. Available at: https://www.croiconference.org/abstract/dapivirine-ring-safety-and-drug-detection-in-breastfeeding-mother-infant-pairs/.
64. Nair G, Celum C, Szydlo D, et al. Adherence, safety, and choice of the monthly dapivirine vaginal ring or oral emtricitabine plus tenofovir disoproxil fumarate for HIV pre-exposure prophylaxis among African adolescent girls and young women: a randomised, open-label, crossover trial. Lancet HIV 2023; S2352-S3018(23):00227–8.
65. Centers for Diseases Control and Prevention. HIV and people who inject drugs. Available at: https://www.cdc.gov/hiv/group/hiv-idu.html.
66. Choopanya K, Martin M, Suntharasamai P, et al. Antiretroviral prophylaxis for HIV infection in injecting drug users in Bangkok, Thailand (the Bangkok Tenofovir Study): a randomised, double-blind, placebo-controlled phase 3 trial. Lancet 2013;381(9883):2083–90.

67. Martin M, Vanichseni S, Suntharasamai P, et al. The impact of adherence to pre-exposure prophylaxis on the risk of HIV infection among people who inject drugs. AIDS 2015;29(7):819–24.

68. Martin M, Vanichseni S, Suntharasamai P, et al. Factors associated with the uptake of and adherence to HIV pre-exposure prophylaxis in people who have injected drugs: an observational, open-label extension of the Bangkok Tenofovir Study. Lancet HIV 2017;4(2):e59–66.

69. Andrews CD, Bernard LS, Poon AY, et al. Cabotegravir long acting injection protects macaques against intravenous challenge with SIVmac251. AIDS 2017; 31(4):461–7.

70. Gandhi RT, Bedimo R, Hoy JF, et al. Antiretroviral drugs for treatment and prevention of HIV infection in adults: 2022 recommendations of the international antiviral society-USA panel. JAMA 2023;329(1):63–84.

71. World Health Organization. Differentiated and simplified pre-exposure prophylaxis for HIV prevention: update to WHO implementation guidance. Geneva: Technical Brief; 2022. Available at: https://iris.who.int/bitstream/handle/10665/360861/9789240053694-eng.pdf?sequence=1.

72. Gibas KM, van den Berg P, Powell VE, et al. Drug resistance during HIV pre-exposure prophylaxis. Drugs 2019;79(6):609–19.

73. Ambrosioni J, Petit E, Liegeon G, et al. Primary HIV-1 infection in users of pre-exposure prophylaxis. Lancet HIV 2021;8(3):e166–74.

74. Landovitz RJ, Tao L, Yang J, et al. HIV-1 incidence, adherence, and drug resistance in individuals taking daily emtricitabine/tenofovir disoproxil fumarate for HIV-1 pre-exposure prophylaxis: pooled analysis from 72 global studies. Clin Infect Dis 2024;14:ciae143.

75. Donnell D, Ramos E, Celum C, et al. The effect of oral preexposure prophylaxis on the progression of HIV-1 seroconversion. AIDS 2017;31(14):2007–16.

76. Eshleman SH, Fogel JM, Piwowar-Manning E, et al. The LEVI syndrome: characteristics of early HIV infection with cabotegravir for PrEP. CROI 2023. February 19-22. Seattle. United States. Available at: https://www.croiconference.org/abstract/the-levi-syndrome-characteristics-of-early-hiv-infection-with-cabotegravir-for-prep/.

77. Eshleman SH, Fogel JM, Halvas EK, et al. HIV RNA screening reduces integrase strand transfer inhibitor resistance risk in persons receiving long-acting cabotegravir for HIV prevention. J Infect Dis 2022;226(12):2170–80.

78. Smith J, Bansi-Matharu L, Cambiano V, et al. Predicted effects of the introduction of long-acting injectable cabotegravir pre-exposure prophylaxis in sub-Saharan Africa: a modelling study. Lancet HIV 2023;10(4):e254–65.

79. Centers for Diseases Control and Prevention. PrEP for HIV prevention in the U.S. Available at: https://www.cdc.gov/hiv/risk/prep/index.html.

80. San Francisco, Department of Public Health, Population Health, Division, HIV Epidemiology Section. HIV Epidemiology Annual Report. 2021. Available at: https://www.sfdph.org/dph/files/reports/RptsHIVAIDS/AnnualReport2021-Red.pdf.

81. Grulich AE, Guy R, Amin J, et al. Population-level effectiveness of rapid, targeted, high-coverage roll-out of HIV pre-exposure prophylaxis in men who have sex with men: the EPIC-NSW prospective cohort study. Lancet HIV 2018;5(11):e629–37.

82. Zhang J, Li C, Xu J, et al. Discontinuation, suboptimal adherence, and reinitiation of oral HIV pre-exposure prophylaxis: a global systematic review and meta-analysis. Lancet HIV 2022;9(4):e254–68.

83. Jourdain H, de Gage SB, Desplas D, et al. Real-world effectiveness of pre-exposure prophylaxis in men at high risk of HIV infection in France: a nested case-control study. Lancet Public Health 2022;7(6):e529–36.

84. Gengiah TN, Abdool Karim Q, Harkoo I, et al. CAPRISA 018: a phase I/II clinical trial study protocol to assess the safety, acceptability, tolerability and pharmacokinetics of a sustained-release tenofovir alafenamide subdermal implant for HIV prevention in women. BMJ Open 2022;12(1):e052880.

85. Young IC, Massud I, Cottrell ML, et al. Ultra-long-acting in-situ forming implants with cabotegravir protect female macaques against rectal SHIV infection. Nat Commun 2023;14(1):708.

86. AVAC. Research Pipeline. The future of ARV-based prevention and more. Available at: https://www.prepwatch.org/research-pipeline/.

87. Corey L, Gilbert PB, Juraska M, et al. Two randomized trials of neutralizing antibodies to prevent HIV-1 acquisition. N Engl J Med 2021;384(11):1003–14.

Human Immunodeficiency Virus Vaccine
Promise and Challenges

Daniel S. Graciaa, MD, MPH, MSc[a,b,*], Stephen R. Walsh, MDCM[c],
Nadine Rouphael, MD, MSc[a,b]

KEYWORDS

- HIV vaccine • Prevention • Broadly neutralizing antibodies • mRNA

KEY POINTS

- Despite multiple efficacy trials of human immunodeficiency virus (HIV) vaccine candidates, none have been adequately protective.
- Current HIV vaccine development is focused on generating broadly neutralizing antibodies to protect against diverse HIV-1 strains.
- Numerous early-stage trials are evaluating vaccine candidates using a variety of platforms.

INTRODUCTION

Over 40 years into the human immunodeficiency virus (HIV)/acquired immunodeficiency syndrome (AIDS) pandemic, there has been substantial progress in treatment and prevention interventions. Globally, an estimated nearly 30 million people are accessing antiretroviral therapy.[1] In addition, antiretrovirals are available as effective pre-exposure prophylaxis (PrEP). Still, over 1.3 million people are newly infected with HIV each year. Due to the extensive global burden of infection and the implementation gap for existing treatment and prevention, a vaccine against HIV is still needed to end the epidemic.[2] The Joint United Nations Programme on HIV/AIDS has set targets for 95% of people with HIV to know their HIV status, 95% of people diagnosed with HIV to receive antiretroviral therapy, and 95% of people on therapy to achieve virologic suppression.[3] Modeling suggests that in addition to achieving these targets for diagnosis and treatment, even a vaccine with 50% efficacy would have an impact

[a] Division of Infectious Diseases, Department of Medicine, Emory University School of Medicine, Atlanta, GA, USA; [b] Hope Clinic of Emory Vaccine Center, 500 Irvin Court, Suite 200, Decatur, GA 30030, USA; [c] Division of Infectious Diseases, Brigham and Women's Hospital, Harvard Medical School, 75 Francis Street, Boston, MA 02115, USA
* Corresponding author.
E-mail address: dsgraci@emory.edu

Infect Dis Clin N Am 38 (2024) 475–485
https://doi.org/10.1016/j.idc.2024.04.004
0891-5520/24/© 2024 Elsevier Inc. All rights reserved.

id.theclinics.com

on new infections.[4] Decades of research have been dedicated to HIV vaccine development; while important and ongoing advances highlight the promise of such a vaccine, significant challenges remain. In this review, the authors discuss the multiple completed or halted efficacy trials of HIV vaccine candidates, of which only 1 showed modest efficacy. The authors give an overview of recent developments and new directions for HIV vaccine research, including ongoing studies, while noting the factors that have added to the immunologic and clinical trial challenge of investigating vaccine candidates.

COMPLETED EFFICACY TRIALS
AIDSVAX (VAX003 and VAX004)

Early approaches to HIV vaccine targeted the HIV-1 envelope protein to generate neutralizing antibodies as correlates of protection for most approved vaccines rely on antibody production. Studies of recombinant envelope glycoprotein subunit (gp120) in non-human primates demonstrated protection from homologous and heterologous HIV-1 viruses, and the recombinant gp120 was shown to be safe and immunogenic in early phase human studies.[5] A bivalent subtype B/B vaccine with alum adjuvant was evaluated among 5095 males and 308 females in the United States and the Netherlands (VAX004, NCT00002441) while a subtype B/E vaccine with alum adjuvant was evaluated among 2546 people who inject drugs in Thailand (VAX003, NCT00006327).[6] Both studies (**Table 1** for a summary of trials) were completed in 2000. Although the vaccines did elicit a robust antibody response, these vaccines did not prevent HIV-1 infection.[7] There was some variation in exploratory subgroup analyses including possible protection in the high-risk group, though this was not statistically significant. Importantly, the successful completion of the trials demonstrated the safety of the AIDSVAX candidates and the feasibility of conducting phase III trials of an HIV vaccine with populations at risk of infection.

Human Immunodeficiency Virus Vaccine Trials Network 502/Human Immunodeficiency Virus Vaccine Trials Network 503

The next evaluated strategy included vectored vaccines aiming to elicit HIV-specific T-cell responses. Vector vaccines are thought to be advantageous as they generate both humoral and cellular responses, which may be superior to an antibody response alone in the context of HIV infection of T-cells. After demonstrating a cell-mediated immune response in phase I trials,[8] the adenovirus type 5 (Ad5) vector vaccine expressing subtype B *gag*, *pol*, and *nef* was evaluated in 2 separate phase IIb trials: HIV Vaccine Trials Network [HVTN] 502/Step[9] (NCT00095576) enrolled 3000 adult men who have sex with men, high-risk men who have sex with women, and women who had unprotected intercourse with high-risk partners in the Americas and Australia and HVTN 503/Phambili[10] (NCT00413725) enrolled 801 sexually active men and women at risk due to the burden of HIV-1 infection in the community in South Africa. At the first independent Data and Safety Monitoring Board (DSMB) review of the Step study in 2007, enrollment into both studies was halted due to pre-determined non-efficacy for the primary endpoints.[11] Further analyses suggested increased incidence of infection in Ad5-seropositive or uncircumcised men who received vaccine in Step, and among those vaccinated in Phambili.[12] These studies raise the possibility of pre-existing immunity to a selected vector influencing susceptibility to HIV in vaccine trials.

Human Immunodeficiency Virus Vaccine Trials Network 505

Building on the lessons regarding Ad5 vectored vaccines from the HIV Vaccine Trials Network (HVTN) 502/Step and HVTN 503/Phambili studies, HVTN 505 (NCT00865566)

Table 1
Completed human immunodeficiency virus vaccine efficacy trials

Study	Sites	Vaccines	Population	Efficacy
VAX004 (NCT00002441)	USA, Netherlands	AIDSVAX B/B gp120 with alum	5095 MSM and 308 women	No
VAX003 (NCT00006327)	Thailand	AIDSVAX B/E gp120 with alum	2546 PWID	No
HVTN 502/Step (NCT00095576)	Americas, Australia	MRKAd5 HIV-1 gag/pol/nef	3000 adults	No
HVTN 503/Phambili (NCT00413725)	South Africa	MRKAd5 HIV-1 gag/pol/nef	801 adults	No
RV144 (NCT00223080)	Thailand	ALVAC-HIV [vCP1521] + AIDSVAX B/E gp120	16,402 adults	31% efficacy at 42 mo
HVTN 505 (NCT00865566)	USA	DNA vaccine + rAd5 vector boost	2504 men or transgender women who have sex with men	No
HVTN 702/Uhambo (NCT02968849)	South Africa	ALVAC-HIV [vCP2438] + bivalent gp120 with MF59	5404 adults	No
HVTN 703/HPTN 084 (NCT02568215)	Sub-Saharan Africa	VRC01 neutralizing antibody infusion	1924 women	Not overall; effective against sensitive HIV-1 strains
HVTN 704/HPTN 085 (NCT02716675)	Americas, Europe	VRC01 neutralizing antibody infusion	2699 men and transgender people	Not overall; effective against sensitive HIV-1 strains
HVTN 705/Imbokodo (NCT03060629)	Sub-Saharan Africa	Ad26 mosaic immunogens + gp140 (clade C) boost	2637 women	No
HVTN 706/Mosaico (NCT03964415)	Americas, Europe	Ad26 mosaic immunogens + bivalent mosaic and gp140 (clade C) boost	3800 men and transgender people	No

Abbreviations: HVTN, HIV vaccine trials network; MSM, men who have sex with men; PWID, people who inject drugs.

studied a regimen of DNA prime with recombinant Ad5 vector boost.[13] This trial enrolled 2504 Ad5-seronegative men and transgender women who have sex with men in the United States. HVTN 505 was also stopped at the first interim analysis in 2013 by the DSMB after finding no difference in infection rates or HIV viral load in those who acquired HIV. The regimen induced a cellular and humoral immune response but was not protective.[14,15] Subsequent trials would focus on different vectored vaccine platforms.

RV144

The RV144 study (NCT00223080) evaluated a "pox-protein" regimen consisting of a canarypox vector expressing *gag*, *pro*, and *env*, boosted with AIDSVAX B/E gp120. A total of 16,402 people at a range of risk of HIV infection were enrolled in Thailand with study completion in 2009.[16] Efficacy was 60% at 12 months after immunization but by 42 months (3.5 years) had decreased to 31.2%. Despite this relatively low efficacy, this strategy remains the only efficacious HIV-1 vaccine trial to date. While the vaccine did not generate neutralizing antibodies, the identification of other immune correlates, including levels and specific subtypes of antibodies binding to the variable region 2 of the envelope protein, informed future trial design.[17]

Human Immunodeficiency Virus Vaccine Trials Network 702

The pox-protein approach from RV144 was further evaluated in the phase I/II study HVTN 100 (NCT02404311) with a regimen targeting the subtype C virus in South Africa: a canarypox vector boosted with bivalent gp120 with a different adjuvant, MF59.[18] While the immunoglobulin (Ig) G response was lower than in RV144, a correlate of protection model still predicted greater than 50% efficacy and the regimen advanced to phase IIb/III evaluation in HVTN 702. Also known as the Uhambo study (NCT02968849), this trial enrolled 5404 adults in South Africa, who were additionally offered local HIV prevention care including access to PrEP.[19] Interim analysis in 2020 showed no evidence of a difference in infection, prompting the DSMB to halt the study. While contrasting results from RV144 may be due to differences in study population and associated risk of HIV acquisition or different vaccine composition and adjuvant, the search for a protective vaccine continued.[20]

Human Immunodeficiency Virus Vaccine Trials Network 705 and Human Immunodeficiency Virus Vaccine Trials Network 706

One of the many immunologic challenges to HIV vaccine development is the global diversity of HIV-1. Investigators approached this problem by creating polyvalent or "mosaic" antigens to generate broader T-cell responses as part of a regimen that also includes Env antigens for antibody responses.[21] Non-human primate studies and the phase I/II APPROACH study (NCT02315703) informed regimen selection of adenovirus 26 (Ad26) vector prime with gp140 boost for subsequent trials.[22] The Ad26 vector was chosen in part due to lower seroprevalence compared to prior adenovirus vectors such as Ad5. The phase I/IIa TRAVERSE study (NCT02788045) demonstrated that a tetravalent Ad26.Mos4.HIV prime resulted in higher antibody response than a trivalent prime; the Ad26.Mos4.HIV prime + clade C gp140 boost was subsequently evaluated in the HVTN 705/Imbokodo phase IIb trial.[23] In parallel, the phase I/IIa ASCENT study (NCT02935686) of the Ad26.Mos4.HIV prime with different boosting regimens resulted in a bivalent subtype C gp140 and mosaic gp140 moving into the HVTN 706/Mosaico phase III trial (NCT03964415). HVTN 705/Imbokodo (NCT03060629) evaluated the tetravalent Ad26.Mos4.HIV + clade C gp140 boost with aluminum phosphate adjuvant among 2637 women in 5 countries in southern Africa through 2021. At a primary analysis 24 months after enrollment, there was no difference in incident infections between vaccine or placebo groups.[24] HVTN 706/Mosaico (NCT03964415) evaluated the tetravalent Ad26.Mos4.HIV + bivalent subtype C gp140 and mosaic gp140 with aluminum phosphate adjuvant among 3800 cisgender men and transgender people in the Americas and Europe. After an interim DSMB review in early 2023, the study was discontinued due to lack of efficacy.[25] While neither the Imbokodo or Mosaico regimens prevented HIV-1 infection, both were found to be safe during the trials. Analyses of antibody response and correlates of risk are pending. While these investigations may provide additional lessons from the Ad26 trials, it is clear that development of a successful HIV vaccine will require improved immunogens.

Antibody-Mediated Prevention Trials

An alternative approach utilizing passive immunization with broadly neutralizing antibodies (bnAbs) has been evaluated in the Antibody- Mediated Prevention (AMP) trials.[26] These studies evaluated the bnAb VRC01, which is directed at the HIV-1 envelope protein CD4-binding site and has broad in vitro coverage against subtype B and subtype C viruses. VRC01 was administered as an infusion in either low dose (10 mg/kg) or high dose (30 mg/kg) and compared to placebo among 1924 women in sub-Saharan Africa in HVTN 703/HIV Prevention Trials Network [HPTN] 084 (NCT02568215) and 2699 men and transgender people in the Americas and Europe in HVTN 704/HPTN 085 (NCT02716675). Participants also had access to PrEP. These studies were completed in 2020 and 2021, respectively. While VRC01 overall did not prevent infection, the pooled prevention efficacy against isolates highly susceptible to VRC01 was 75.4% (95% CI, 45.5–88.9).[26] The AMP trials provide proof of concept for the use of bnAb to prevent HIV infection and data that have informed potential biomarkers for evaluation of other bnAb regimens and candidate vaccines.[27]

CURRENT APPROACHES

Based on the lack of efficacy with prior vaccine approaches despite vaccine candidates generating an immune response and the proof of concept of bnAbs, current HIV vaccine development is focused on the generation of bnAbs that protect against diverse HIV-1 strains. While it is known that some people with HIV (PWH) produce bnAbs in response to chronic infection, there are multiple virus and host factors that make induction of protective bnAb challenging, including HIV-1 sequence diversity, features of the envelope protein, and immune tolerance limiting bnAb development.[28] Some early success on this pathway has been described in the phase I HVTN 133 trial (NCT03934541) in which a gp41 membrane proximal external region (MPER) peptide-liposome vaccine induced MPER bnAb precursors and heterologous neutralizing antibodies.[29,30] The phase I International AIDS Vaccine Initiative (IAVI) G001 trial (NCT03547245) found that the nanoparticle eOD-GT8 60mer (gp120 engineered outer domain germline-targeting) with AS01 adjuvant induced CD4 binding site bnAb precursors.[31] These results support the concept of germline-targeting vaccine priming as part of a sequential vaccination program that would then use boost immunogens to guide maturation of bnAbs (**Fig. 1**).[32] Investigators are probing this approach with a focus on early phase trials for immunogen discovery and evaluation—also known as discovery medicine—to move the field iteratively forward compared to traditional phase I/II/III clinical trials by allowing the parallel investigation of multiple strategies to elicit neutralizing antibodies.[33–35]

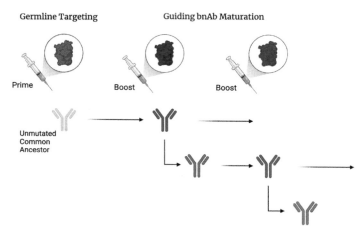

Fig. 1. Overview of sequential vaccination strategy to induce broadly neutralizing antibodies (bnAbs) against human immndefiociency virus (HIV)-1. Multiple strategies are used to design immunogens to guide this process including computationally inferring an undifferentiated common ancestor (UCA) and intermediates on the pathway to bnAbs. Immunogens designed to bind to UCA are given as a priming vaccination to activate precursor B cells. Distinct subsequent boost immunogens are designed to select for increasing affinity for the target region on HIV-1 in steps known as "shaping" and "polishing" to guide the maturation of bnAb. Created with BioRender.com.

Envelope Trimers

Native-like envelope trimers are designed to mimic the structure of the HIV-1 envelope spike, which is the target for neutralizing antibodies, providing a potential mechanism for the induction of bnAbs, similar to the successes seen with development of vaccines for respiratory syncytial virus and severe acute respiratory syndrome coronavirus 2 (SARS-CoV-2) based on structural biology.[36,37] The BG505 SOSIP.644 and related native-like soluble trimers with different adjuvants are being evaluated in several clinical trials by IAVI and in HVTN protocols including HVTN 137 (NCT04177355) and HVTN 300 (NCT04915768).

Messenger RNA

Messenger RNA (mRNA) vaccines utilize host cellular processes to generate protein antigens that induce antibody and cellular immune responses.[38] Decades of research into mRNA design, effective delivery mechanisms such as lipid nanoparticles (LNP), and platform flexibility to cover a wide array of antigens allowed the accelerated development and safe, effective implementation of this approach against SARS-CoV-2; this success has renewed interest in the development of mRNA vaccines for HIV.[39] Animal studies have demonstrated immunogenicity of an mRNA-LNP encoding envelope gp120 in non-human primates, generating durable humoral and cellular responses in macaques.[40,41]

Phase I trials of mRNA platform HIV vaccines are currently underway. HVTN 302 (NCT05217641) is evaluating the safety and immunogenicity of trimer mRNA based on the BG505 MD39 native-like trimer and includes lymph node fine-needle aspiration for tissue immunologic studies, which is an important growth area for evaluation of vaccines. IAVI G002 (NCT05001373) is using eOD-GT8 60mer mRNA and Core-g28v2 60mer to evaluate the safety and immunogenicity of sequential vaccination of a germline-targeting prime and directional boost to guide generation of bnAbs. Both HVTN 302 and IAVI G002 have completed enrollment with results expected in 2024. As demonstrated by production of multiple variants and updated vaccines for SARS-CoV-2, the mRNA platform allows rapid iteration of vaccine products, dramatically shortening the timeline from antigen identification to clinical trial and providing an exciting new tool in HIV vaccine development.

Cytomegalovirus Vector Vaccines

While adenovirus vector vaccines have not been successful, human cytomegalovirus (HCMV) has been of interest as a potential vector due to the persistence of infecting virus in the human host despite its immunogenicity, which when deployed as a vector could allow persistent expression of HIV antigens.[42] In a rhesus macaque model, a rhesus CMV vector expressing simian immunodeficiency virus (SIV) proteins demonstrated durable control of SIV challenge with about 50% of macaques remaining aviremic for up to 3 years.[43] This cell-mediated immune control of SIV infection is similar to that of some elite controllers with HIV infection.[44] This led to the design of HCMV vaccine candidates for HIV including VIR-1388, which is currently being evaluated in the phase I trial HVTN 142 (NCT05854381) with initial results expected in 2024.

CHALLENGES

As noted in the review of completed and ongoing trials investigating HIV vaccine candidates, there are multiple challenges impeding development of a safe and effective vaccine. Features of the HIV-1 virus and its interaction with the host that present barriers include sequence diversity, multiple transmission routes, viral reservoirs, integration with the host genome that sustains infection, and immune evasion processes.[45] The current focus on generation of bnAbs brings with it myriad additional obstacles including features of bnAbs themselves that can be impacted by immune tolerance mechanisms, the rarity of precursors of immune cells capable of producing relevant antibodies, and the need for multiple types of antibodies to achieve the needed breadth and durability of neutralization.[28]

Developing and evaluating vaccine candidates requires complex immunology and clinical trial expertise that has been made possible by collaborative networks. The impact of treatment and effective HIV prevention interventions such as PrEP and barrier methods adds complexity to efficacy trial design due to changing incidence and ethical considerations to address access to existing recommended prevention methods.[46] Offering PrEP to study participants, as has been done in multiple trials including HVTN 702/Uhambo, HVTN 705/Imbokodo, HVTN 706/Mosaico, and the AMP studies, may make it difficult to demonstrate vaccine efficacy.[47] Variation in efficacy across geographic settings, as seen with RV144 constructs in Thailand compared to South Africa and in many SARS-CoV-2 vaccine trials, may be due to viral or population differences and is another factor for consideration in trial design and interpretation. If and when a safe and effective vaccine is developed, there will be additional challenges with regard to funding, manufacturing, and delivery to ensure equitable deployment for populations most impacted by HIV.[48] These obstacles should not discourage the continued quest for an HIV vaccine but illustrate the importance of planning and collaboration to realize the promise of such an essential vaccine.

FUTURE DIRECTIONS

While there are promising avenues under investigation for HIV vaccine development, the inherent challenges and timeline require innovation to advance the field. Two such strategies are vaccinating people with HIV and analytical treatment interruption. It is possible that vaccinating PWH who are virologically suppressed on antiretrovirals would allow immune profiling to identify which immunogens boost relevant bnAb, potentially with a single trimer immunization rather than the multiple doses required in HIV-naïve individuals.[49] Additionally, post-vaccination analytical treatment interruption in which antiretroviral administration is suspended with close monitoring would provide an opportunity to associate a neutralization titer with viral replication, among other immunologic questions.[50] These strategies may also widen the population of potential participants in vaccine trials in the context of effective treatment and inform the development of therapeutic vaccines to control HIV infection, though these remain on the distant horizon.

SUMMARY

Development of a safe and effective HIV vaccine is a persistent immunology challenge despite decades of foundational and clinical research. Previous strategies utilizing protein subunit and viral vector vaccines generated antibody responses in early phase trials and were safe but not protective. Lessons learned from passive immunization studies and other investigations have shifted focus to strategies to induce bnAbs through sequential vaccination. Multiple early phase trials are in progress to advance this approach in addition to potential mRNA or CMV-vectored vaccines. Given the ongoing challenges facing investigators seeking to create an HIV vaccine, parallel development of multiple candidate immunogens and vaccine platforms is necessary for eventual success. A safe and effective vaccine is crucial to achieving the promise of ending the HIV epidemic.

CLINICS CARE POINTS

- There is no preventive or therapeutic HIV vaccine currently available.
- Passive immunization with bnAbs provided proof of concept for this approach to prevention of HIV infection and informed subsequent vaccine design.
- Current HIV vaccine development is focused on generation of bnAb through a variety of approaches.
- Future studies will involve vaccination of people with HIV and include analytical treatment interruption.

DISCLOSURE

This work was supported by National Institutes of Health, United States (NIH)/National Institute of Allergy and Infectious Diseases (NIAID) grants UM1AI069412 (S.R. Walsh) and UM1AI148576 (N. Rouphael) and by Infectious Diseases Clinical Research Consortium through NIH/NIAID under award number UM1AI148684 (D.S. Graciaa). S.R. Walsh has received institutional funding from NIH/NIAID; and institutional grants or contracts from Sanofi Pasteur, Janssen Vaccines/Johnson & Johnson, Moderna Tx, Pfizer, Vir Biotechnology, and Worcester HIV Vaccine; has participated on data safety monitoring or advisory boards for Janssen Vaccines/Johnson & Johnson and BioNTech; and his spouse holds stock/stock options in Regeneron Pharmaceuticals. N. Rouphael serves as safety consultant for ICON, CyanVac and EMMES. She serves or has served on the advisory boards for Sanofi, Seqirus, Pfizer and Moderna. Emory receives funds for N. Rouphael to conduct research from Sanofi, Lilly, Merck, Quidel, Immorna, Vaccine Company and Pfizer.

REFERENCES

1. UNAIDS. Global HIV & AIDS statistics — Fact sheet. Available at: https://www.unaids.org/en/resources/fact-sheet. [Accessed 20 November 2023].
2. Fauci AS. An HIV vaccine is essential for ending the HIV/AIDS pandemic. JAMA 2017;318(16):1535–6.
3. Frescura L, Godfrey-Faussett P, Feizzadeh AA, et al. Achieving the 95 95 95 targets for all: a pathway to ending AIDS. PLoS One 2022;17(8):e0272405.
4. Medlock J, Pandey A, Parpia AS, et al. Effectiveness of UNAIDS targets and HIV vaccination across 127 countries. Proc Natl Acad Sci USA 2017;114(15):4017–22.
5. Flynn NM, Forthal DN, Harro CD, et al. Placebo-controlled phase 3 trial of a recombinant glycoprotein 120 vaccine to prevent HIV-1 infection. J Infect Dis 2005;191(5):654–65.
6. Pitisuttithum P, Gilbert P, Gurwith M, et al. Randomized, double-blind, placebo-controlled efficacy trial of a bivalent recombinant glycoprotein 120 HIV-1 vaccine among injection drug users in Bangkok, Thailand. J Infect Dis 2006;194(12):1661–71.
7. Gilbert P, Wang M, Wrin T, et al. Magnitude and breadth of a nonprotective neutralizing antibody response in an efficacy trial of a candidate HIV-1 gp120 vaccine. J Infect Dis 2010;202(4):595–605.
8. Priddy FH, Brown D, Kublin J, et al. Safety and immunogenicity of a replication-incompetent adenovirus type 5 HIV-1 clade B gag/pol/nef vaccine in healthy adults. Clin Infect Dis 2008;46(11):1769–81.
9. Buchbinder SP, Mehrotra DV, Duerr A, et al. Efficacy assessment of a cell-mediated immunity HIV-1 vaccine (the Step Study): a double-blind, randomised, placebo-controlled, test-of-concept trial. Lancet 2008;372(9653):1881–93.
10. Gray GE, Allen M, Moodie Z, et al. Safety and efficacy of the HVTN 503/Phambili study of a clade-B-based HIV-1 vaccine in South Africa: a double-blind, randomised, placebo-controlled test-of-concept phase 2b study. Lancet Infect Dis 2011;11(7):507–15.
11. Gray G, Buchbinder S, Duerr A. Overview of STEP and phambili trial results: two phase IIb test-of-concept studies investigating the efficacy of MRK adenovirus type 5 gag/pol/nef subtype B HIV vaccine. Curr Opin HIV AIDS 2010;5(5):357–61.
12. Gray GE, Moodie Z, Metch B, et al. Recombinant adenovirus type 5 HIV gag/pol/nef vaccine in South Africa: unblinded, long-term follow-up of the phase 2b HVTN 503/Phambili study. Lancet Infect Dis 2014;14(5):388–96.
13. Hammer SM, Sobieszczyk ME, Janes H, et al. Efficacy trial of a DNA/rAd5 HIV-1 preventive vaccine. N Engl J Med 2013;369(22):2083–92.
14. Janes HE, Cohen KW, Frahm N, et al. Higher T-cell responses induced by DNA/rAd5 HIV-1 preventive vaccine are associated with lower HIV-1 infection risk in an efficacy trial. J Infect Dis 2017;215(9):1376–85.
15. Fong Y, Shen X, Ashley VC, et al. Modification of the association between T-cell immune responses and human immunodeficiency virus type 1 infection risk by vaccine-induced antibody responses in the HVTN 505 trial. J Infect Dis 2018;217(8):1280–8.

16. Rerks-Ngarm S, Pitisuttithum P, Nitayaphan S, et al. Vaccination with ALVAC and AIDSVAX to prevent HIV-1 infection in Thailand. N Engl J Med 2009;361(23): 2209-20.

17. Haynes BF, Gilbert PB, McElrath MJ, et al. Immune-correlates analysis of an HIV-1 vaccine efficacy trial. N Engl J Med 2012;366(14):1275-86.

18. Bekker LG, Moodie Z, Grunenberg N, et al. Subtype C ALVAC-HIV and bivalent subtype C gp120/MF59 HIV-1 vaccine in low-risk, HIV-uninfected, South African adults: a phase 1/2 trial. Lancet HIV 2018;5(7):e366-78.

19. Gray GE, Bekker LG, Laher F, et al. Vaccine efficacy of ALVAC-HIV and bivalent subtype C gp120-MF59 in adults. N Engl J Med 2021;384(12):1089-100.

20. Moodie Z, Dintwe O, Sawant S, et al. Analysis of the HIV vaccine trials network 702 Phase 2b-3 HIV-1 vaccine trial in south africa assessing RV144 antibody and T-cell correlates of HIV-1 acquisition risk. J Infect Dis 2022;226(2):246-57.

21. Fischer W, Perkins S, Theiler J, et al. Polyvalent vaccines for optimal coverage of potential T-cell epitopes in global HIV-1 variants. Nat Med 2007;13(1):100-6.

22. Barouch DH, Tomaka FL, Wegmann F, et al. Evaluation of a mosaic HIV-1 vaccine in a multicentre, randomised, double-blind, placebo-controlled, phase 1/2a clinical trial (APPROACH) and in rhesus monkeys (NHP 13-19). Lancet 2018; 392(10143):232-43.

23. Baden LR, Stieh DJ, Sarnecki M, et al. Safety and immunogenicity of two heterologous HIV vaccine regimens in healthy, HIV-uninfected adults (TRAVERSE): a randomised, parallel-group, placebo-controlled, double-blind, phase 1/2a study. Lancet HIV 2020;7(10):e688-98.

24. NIH. HIV vaccine candidate does not sufficiently protect women against HIV infection. Available at: https://www.nih.gov/news-events/news-releases/hiv-vaccine-candidate-does-not-sufficiently-protect-women-against-hiv-infection. [Accessed 15 November 2023].

25. NIH. Experimental HIV vaccine regimen safe but ineffective, study finds. Available at: https://www.nih.gov/news-events/news-releases/experimental-hiv-vaccine-regimen-safe-ineffective-study-finds. [Accessed 15 November 2023].

26. Corey L, Gilbert PB, Juraska M, et al. Two randomized trials of neutralizing antibodies to prevent HIV-1 acquisition. N Engl J Med 2021;384(11):1003-14.

27. Gilbert PB, Huang Y, deCamp AC, et al. Neutralization titer biomarker for antibody-mediated prevention of HIV-1 acquisition. Nat Med 2022;28(9):1924-32.

28. Haynes BF, Wiehe K, Borrow P, et al. Strategies for HIV-1 vaccines that induce broadly neutralizing antibodies. Nat Rev Immunol 2023;23(3):142-58.

29. Haynes BF, Wiehe K, Alam SM, et al. Progress with induction of HIV broadly neutralizing antibodies in the Duke Consortia for HIV/AIDS Vaccine Development. Curr Opin HIV AIDS 2023;18(6):300-8.

30. Williams WB, Alam SM, Ofek G, et al. Vaccine induction of heterologous HIV-1 neutralizing antibody B cell lineages in humans. medRxiv 2023;2009:23286943.

31. Leggat DJ, Cohen KW, Willis JR, et al. Vaccination induces HIV broadly neutralizing antibody precursors in humans. Science 2022;378(6623):eadd6502.

32. Burton DR. Advancing an HIV vaccine; advancing vaccinology. Nat Rev Immunol 2019;19(2):77-8.

33. Martin TM, Robinson ST, Huang Y. Discovery medicine - the HVTN's iterative approach to developing an HIV-1 broadly neutralizing vaccine. Curr Opin HIV AIDS 2023;18(6):290-9.

34. Prudden H, Tatoud R, Slack C, et al. Experimental medicine for HIV vaccine research and development. Vaccines (Basel) 2023;11(5):970.

35. Koff WC, Burton DR, Johnson PR, et al. Accelerating next-generation vaccine development for global disease prevention. Science 2013;340(6136):1232910.
36. Sanders RW, Moore JP. Native-like Env trimers as a platform for HIV-1 vaccine design. Immunol Rev 2017;275(1):161–82.
37. Graham BS. The journey to RSV vaccines - heralding an era of structure-based design. N Engl J Med 2023;388(7):579–81.
38. Matarazzo L, Bettencourt PJG. mRNA vaccines: a new opportunity for malaria, tuberculosis and HIV. Front Immunol 2023;14:1172691.
39. Mu Z, Haynes BF, Cain DW. HIV mRNA vaccines-progress and future paths. Vaccines (Basel) 2021;9(2):134.
40. Pardi N, Hogan MJ, Naradikian MS, et al. Nucleoside-modified mRNA vaccines induce potent T follicular helper and germinal center B cell responses. J Exp Med 2018;215(6):1571–88.
41. Pardi N, LaBranche CC, Ferrari G, et al. Characterization of HIV-1 nucleoside-modified mRNA vaccines in rabbits and rhesus macaques. Mol Ther Nucleic Acids 2019;15:36–47.
42. Abad-Fernandez M, Goonetilleke N. Human cytomegalovirus-vectored vaccines against HIV. Curr Opin HIV AIDS 2019;14(2):137–42.
43. Hansen SG, Marshall EE, Malouli D, et al. A live-attenuated RhCMV/SIV vaccine shows long-term efficacy against heterologous SIV challenge. Sci Transl Med 2019;11(501):eaaw2607.
44. Kwaa AK, Blankson JN. Immune responses in controllers of HIV infection. Annu Rev Immunol 2023. https://doi.org/10.1146/annurev-immunol-083122-035233.
45. Kim J, Vasan S, Kim JH, et al. Current approaches to HIV vaccine development: a narrative review. J Int AIDS Soc 2021;24(Suppl 7):e25793.
46. Janes H, Donnell D, Gilbert PB, et al. Taking stock of the present and looking ahead: envisioning challenges in the design of future HIV prevention efficacy trials. Lancet HIV 2019;6(7):e475–82.
47. Janes H, Buchbinder S. Control groups for HIV prevention efficacy trials: what does the future hold? Curr Opin HIV AIDS 2023;18(6):349–56.
48. Bekker LG, Tatoud R, Dabis F, et al. The complex challenges of HIV vaccine development require renewed and expanded global commitment. Lancet 2020; 395(10221):384–8.
49. Trkola A, Moore PL. Vaccinating people living with HIV: a fast track to preventive and therapeutic HIV vaccines. Lancet Infect Dis 2024;24(4):e252–5.
50. Stamatatos L. Immunization during ART and ATI for HIV-1 vaccine discovery/ development. Curr Opin HIV AIDS 2023;18(6):309–14.

Advancing Toward a Human Immunodeficiency Virus Cure

Initial Progress on a Difficult Path

David M. Margolis, MD[a,b,c,*]

KEYWORDS

- HIV infection • Latency • Persistence • Eradication • Clinical trials

KEY POINTS

- Continued effort toward the development of deployable therapies that could eradicate human immunodeficiency virus (HIV) infection should be pursued in parallel to continued efforts toward prevention, diagnosis, and treatment of HIV infection.
- The strategy of exposing the latent HIV reservoir using latency reversal agents, paired with interventions to clear infected cells, has made steady progress but still requires a successful clinical proof-of-concept trial.
- While improvements in latency reversal modalities and antiviral immunotherapies are brought forward for clinical testing, new concepts toward HIV cure are in pre-clinical development.

INTRODUCTION

Following the emergence of the human immunodeficiency virus (HIV) pandemic, more than 2 decades of intense effort and investment was required to develop and implement antiretroviral therapy (ART). As has been reviewed earlier in this volume, modern ART is a nearly-optimal treatment tool[1] that can halt the progression of HIV infection, reverse immune deficiency, and reduce the spread of new infection. Refinement of antivirals continues, with the promise of long-acting therapies that might require only a few treatments per year.[2]

In parallel with the effort to develop ART, for 40 years an equally broad research portfolio has sought to develop a critical tool to end the HIV pandemic: a scalable prophylactic vaccine that can effectively prevent HIV infection. A number of different HIV vaccine concepts have been developed, and in 4 decades 8 have reached advanced testing in clinical

[a] Medicine, Microbiology & Immunology, Epidemiology; [b] UNC HIV Cure Center; [c] University of North Carolina at Chapel Hill, 2016 Genetic Medicine Building, 120 Mason Farm Road, CB 7042, Chapel Hill, NC 27599-7042, USA
* Corresponding author. University of North Carolina at Chapel Hill, 2016 Genetic Medicine Building, 120 Mason Farm Road, CB 7042, Chapel Hill, NC 27599-7042.
E-mail address: dmargo@med.unc.edu

Infect Dis Clin N Am 38 (2024) 487–497
https://doi.org/10.1016/j.idc.2024.06.001   **id.theclinics.com**

efficacy trials, but none have shown adequate clinical efficacy.[3] Efforts to replicate the modest success of RV144[4] failed with the early closure of HVTN 702,[5] and a more recent study of a promising vaccine candidate was also terminated prematurely for lack of efficacy.[6] It is hoped that a strategy of sequential prime and boost vaccinations might accelerate the evolution of broadly neutralizing antibodies (bnAbs),[7,8] but this complex prophylactic strategy may be difficult to deploy, and years of effort are still needed.

However, while the groundbreaking advances of ART can be effectively implemented across the globe, there is continuing concern that the investment needed for this effort may not be as persistent as the virus. Even if both treatment-as-prevention and pre-exposure ART prophylaxis are widely deployed, for the foreseeable future millions of people with HIV (PWH) will still be burdened by decades of chronic drug therapy, and its attendant medical care. And, perhaps a greater cost than the burden of lifelong ART for the health care systems of the world, these millions will inevitably face the stigma of chronic HIV-1 infection.[9]

Therefore, just as further effort is needed toward the distant goal of an effective HIV vaccine, so is research toward therapies that could yield a cure for HIV infection. As an intermediate goal, interventions that could allow durable immunologic control without the need for medication ("drug-free remission") would also be transformative for the millions with HIV. For over a decade, there has been significant concern about ongoing inflammation associated with persistent HIV infection, despite successful ART.[10] It should therefore be noted that in the setting of an ongoing battle between the immune system and HIV, it is unclear that drug-free control of HIV infection without cure will yield optimal health outcomes. Neither is it clear that eradication of HIV infection will eliminate concern about ongoing immune dysfunction and inflammation. Nevertheless, recent advances give some hope that progress toward viral eradication is possible.

PERSISTENT HUMAN IMMUNODEFICIENCY VIRUS INFECTION

The major barrier to HIV cure is a population of infected, long-lived cells containing persistent and latent viral genomes that cannot be detected or eliminated by host defenses. At the onset of the era of potent ART, it was briefly hoped that potent and early therapy might eradicate HIV infection. But the discovery and documentation of the HIV latent reservoir put those hopes to rest.[11] The past decade of research has resulted in deeper understanding of the molecular and cellular mechanisms of persistent HIV infection, with the discovery that viral persistence is highly complex and multidimensional. Replication-competent integrated HIV viral genomes survive despite years of ART, but persistence is driven only in part by the state of viral latency, or the absence of viral expression. It has become clear that HIV can persist despite decades of clinically successful ART for at least 3 reasons (**Fig. 1**).

First, the last decades of study have described several molecular mechanisms that establish and enforce post-integration latency of this retrovirus.[12–14] The elucidation of cellular factors that are required to establish and maintain proviral latency led to efforts to manipulate these host pathways as a way to therapeutically attack latent, persistent viral infection. HIV latency reversal agents (LRAs) have been proposed to allow the expression of virus within reservoirs by either providing inductive signals to the viral genome, or by removing obstacles to viral expression that contribute to latency once it is established. As these processes are driven, at least in the first instance, by host cell pathways and factors, LRAs are by definition host-targeted, and so must be carefully developed with an eye on safety and tolerability.

A second major force that allows the survival of the persistent viral reservoir is clonal proliferation, or clonal expansion. Surprisingly, populations of clonal proviruses seem

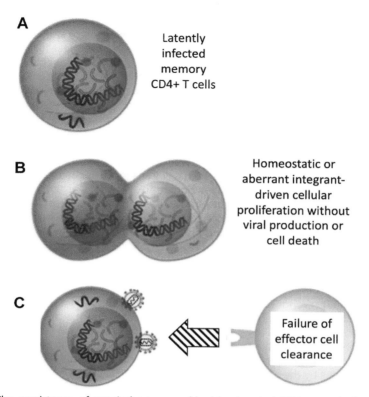

A Latently infected memory CD4+ T cells

B Homeostatic or aberrant integrant-driven cellular proliferation without viral production or cell death

C Failure of effector cell clearance

Fig. 1. The persistence of proviral genomes (double stranded DNA, green) that encode replication-competent HIV is due to multiple factors: (*A*) within cell populations, primarily a pool of memory CD4 + T cells that are in the resting state, viral genomes persist with minimal or intermittent viral gene expression (viral RNA strand, green), and minimal or absent viral protein expression or particle production; (*B*) Intermittently latently infected cells divide without resultant viral expression, yielding 2 infected daughter cells; (*C*) rarely but stably in the tissue of people with HIV (PWH) on long-term ART cells can be detected expressing viral RNAs and/or particles, implying a host defect in the ability to rapidly and effectively clear infected cells in the setting of low, rare, and anatomically diffuse presentation of viral target. (Figure modified with permission from[72]).

to be able to expand as silent passengers carried forward in T cell populations undergoing natural homeostatic proliferation. This key process is required to maintain pools of antigen-specific T cells, immune cell response, function, and immunologic memory. Long lived, stable pools of cells containing clones of identical integrated proviruses have been described.[15-18] While many persistent proviruses encode mutations or deletions rendering them defective,[19] replication-competent clones[20-22] also persist within the latent reservoir.

Finally, a third factor allowing HIV persistence appears to rest in the properties of the host cells that harbor the durable viral reservoir. Initial studies that described the latent HIV reservoir were undertaken in resting memory CD4 + T cells, lacking activation markers.[23-26] This central memory CD4 T cell compartment has been the most carefully and rigorously characterized in longitudinal studies, with an estimated half-life of 3.7 years.[27,28] However, many other populations of naïve (TN), transitional, memory

(TTM), effector memory (TEM), T memory stem cell (TSCM), gamma/delta T cells, and T regulatory T cells (Tregs) have been described as latent reservoirs,[29-33] although the stability of replication-competent provirus in these cells has been less fully quantitated over years of continuous ART administration. The natural differentiation process of T cells into various compartments (eg, central memory to or from effector memory), and the likelihood that a latent proviral genome may sometimes remain quiescent as an infected cell transitions into the effector pool or returns to the memory pool, complicates the longitudinal quantitation of the latent reservoir, but also speaks to the central contribution of the host cell environment to viral persistence.

In addition to the contribution of the infected host cell phenotype to both the entrance of the provirus into latency, and the maintenance of viral quiescence, it has recently been recognized that the host cell transcriptome, as exemplified by the expression of survival genes, likely contributes to the ability of an infected cell to persist. Such cells may better tolerate transient, intermittent expression of the viral genome.[34,35] A more durable cell appears more likely to carry a latent provirus, undergo clonal expansion over time, and may be more resistant to immune clearance if its resident provirus leaves latency.

INITIAL STRATEGIES TO ERADICATE HUMAN IMMUNODEFICIENCY VIRUS

The first concept proposed to clear HIV infection,[36] and the first human trial that sought to achieve this goal aimed to activate T cells using the anti-CD3 antibody OKT3 and interleukin 2.[37] However, the attempt to shock and kill the viral reservoir failed as global T cell activation yielded profound T cell depletion, substantial increase in inflammatory cytokine production, and severe toxicities. Attempts to purge the viral reservoir then fell by the wayside for a time.

Subsequently, leveraging the emerging understanding of molecular mechanisms that underpin proviral latency, agents that target those process were developed and tested, termed LRAs. Initially, these were histone deacetylase inhibitors such as valproic acid, vorinostat, panobinostat, romidepsin, and chidamide, which alter chromatin structure and thereby neighboring gene expression.[38-43] These LRAs were shown to be capable of inducing expression of HIV RNA or viral protein from latent viral genomes in vitro and in vivo.

Unfortunately, the flashy slogans ("Shock and Kill," "Kick and Kill") attached to these efforts proved to be an overpromise. Although some initially hoped that poking the latent reservoir in this way would be enough to cause cell death, no studies using single LRAs induced a measurable, reproducible depletion of the viral reservoir.[44] In retrospect, as the complexity of factors that restrict proviral expression, and the proliferative capacity of reservoir cells was appreciated, these failures were not surprising.

Subsequently, other approaches to signal latently infected cells and induce quiescent proviruses to leave the latent state were developed and tested in the clinic. Toll-like receptor agonists were reported to reverse latency and shown to be immune stimulants.[45] The protein kinase C agonist bryostatin was safely deployed but failed to show LRA activity.[46] The IL-15 superagonist was tested and found to be safe, with some evidence of increased proviral expression after treatment.[47] The BAF complex regulates human gene expression and may play a role in HIV latency as well. Pyrimethamine is an inhibitor of BAF complex activity, and its administration was safe and associated with significant increase in cell-associated HIV-1 RNA expression in PWH on ART.[48] Pyrimethamine did not result in a reduction of viral reservoir measures but may represent a new LRA approach.

Immune checkpoint blockers (ICBs), widely used to augment the anti-cancer immune response, have also been explored in the setting of HIV infection for their potential to act as LRAs, as well as potentially augment the anti-viral immune response. Pembrolizumab (anti-PD-1) reversed latency in 32 PWH and cancer on ART.[49] In a small observational study, various ICBs given for cancer to 3 PWH on ART were observed to variably activate latent HIV and enhance HIV-specific T cell function.[50] And in study of 33 PWH on ART with cancer, nivolumab (anti-PD-1) alone (n = 33) failed to show an effect of latent HIV, while nivolumab with ipilimumab (anti-CTLA-4; n = 4) had a modest effect on latent viral expression.[51] ICBs deserve further study, but their known severe toxicities may make it difficult to employ in the absence of a concurrent oncology indication.

A promising new LRA approach, at least as judged by activity in animal models, is the induction of NF-kB signaling via the non-canonical pathway. SMAC mimetics, or IAP inhibitors, were initially developed within oncology research programs, but shown to robustly reverse HIV and simian immunodeficiency virus (SIV) latency, alone and in combination with other agents, in both the non-human primate (SIV) and humanized mouse (HIV) model systems.[52,53] Efforts are ongoing to develop an acceptable IAP inhibitor for human studies to test this approach in a pilot trial.

To improve the activity of LRAs, it has long been hypothesized that combinations of agents with synergistic activity will be required. Although a handful of combination approaches have been found to be potent in animal model studies, few have entered the clinic. An attempt to augment the activity of vorinostat using tamoxifen, based on in vitro modeling, was not successful in one clinical trial.[54] In a heroic study in which ART was initiated at acute infection, higher levels of viremia were seen when vorinostat, hydroxychloroquine, and maraviroc were added to ART, and while reservoir size was not definitively measured, no change in viral rebound was seen following ART interruption.[55]

MOVING TO COMBINATION LATENCY REVERSAL AND CLEARANCE STRATEGIES

Given the lack of impact on the latent reservoir on single LRA approaches, clinical studies were initiated to test the capacity of an LRA when paired with immune therapies to assist in the clearance of infection. A major challenge to efforts to develop latency reversal and reservoir clearance strategies is that the paired approaches are co-dependent. It is difficult to know if latency reversal is functionally active without an immunotherapeutic clearance mechanism in place. And it is difficult to know if an immunotherapeutic clearance mechanism is efficacious without an effective LRA. There are not yet gold standards for either modality.

3 pilot studies tested the serial administration of HDAC inhibitors, shown to upregulate viral RNA expression within cells, with a variety of HIV vaccine platforms.[56-58] While latency reversal activity appeared measurable as an increase of HIV RNA expression within circulating lymphocytes, it is still unclear if this response will translate to sufficiently robust and durable HIV-1 protein expression to enable immune clearance of infected cells. In these studies, increases in cell-associated HIV RNA were indeed seen, but depletion of latent, persistent infection could not be measured. As only a minority of the latent reservoir may have become vulnerable to immune clearance following each LRA dose, the immune responses induced in these studies may have been insufficient to identify and clear such challenging, and likely transient, targets. A fourth study using romidepsin, GM-CSF, and an HIV gag peptide vaccination appeared to have a very modest effect in reducing the frequency of latent infection, but no effect on viral rebound after a treatment interruption.[59]

As an alternative immunotherapy to vaccination, broadly neutralizing antibodies have been tested swith histone deacetylase (HDAC) inhibitors have been tested with broadly neutralizing HIV antibodies. In the ROADMAP study, romedepsin was combined with 3BNC117, an antibody targeting the CD4 binding site of the HIV-1 Env protein, highly active in clinical studies.[60] Again, latency reversal was measured, but no reduction in persistent infection, and no effect on viral rebound after a treatment interruption, was seen. At the same time, a study testing vorinostat with the bnAb VRC-07 to 523-LS, also found no reduction of persistent infection, despite repeatedly measurable latency reversal, and the lack of viruses resistant to VRC-07 within the viral reservoir.[61] Similarly, the TITAN trial combined a TLR9 agonist with the bnAbs 3BNC117 and 10 to 1074, could not measure an effect on the latent reservoir prior to treatment interruption.[62] In this study, and others there has been an effect in some participants following the administration of bnAbs, with a delay in viral rebound seen despite the absence of evidence of reservoir depletion. The mechanism for this increased ability to control viremia, at least to some extent and for some time, is not understood, certainly deserves further study, but appears to be mediating control of persistent infection rather than elimination of it.

CURRENT CHALLENGES AND FUTURE DIRECTIONS

What is most needed for current approaches is clear evidence that the latent, persistent reservoir of HIV infection that is the source of viral rebound after treatment interruption can be measurably depleted. This would signal that a path forward has been identified. 2 recent studies leave some room for optimism.

In a primate study, recently developed LRA strategies led to robust latency reversal, and when given with a combination of bnAbs, evidence of reservoir depletion could be measured in the tissues.[63] If these advanced LRAs can be brought to human testing, this could be a tractable approach. And in a pilot human clinical trial, ART-suppressed PWH received the widely tested first-generation LRA, vorinostat, in combination with autologous HIV-1 antigen-specific T cells that had been expanded ex vivo and readministered during vorinostat dosing.[64] In the group of PWH who received the higher dose of T cells, declines of integrated proviral DNA were seen (in 3 of 3 high dose vs 1 of 6 receiving lower dose). A second recent human pilot trial administered panobinistat as an LRA in combination with interferon as an antiviral immunotherapy.[65] While depletion of the latent reservoir was not measured, the investigators used elegant molecular studies to suggest that latency reversal can sensitize HIV-1 proviruses to immune clearance. Foreseeable improvements in these strategies may allow clinically relevant inroads into the persistent viral reservoir.

Numerous other approaches that may yield durable control, if not viral elimination, are also under earlier phases of study. The infusion of bnAbs with early ART may lead to post-ART control, an acceptable outcome if the clinical benefits can be shown to be equal to ART. Agents to induce the death of HIV-infected cells are entering pre-clinical or clinical testing.[66,67] CRISPR gene editing approaches are being tested in animal models, although are likely years away from clinical testing, and long-term safety concerns for CRISPR technology have yet to be addressed.[68,69] Strategies to permanently silence viral genomes are under study, but concerns of how durable silencing will be without repeated treatments are still to be vetted.[70] As ART is further developed toward ultra-long-acting drug formulations,[2] it could be replaced by genetic therapy that delivers a stably produced antiviral molecule.[71]

SUMMARY

Eradication of infection in PWH is a cherished optimal goal, but it is still far from being practically achievable. In the fifth decade of the AIDS pandemic, huge advances have been made in clinical care and prevention methods, but a cure or effective vaccine is not at hand. However, we mark more than 10 years of scientific effort refocused toward the goal of viral eradication, and this has yielded a better understanding of the many mechanisms of viral persistence and expanding tools to measure persistence and test therapies. Efforts to disrupt latency and target reservoirs for clearance are advancing toward clinical testing.

Like many of the most challenging problems facing society, the response to the HIV pandemic must be multifaceted. Among the many important goals for future research is the development of temporally contained therapies capable of eradicating HIV infection. A paradigm for this effort is found in the decades-long effort in searching for a "cure" for cancer. Our progress made so far in deciphering HIV pathogenesis and developing treatment strategies gives hope that eradication of established HIV infection is an attainable goal if we maintain persistent effort against a persistent pathogen.

CLINICS CARE POINTS

- The strategy of exposing the latent HIV reservoir using LRAs, paired with interventions to clear infected cells, has made steady progress.

- In addition to the many clinical benefits of early and effective antiviral treatment of HIV infection, durably treated PLH may benefit from future HIV cure strategies.

- Continued effort toward the development of deployable therapies that could eradicate HIV infection should be pursued in parallel to continued efforts toward prevention, diagnosis, and treatment of HIV infection.

ACKNOWLEDGMENTS

This work was supported by National Institutes of Health, United States UM1 AI164567 to DMM. We thank the many investigators who have contributed, and the many study participants who have advanced the field.

DISCLOSURE

The author owns common stock in Gilead Sciences.

REFERENCES

1. Gandhi RT, Bedimo R, Hoy JF, et al. Antiretroviral drugs for treatment and prevention of HIV infection in adults: 2022 Recommendations of the International Antiviral Society–USA Panel. JAMA 2023;329:63–84.
2. Flexner C, Thomas DL, Clayden P, et al. What clinicians need to know about the development of long-acting formulations. Clin Infect Dis 2022;75. S487-s9.
3. Nkolola JP, Barouch DH. Prophylactic HIV-1 vaccine trials: past, present, and future. Lancet HIV 2023. https://doi.org/10.1016/S2352-3018(23)00264-3.
4. Kim JH, Excler JL, Michael NL. Lessons from the RV144 Thai phase III HIV-1 vaccine trial and the search for correlates of protection. Annu Rev Med 2015;66: 423–37.

5. Gray GE, Bekker LG, Laher F, et al. Vaccine Efficacy of ALVAC-HIV and Bivalent Subtype C gp120-MF59 in Adults. N Engl J Med 2021;384:1089–100.

6. Phase 3 Mosaic-Based Investigational HIV Vaccine Study Discontinued Following Disappointing Results of Planned Data Review. https://www.nih.gov/news-events/news-releases/experimental-hiv-vaccine-regimen-safe-ineffective-study-finds.

7. Eisinger RW, Fauci AS. Ending the HIV/AIDS Pandemic(1). Emerg Infect Dis 2018;24:413–6.

8. Saunders KO, Counts J, Thakur B, et al. Vaccine induction of CD4-mimicking HIV-1 broadly neutralizing antibody precursors in macaques. Cell 2024;187:79–94.e24.

9. Ferguson L, Gruskin S, Bolshakova M, et al. Systematic review and quantitative and qualitative comparative analysis of interventions to address HIV-related stigma and discrimination. AIDS 2023;37:1919–39.

10. Deeks SG, Tracy R, Douek DC. Systemic effects of inflammation on health during chronic HIV infection. Immunity 2013;39:633–45.

11. Siliciano JD, Siliciano RF. In vivo dynamics of the latent reservoir for HIV-1: new insights and implications for cure. Annu Rev Pathol 2022;17:271–94.

12. Rodari A, Darcis G, Van Lint CM. The current status of latency reversing agents for HIV-1 remission. Annu Rev Virol 2021;8:491–514.

13. Mbonye U, Karn J. The molecular basis for human immunodeficiency virus latency. Annu Rev Virol 2017;4:261–85.

14. Lewis CA, Margolis DM, Browne EP. New concepts in therapeutic manipulation of HIV-1 transcription and latency: latency reversal versus latency prevention. Viruses 2023;15.

15. Bailey JR, Sedaghat AR, Kieffer T, et al. Residual human immunodeficiency virus type 1 viremia in some patients on antiretroviral therapy is dominated by a small number of invariant clones rarely found in circulating CD4+ T cells. J Virol 2006;80:6441–57.

16. Maldarelli F, Wu X, Su L, et al. Specific HIV integration sites are linked to clonal expansion and persistence of infected cells. Science 2014;345:179–83.

17. Tobin NH, Learn GH, Holte SE, et al. Evidence that low-level viremias during effective highly active antiretroviral therapy result from two processes: expression of archival virus and replication of virus. J Virol 2005;79:9625–34.

18. Wagner TA, McLaughlin S, Garg K, et al. Proliferation of cells with HIV integrated into cancer genes contributes to persistent infection. Science 2014;345:570–3.

19. Bruner KM, Wang Z, Simonetti FR, et al. A quantitative approach for measuring the reservoir of latent HIV-1 proviruses. Nature 2019;566:120–5.

20. Bui JK, Sobolewski MD, Keele BF, et al. Proviruses with identical sequences comprise a large fraction of the replication-competent HIV reservoir. PLoS Pathog 2017;13:e1006283.

21. Hosmane NN, Kwon KJ, Bruner KM, et al. Proliferation of latently infected CD4(+) T cells carrying replication-competent HIV-1: Potential role in latent reservoir dynamics. J Exp Med 2017;214:959–72.

22. Simonetti FR, Sobolewski MD, Fyne E, et al. Clonally expanded CD4+ T cells can produce infectious HIV-1 in vivo. Proc Natl Acad Sci U S A 2016;113:1883–8.

23. Chun TW, Finzi D, Margolick J, et al. In vivo fate of HIV-1-infected T cells: quantitative analysis of the transition to stable latency. Nat Med 1995;1:1284–90.

24. Chun TW, Stuyver L, Mizell SB, et al. Presence of an inducible HIV-1 latent reservoir during highly active antiretroviral therapy. Proc Natl Acad Sci U S A 1997;94:13193–7.

25. Finzi D, Hermankova M, Pierson T, et al. Identification of a reservoir for HIV-1 in patients on highly active antiretroviral therapy. Science 1997;278:1295–300.

26. Wong JK, Hezareh M, Gunthard HF, et al. Recovery of replication-competent HIV despite prolonged suppression of plasma viremia. Science 1997;278:1291–5.

27. Crooks AM, Bateson R, Cope AB, et al. Precise quantitation of the latent HIV-1 reservoir: implications for eradication strategies. JID (J Infect Dis) 2015;212: 1361–5.

28. Siliciano JD, Kajdas J, Finzi D, et al. Long-term follow-up studies confirm the stability of the latent reservoir for HIV-1 in resting CD4(+) T cells. Nat Med 2003;9: 727–8.

29. Chomont N, El-Far M, Ancuta P, et al. HIV reservoir size and persistence are driven by T cell survival and homeostatic proliferation. Nat Med 2009;15:893–900.

30. Zerbato JM, McMahon DK, Sobolewski MD, et al. Naive CD4+ T Cells Harbor a Large Inducible Reservoir of Latent, Replication-competent Human Immunodeficiency Virus Type 1. Clin Infect Dis 2019;69:1919–25.

31. Tran TA, de Goër de Herve MG, Hendel-Chavez H, et al. Resting regulatory CD4 T cells: a site of HIV persistence in patients on long-term effective antiretroviral therapy. PLoS One 2008;3:e3305.

32. Soriano-Sarabia N, Bateson RE, Dahl NP, et al. Quantitation of replication-competent HIV-1 in populations of resting CD4+ T cells. J Virol 2014;88:14070–7.

33. Buzon MJ, Sun H, Li C, et al. HIV-1 persistence in CD4+ T cells with stem cell-like properties. Nat Med 2014;20:139–42.

34. Sun W, Gao C, Hartana CA, et al. Phenotypic signatures of immune selection in HIV-1 reservoir cells. Nature 2023;614:309–17.

35. Clark IC, Mudvari P, Thaploo S, et al. HIV silencing and cell survival signatures in infected T cell reservoirs. Nature 2023;614:318–25.

36. Hamer DH. Can HIV be Cured? Mechanisms of HIV persistence and strategies to combat it. Curr HIV Res 2004;2:99–111.

37. Prins JM, Jurriaans S, van Praag RM, et al. Immuno-activation with anti-CD3 and recombinant human IL-2 in HIV-1-infected patients on potent antiretroviral therapy. AIDS 1999;13:2405–10.

38. Lehrman G, Hogue IB, Palmer S, et al. Depletion of latent HIV-1 infection in vivo: a proof-of-concept study. Lancet 2005;366:549–55.

39. Archin NM, Liberty AL, Kashuba AD, et al. Administration of vorinostat disrupts HIV-1 latency in patients on antiretroviral therapy. Nature 2012;487:482–5.

40. Elliott JH, Wightman F, Solomon A, et al. Activation of HIV transcription with short-course vorinostat in HIV-infected patients on suppressive antiretroviral therapy. PLoS Pathog 2014;10:e1004473.

41. Søgaard OS, Graversen ME, Leth S, et al. The Depsipeptide Romidepsin Reverses HIV-1 Latency In Vivo. PLoS Pathog 2015;11:e1005142.

42. Rasmussen TA, Tolstrup M, Brinkmann CR, et al. Panobinostat, a histone deacetylase inhibitor, for latent-virus reactivation in HIV-infected patients on suppressive antiretroviral therapy: a phase 1/2, single group, clinical trial. Lancet HIV 2014;1:e13–21.

43. Li JH, Ma J, Kang W, et al. The histone deacetylase inhibitor chidamide induces intermittent viraemia in HIV-infected patients on suppressive antiretroviral therapy. HIV Med 2020;21:747–57.

44. Rasmussen TA, Sogaard OS. Clinical Interventions in HIV Cure Research. Adv Exp Med Biol 2018;1075:285–318.

45. Vibholm LK, Konrad CV, Schleimann MH, et al. Effects of 24-week Toll-like receptor 9 agonist treatment in HIV type 1+ individuals. AIDS 2019;33:1315–25.

46. Gutiérrez C, Serrano-Villar S, Madrid-Elena N, et al. Bryostatin-1 for latent virus reactivation in HIV-infected patients on antiretroviral therapy. AIDS 2016;30: 1385–92.

47. Miller JS, Davis ZB, Helgeson E, et al. Safety and virologic impact of the IL-15 superagonist N-803 in people living with HIV: a phase 1 trial. Nat Med 2022;28: 392–400.

48. Prins HAB, Crespo R, Lungu C, et al. The BAF complex inhibitor pyrimethamine reverses HIV-1 latency in people with HIV-1 on antiretroviral therapy. Sci Adv 2023;9:eade6675.

49. Uldrick TS, Adams SV, Fromentin R, et al. Pembrolizumab induces HIV latency reversal in people living with HIV and cancer on antiretroviral therapy. Sci Transl Med 2022;14:eabl3836.

50. Lau JSY, McMahon JH, Gubser C, et al. The impact of immune checkpoint therapy on the latent reservoir in HIV-infected individuals with cancer on antiretroviral therapy. AIDS 2021;35:1631–6.

51. Rasmussen TA, Rajdev L, Rhodes A, et al. Impact of Anti-PD-1 and Anti-CTLA-4 on the Human Immunodeficiency Virus (HIV) Reservoir in People Living With HIV With Cancer on Antiretroviral Therapy: The AIDS Malignancy Consortium 095 Study. Clin Infect Dis 2021;73:e1973–81.

52. Nixon CC, Mavigner M, Sampey GC, et al. Systemic HIV and SIV latency reversal via non-canonical NF-kappaB signalling in vivo. Nature 2020. https://doi.org/10. 1038/s41586-020-1951-3.

53. Mavigner M, Liao LE, Brooks AD, et al. CD8 lymphocyte depletion enhances the latency reversal activity of the SMAC mimetic AZD5582 in ART-suppressed SIV-infected rhesus macaques. J Virol 2021;95.

54. Scully EP, Aga E, Tsibris A, et al. Impact of tamoxifen on vorinostat-induced human immunodeficiency virus expression in women on antiretroviral therapy: AIDS clinical trials group A5366, The MOXIE Trial. Clin Infect Dis 2022;75: 1389–96.

55. Kroon E, Ananworanich J, Pagliuzza A, et al. A randomized trial of vorinostat with treatment interruption after initiating antiretroviral therapy during acute HIV-1 infection. J Virus Erad 2020;6:100004.

56. Gay CL, Kuruc JD, Falcinelli SD, et al. Assessing the impact of AGS-004, a dendritic cell-based immunotherapy, and vorinostat on persistent HIV-1 Infection. Sci Rep 2020;10:5134.

57. Fidler S, Stohr W, Pace M, et al. Antiretroviral therapy alone versus antiretroviral therapy with a kick and kill approach, on measures of the HIV reservoir in participants with recent HIV infection (the RIVER trial): a phase 2, randomised trial. Lancet 2020. https://doi.org/10.1038/s41586-020-1951-3.

58. Mothe B, Rosás-Umbert M, Coll P, et al. HIVconsv vaccines and romidepsin in early-treated HIV-1-infected individuals: safety, immunogenicity and effect on the viral reservoir (Study BCN02). Front Immunol 2020;11:823.

59. Leth S, Schleimann MH, Nissen SK, et al. Combined effect of Vacc-4x, recombinant human granulocyte macrophage colony-stimulating factor vaccination, and romidepsin on the HIV-1 reservoir (REDUC): a single-arm, phase 1B/2A trial. Lancet HIV 2016;3:e463–72.

60. Gruell H, Gunst JD, Cohen YZ, et al. Effect of 3BNC117 and romidepsin on the HIV-1 reservoir in people taking suppressive antiretroviral therapy (ROADMAP): a randomised, open-label, phase 2A trial. Lancet Microbe 2022;3:e203–14.

61. Gay CL, James KS, Tuyishime M, et al. Stable latent HIV infection and low-level viremia despite treatment with the broadly neutralizing antibody VRC07-523LS and the latency reversal agent vorinostat. J Infect Dis 2022;225:856–61.
62. Gunst JD, Højen JF, Pahus MH, et al. Impact of a TLR9 agonist and broadly neutralizing antibodies on HIV-1 persistence: the randomized phase 2a TITAN trial. Nat Med 2023;29:2547–58.
63. Dashti A, Sukkestad S, Horner AM, et al. AZD5582 plus SIV-specific antibodies reduce lymph node viral reservoirs in antiretroviral therapy-suppressed macaques. Nat Med 2023;29:2535–46.
64. Gay CLHP, Archin NM, Pedersen SM, et al. The effects of HIV-1 antigen expanded specific T Cell Therapy (HXTC) and Vorinostat on Persistent HIV-1 in People Living with HIV on Antiretroviral Therapy. J Infect Dis 2024;229(3):743–52.
65. Armani-Tourret M, Gao C, Hartana CA, et al. Selection of epigenetically privileged HIV-1 proviruses during treatment with panobinostat and interferon-α2a. Cell 2024;187:1238–54.e14.
66. Cummins NW, Baker J, Chakraborty R, et al. Single center, open label dose escalating trial evaluating once weekly oral ixazomib in ART-suppressed, HIV positive adults and effects on HIV reservoir size in vivo. EClinicalMedicine 2021;42:101225.
67. Balibar CJ, Klein DJ, Zamlynny B, et al. Potent targeted activator of cell kill molecules eliminate cells expressing HIV-1. Sci Transl Med 2023;15:eabn2038.
68. Dash PK, Kaminski R, Bella R, et al. Sequential LASER ART and CRISPR Treatments Eliminate HIV-1 in a Subset of Infected Humanized Mice. Nat Commun 2019;10:2753.
69. Liu Y, Binda CS, Berkhout B, et al. CRISPR-Cas attack of HIV-1 proviral DNA can cause unintended deletion of surrounding cellular DNA. J Virol 2023;97.013344-e1423.
70. Lyons DE, Kumar P, Roan NR, et al. HIV-1 Remission: Accelerating the Path to Permanent HIV-1 Silencing. Viruses 2023;15.
71. Joshi LR, Gálvez NMS, Ghosh S, et al. Delivery platforms for broadly neutralizing antibodies. Curr Opin HIV AIDS 2023;18:191–208.
72. Margolis DM, Garcia JV, Hazuda DJ, et al. Latency reversal and viral clearance to cure HIV-1. Science 2016;353:aaf6517.

Weight Gain and Antiretroviral Therapy

Samuel S. Bailin, MD, MSCI*, John R. Koethe, MD, MSCI

KEYWORDS

- Weight gain • Obesity • Antiretroviral therapy • Metabolism • HIV

KEY POINTS

- The proportion of persons with human immunodeficiency virus (PWH) who are overweight or have obesity both before and after antiretroviral therapy initiation has substantially increased over the past decades and mirrors long-standing trends in the general population.
- Substantial evidence from pharmacokinetic and pre-exposure prophylaxis studies suggests efavirenz and tenofovir disoproxil fumarate are weight suppressing in some individuals.
- Weight gain on ART is mainly fat mass, preferentially occurs at visceral sites, and begins early after treatment initiation.
- Ongoing studies evaluating newer weight loss medications, bariatric surgery, and antiretroviral switches will shed light on the use of these interventions in PWH with excess weight gain.

INTRODUCTION

In the era of modern antiretroviral therapy (ART), persons with HIV (PWH) have significantly improved longevity that now approaches that of HIV-negative individuals.[1,2] However, as the population ages, cardiometabolic diseases and other comorbidities have emerged as significant contributors to reduced quality of life and mortality.[3–6] Excess adiposity and altered body fat distribution is a major risk factor for the development of metabolic diseases, and an increasing prevalence of obesity in PWH mirrors the trend observed in the general population.[7] Understanding and treating factors that contribute to excess adiposity could reduce weight-associated comorbidities including diabetes, cardiovascular disease (CVD), liver disease, and neurocognitive impairments in an aging PWH population.

While obesity is a complex multifactorial disease, the role of ART agents as a determinant of body weight is an evolving area of research.[8] Newer ART regimens, particularly

Division of Infectious Diseases, Vanderbilt University Medical Center, 1161 21st Avenue South, A2200 Medical Center North, Nashville, TN 37232, USA
* Corresponding author.
E-mail address: Samuel.bailin@vumc.org

Infect Dis Clin N Am 38 (2024) 499–515
https://doi.org/10.1016/j.idc.2024.04.005
0891-5520/24/© 2024 Elsevier Inc. All rights reserved.

id.theclinics.com

those including tenofovir alafenamide (TAF) and integrase strand transfer inhibitors (INSTIs), have been associated with greater weight gain in clinical trials,[8,9] and implicated in the rise in weight-associated comorbidities.[10,11] Recent studies in both PWH and HIV-negative persons on pre-exposure prophylaxis (PrEP) have provided important insights into whether some agents may be weight suppressing versus weight promoting, and an ongoing reassessment of weight change in prior studies of ART-naïve and ART-experienced participants focuses on how to define "weight neutral" agents given the diversity of observed effects among ART classes and individual drugs. Efforts to elucidate the mechanisms for weight gain on ART, reverse ART-associated weight gain, ameliorate the effect on cardiometabolic health, and identify the individuals most susceptible to weight gain is an area of continuing research.

DISCUSSION
Weight Trends in Persons with Human Immunodeficiency Virus and in the General Population

Obesity is a complex trait of excess fat accumulation that involves interactions between genetic, socioeconomic, psychological, and environmental factors. Greater physical activity has been linked to a lower risk of obesity,[12] may reduce visceral adipose tissue (VAT) volume even in absence of overall weight loss,[13] and can modify effect size of obesity-risk genetic loci.[14] However, twin studies have estimated a 40% to 70% heritability of obesity, which is illustrated in the varying effectiveness of lifestyle modification across individuals.[15] Racial inequalities and socioeconomic status are also associated with obesity,[16] and exposure to psychological stressors, which is greater among Black and US-born Hispanic individuals, may also contribute to the development of obesity and partially explain differences in obesity rates compared to White individuals.[17]

To accurately interpret and make informed clinical decisions about weight gain in PWH on ART, the data must be interpreted within the context of population changes in weight during the same era. Globally from 1975 to 2014, the proportion of underweight (body mass index [BMI] <18.5 kg/m^2) individuals decreased, and the prevalence of obesity (BMI $\geq$30 kg/m^2) substantially increased in most regions of the world.[18] Though the prevalence of underweight individuals remains persistently high in East and Central Africa and other resource-constrained areas, higher-income, predominately English-speaking countries, including the United States, have seen a disproportionate growth of individuals with obesity and severe obesity. In the 2018 National Health and Nutrition Examination Survey (NHANES), the prevalence of obesity among US adults aged 20 and over was 42.4%, and another 30.7% were overweight (BMI 25–29.9 kg/m^2).[19] Individuals who self-identified as non-Hispanic Black or Hispanic had higher rates of obesity than non-Hispanic Whites. This increasing prevalence is accompanied by an increasing burden of weight-associated diseases, including CVD, diabetes mellitus, chronic kidney diseases, and neoplasms that contribute to substantial morbidity and mortality.[20]

Similar population-based data in PWH are limited and confounded by rapid weight gain after ART initiation. In the North America AIDS Cohort Collaboration on Research and Design (NA-ACCORD), the proportion of individuals with obesity at ART initiation in the United States and Canada increased from 11% (1998–2000) to 17% (2007–2010), which may reflect earlier identification of HIV and earlier initiation of ART, but may also reflect increasing background obesity rates.[7] Compared to matched NHANES individuals from the same era, mean BMI among PWH after 3 years of ART did not differ from the general population, and was significantly higher for self-identified non-Hispanic White women with HIV. Recent clinical trials in South Africa demonstrate high rates of obesity in ART-naïve PWH.[21] Thus, obesity in PWH on long-term ART is a multifactorial disease with many shared causes with the general population that include genetic, socioeconomic, psychological, and environmental factors (**Fig. 1**).

Measurements of Weight

BMI is defined as total body weight in kilograms (kg) divided by height in meters, squared.[22] This method is most widely used in the clinical setting due to the ease of use, low cost, and high reproducibility. Elevated BMI is linked to the development of diabetes, liver disease, neurocognitive disease, and, to a lesser extent, CVD in both the general population and in PWH.[20,23–25] However, there are several pitfalls to using BMI as an indicator of adiposity. First, BMI poorly discriminates between muscle mass and fat mass and does not discriminate between subcutaneous adiposity and visceral adiposity.[22] VAT volume is most strongly associated with insulin resistance and CVD development in the general population, even after adjusting for BMI.[26] Second, there is significant heterogeneity in body composition and body shape across different racial/ethnic groups, and by sex, and age.[27] This is particularly problematic since the "normal" distribution for BMI was derived from largely non-Hispanic White individuals. Given these limitations, other simple-to-obtain anthropometric measures have been proposed, including waist circumference and waist-to-hip ratio. VAT is more difficult to measure without imaging, though waist circumference has been proposed as a rough approximation.[28] Currently, the gold standard is measuring VAT volume through computed tomography (CT) or MRI. While dual x-ray absorptiometry (DEXA) scanning can compute VAT using image density and software algorithms, DEXA may be less accurate in some individuals.[29,30] Beyond VAT, MRI may be better

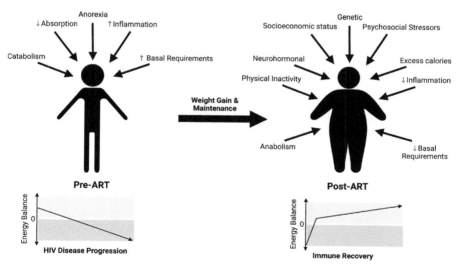

Fig. 1. Untreated human immunodeficiency virus is characterized by anorexia, decreased nutrient absorption, increased inflammatory cytokines, increased basal metabolic requirements in the setting of opportunistic infections, and an overall catabolic state that results in a negative energy balance and weight loss as HIV progresses. After antiretroviral therapy (ART) initiation, basal metabolic rate decreases, inflammatory cytokines decrease, and metabolism is shifted toward an overall anabolic state. Complex contributions of genetic, psychological stressors, socioeconomic status, neurohormonal regulation of energy intake and usage, physical inactivity, and access to food contribute to net positive energy balance and overall maintenance of weight.

at discerning liver steatosis than CT.[31] However, these imaging technologies are expensive and primarily limited to clinical research. In summary, BMI is an imperfect measure of adiposity and poor predictor for the development of metabolic disease, which emphasizes the need to supplant this measure with other clinical measures (**Fig. 2**).

Weight Gain in Antiretroviral Therapy-Naïve Persons with Human Immunodeficiency Virus

Early in the epidemic, HIV-associated wasting disease was a frequent presenting condition in advanced HIV disease and characterized by weight loss accompanying $CD4^+$ T cell depletion and an overall catabolic state.[32] ART rapidly reverses this catabolic state. Lower baseline $CD4^+$ T cell count, a surrogate for disease severity, is associated with greater weight gain.[33] Importantly, weight gain with ART initiation in underweight individuals has been associated with reduced mortality in both high-income and resource-constrained countries.[33,34] In contrast, weight gain in PWH who are overweight or have obesity at baseline does not improve mortality compared with normal BMI, and increases the risk for the development of metabolic diseases.[25]

Concern about weight gain associated with specific ART emerged early after the introduction of INSTI-based regimens in observational cohorts, demonstrating excess weight gain in PWH initiated on INSTI-based or protease inhibitor (PI)-based regimens compared with non-nucleoside reverse transcriptase inhibitor (NNRTI)-based regimens.[35,36] ART-specific weight gain risk was assessed in a pooled analysis of 8 randomized controlled trials of 5680 ART-naïve PWH initiating ART between 2003 and 2015.[8] PWH on INSTI-based regimens gained 3.24 kg at 96 weeks, which was significantly greater than PI-based (1.72 kg) and NNRTIs-based regimens (1.93 kg). Among the INSTI-based regimens, bictegravir (BIC) and dolutegravir (DTG) had similar weight gain, which was greater than cobicistat-boosted elvitegravir (EVG/c). Within the NNRTI class, rilpivirine (RVP) had greater weight gain compared with efavirenz (EFV). Among nucleoside reverse transcriptase inhibitors (NRTIs), TAF was associated with the greatest weight gain followed by abacavir (ABC) and tenofovir disoproxil fumarate (TDF) (**Table 1**). While these studies were predominantly conducted in high-income countries

Metabolically Healthy   **Metabolically Unhealthy**

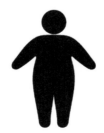   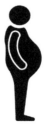

BMI: 30.0 kg/m²   **BMI**: 30.0 kg/m²
Waist Circ: 92 cm   **Waist Circ**: 106 cm
VAT Volume: 100 cm³   **VAT Volume**: 366 cm³
HOMA-IR: 0.5   **HOMA-IR**: 5.0

Fig. 2. Example of the limitations of body mass index (BMI) in predicting metabolic disease. Despite the same BMI, the person on the left has a smaller waist circumference, smaller visceral adipose tissue (VAT) volume, and no evidence of insulin resistance whereas the person on the right has a larger waist circumference, larger VAT volume, and significant evidence of insulin resistance.

and included majority male and non-Hispanic White participants, the results have largely been replicated in African cohorts.

Some of the most compelling data for weight gain with ART in African populations comes from the 96-week outcomes of the ADVANCE trial, a randomized, open-label, non-inferiority phase 3 clinical trial conducted in South Africa that enrolled 1053 ART-naïve PWH who were randomly assigned 1:1:1 to TAF/emtricitabine (FTC)+DTG, TDF/FTC + DTG, or EFV/TDF/FTC.[21] Greater weight gain was observed in PWH on TAF/FTC + DTG (7.1 kg) compared with TDF/FTC + DTG (4.3 kg) and EFV/TDF/FTC (2.3 kg). Weight gain was greatest in Black women and the emergence of obesity was significantly higher in women at 96 weeks, reaching 28% in the TAF/FTC + DTG group compared with only 5% in men.

The 2-drug regimen DTG/lamivudine (3 TC) is now a recommended first-line therapy in the Department of Health and Human Services (HHS) and the International Antiviral Society (IAS)-USA guidelines.[37,38] In GEMINI-1 and GEMINI-2, ART-naïve PWH were randomized to either DTG/3TC or TDF/FTC + DTG. Over 96 weeks, weight gain was similar between the 2 arms.[39] There are fewer data on newer NNRTI agents, though in the DRIVE-AHEAD phase 3, trial in 728 ART-naïve PWH who were randomized to either doravirine (DOR)/TDF/3TC or EFV/TDF/FTC for 96 weeks, weight gain was not different between the arms.[40] In summary, recent large observational retrospective cohorts and randomized clinical trials across diverse populations show differential weight gain with ART initiation, with the largest gains in INSTI-based and TAF-based regimens, and greater gains among Black women compared with other populations.

Weight Gain in Antiretroviral Therapy-Experienced Persons with Human Immunodeficiency Virus

Studies evaluating weight gain in ART-naïve PWH must be interpreted in the context of the "return to health" phenomenon, or the varying degrees of reversal from a catabolic to anabolic state that occur with the suppression of plasma viremia. ART switch

Table 1
Weight gain risk and the overall effect of agent on weight gain in antiretroviral-naïve persons with human immunodeficiency virus

ART Agent	Weight Change	Overall Effect
Efavirenz	↑[a]	Weight suppressing
Rilpivirine	↑↑	
TDF	↑	Weight suppressing
TAF	↑↑↑	
Abacavir	↑↑	
DRV/ATV	↑↑[b]	
Bictegravir	↑↑↑	
Dolutegravir	↑↑↑	
Elvitegravir	↑↑	
Raltegravir	↑↑↑	

Abbreviations: ATV, atazanavir; DRV, darunavir; NNRTIs, non-nucleoside reverse transcriptase inhibitors; NRTIs, nucleoside reverse transcriptase inhibitors; TAF, tenofovir alafenamide; TDF, tenofovir disoproxil fumarate.

Combination of agents, for example, dolutegravir and TAF, can further modify weight gain risk.

[a] The amount of weight gain is dependent on the CYP2B6 genotype.

[b] The estimates for atazanavir and darunavir are less clear, though studies hint that weight gain might be greater with darunavir.

studies in virologically suppressed PWH are not confounded by the "return to health" phenomenon. However, recent data increasingly demonstrate that the pre-switch ART regimen is a substantial determinant of post-switch weight gain on an INSTI-based or TAF-based regimen (**Table 2**). Whereas it was previously assumed that weight gain with these regimens was due to their tendency to promote weight, compelling evidence from pre-exposure prophylaxis (PrEP),[41–43] pharmacokinetic,[44] and randomized switch studies suggest that efavirenz and TDF are weight suppressants in many individuals. Therefore, it is necessary to consider the baseline ART regimen to interpret weight gain in the context of ART regimen changes.

A pooled analysis of 12 clinical trials evaluating ART switch versus stable regimen (SBR) in virologically suppressed PWH provides some of the most rigorous data on weight changes.[9] Overall, the median weight change was 2.0 kg (switch) compared with 0.5 kg (SBR), though it is important to note that 28% of switch and 43% of SBR participants lost weight by 96 weeks. There was no difference in weight gain at 48 weeks between those staying on a PI compared with those who changed to BIC or EVG/c, those remaining on DTG compared with those changed to BIC, or those who remained on nevirapine (NVP) compared with those changed to EVG/c. However, on average, there was a 0.7 kg weight gain at 48 weeks switching to BIC compared with staying on EVG/c, which is consistent with findings in ART-naïve PWH.[8] The greatest changes in weight occurred when comparing those who stayed on EFV with those who changed to RPV (+1.5 kg) or EVG/c (+0.9 kg). Among NRTIs, a switch from TDF to TAF (+1.6 kg) or ABC to TAF was associated with increased weight gain. Those who remained on TDF, TAF, or ABC had similar weight trajectories, suggesting that despite initial weight gain differences between agents, individuals adapt to weight set points regardless of the ART agent. A similar study pooling data from advancing clinical therapeutics globally for HIV/AIDS and other infections (ACTG) cohorts A5001 and A5322 found that compared with baseline PI, switching to DTG but not raltegravir (RAL) or EVG/c was associated with weight gain.[45] In contrast, switching from an NNRTI was associated with significant weight gain in both DTG and EVG/c but not RAL. Similar to other studies, switch to INSTI with ABC or TAF was associated with greater weight gain than a switch with TDF. These results were largely reproduced in observational cohorts in African populations.[46,47] Importantly, EVF-based regimens were the first-line recommended therapies in African countries until recently,[48] which, in part, likely underlies the significant weight changes observed in these cohorts.

Switching from TDF-based to TAF-based regimen is associated with weight gain.[49–52] However, there are conflicting findings on when this weight gain occurs after

Table 2
Weight gain risk in antiretroviral switches (experienced)

Baseline Agent	Switch Agent	Weight Gain Risk
Efavirenz	INSTI	↑↑↑[a]
Efavirenz	Rilpivirine	↑↑↑[a]
TDF	TAF	↑↑↑
Abacavir	TAF	-↑
Protease Inhibitor	INSTI	↑[b]
EVG/c	BIC/DTG	↑

Abbreviations: BIC, bictegravir; DTG, dolutegravir; EVG/c, boosted elvitegravir; INSTI, integrase strand transfer inhibitor; TAF, tenofovir alafenamide; TDF, tenofovir disoproxil fumarate.
[a] Weight gain is dependent on CYP2B6 genotype and is typically less with EVG/c switches.
[b] Some studies have suggested statistically but not clinically significant weight gain.

the switch. In the US OPERA (Observational Pharmco-Epidemiology Research and Analysis) cohort in PWH who switched from TDF to TAF, weight gain accelerated from 0.48 kg/year (prior to switch) to 2.43 kg/year between 0 and 9 months, then stabilized near pre-switch levels after 9 months (0.24 kg/year).[51] In contrast, in the HIV Outpatient Study that included INSTI-naïve and virologically suppressed PWH switched to an INSTI-based or non-INSTI-based regimen, INSTIs were associated with 87% of the weight gain during the first 8 months after switch, whereas TAF was associated with 73% of the weight gain after 8 months.[52]

Much of the apparent weight gain observed with TAF may not be a direct effect of TAF, but rather the loss of weight-suppressing effects of TDF, which is discussed in more detail later. Switch studies assessing DTG/3TC provide insight into the effect of removing TAF from a regimen entirely without substitution of another NRTI (with the caveat that many participants changed from FTC to the chemically similar 3TC). The TANGO trial was a phase 3, randomized, non-inferiority trial evaluating a switch to DTG/3TC versus continuation of TAF-based regimens in PWH who were virologically suppressed. Weight change at 144 weeks was similar, as was the proportion of individuals with ≥5% or ≥10% weight gain from baseline showing no impact on weight when removing TAF from the regimen.[53] The SALSA trial randomized mostly cis-gender males virologically suppressed on any 3-/4-drug regimens to either DTG/3TC or continuation of baseline regimen.[54] In contrast to TANGO, baseline regimens included TDF (44%) and DTG was the most common INSTI. After 48 weeks, the change in weight for the DTG/3TC arm (2.1 kg) was significantly greater than in the continuation of baseline regimen arm (0.6 kg). Importantly, weight gain was most dependent on whether the baseline ART regimen contained TDF. Finally, the SOLAR trial randomized virologically suppressed PWH to either cabotegravir (CAB) + RPV versus continuing BIC/TAF/FTC and found no difference in weight change between the 2 arms at 1 year.[55] Thus, INSTI ± TAF are likely similar with regards to weight trajectories.

Efavirenz is Weight Suppressing

Pharmacokinetic studies suggest EFV is weight suppressing. EFV is metabolized by $CYP2B6$,[56] and 3 polymorphisms explain one-third of interindividual variability in plasma efavirenz concentration.[57] In a single-center study, weight gain after switching from EFV to an INSTI was highly dependent on $CYP2B6$ genotype with greater weight gain observed in the slow (+2.0 kg) and intermediate (+2.6 kg) metabolizers compared with normal (+0.1 kg), likely due to higher pre-switch EFV exposure.[44] In ADVANCE, slow metabolizers of EFV (those with higher EFV levels) gained significantly less weight than normal metabolizers in the EFV/TDF/FTC arm, and the weight gain among normal metabolizers was similar to the DTG/TDF/FTC arm.[58]

Tenofovir Disoproxil Fumarate is Weight Suppressing in Pre-Exposure Prophylaxis Studies

Weight gain studies in PWH necessarily occur in the context of HIV, which can alter metabolism and change weight trajectories. PrEP studies offer a way to investigate weight changes associated with antiretrovirals independent of HIV. In the iPrEx study that included HIV-negative participants who were assigned male sex at birth, weight gain was significantly less at 24 weeks in the TDF/FTC group compared with placebo, but not at 96 weeks.[42] A subsequent meta-analysis of PrEP studies found persons randomized to TDF compared to placebo or CAB + RPV had an odds of 1.44 for ≥5% weight loss.[59] In the DISCOVER trial that included cisgender men and transgender women who have sex with men and assigned male sex at birth, the TDF arm (+0.5 kg) had significantly reduced weight gain compared with TAF (+1.7 kg).[60]

Long-acting injectable CAB + RPV has shown superior efficacy in HIV prevention compared with TDF/FTC.[61] In the HIV Prevention Trials Network (HPTN) 077 phase 2 clinical trial that randomized HIV-negative individuals to CAB + RPV or placebo, there was no significant difference in weight at 41 weeks in this small study.[43] In contrast, the Phase 3 clinical trial HPTN 083 that randomized at-risk cisgender men and transgender women who have sex with men to either CAB + RPV or TDF/FTC, weight was significantly greater through 40 weeks in the CAB + RPV arm compared with the TDF/FTC arm, though weight changes were similar after 40 weeks.[61] The results from HPTN 084 that randomized at-risk women or transgender males in sub-Saharan Africa to CAB + RPV or TDF/FCT were similar, though the difference in weight gain remained significant during the following 3 years.[41] In summary, PrEP trials that are not confounded by HIV demonstrate that TDF is weight suppressing and that the majority of weight gain observed with TAF or CAB + RPV is likely due to the lack of weight suppressing effects of TDF.

Identifying Individuals at Risk for Weight Gain

Risk factors for weight gain in ART-naïve PWH include low baseline $CD4^+$ T cell count, higher baseline HIV-1 viral load, lower baseline BMI, the presence of opportunistic infections or other AIDS-defining conditions, female sex, Black race, and younger age.[8,35,36] The risk factors for weight gain in ART-experienced PWH who are switching therapy are largely the same and include younger age, female sex, Black race, and lower BMI.[9,46,50,53]

Tissue Type and Distribution of Weight Gain

In ADVANCE, increase in fat mass in the trunk and limbs, measured by DEXA, was greater than lean mass increase across all groups, and fat mass increase was greater in women compared with men.[21] Furthermore, VAT significantly increased by mass and volume in the TAF/FTC + DTG arm compared with other groups, including an astounding 51% rise in women.[21] In another study comparing ART-naïve PWH starting INSTI-based ART, waist circumference increased and was not different between DTG-containing and BIC-containing regimens.[62] ACTG A5260s, a substudy of A5272 that randomized ART-naïve PWH to TDF/FTC and either boosted atazanavir or darunavir, or RAL, found significant increases in VAT and subcutaneous adipose tissue (SAT) fat gain at 96 weeks, which was not different between the arms, but did show wide variability in the degree of VAT change.[63] In the Women's Interagency HIV Study, women switching to an INSTI compared to those remaining on non-INSTI ART had greater increase in percent body fat, and waist, hip, arm, and thigh circumferences.[64] PWH on long-term ART have continual increase in trunk fat mass, which was greater with female sex, higher BMI, and older age.[65] In the iPrEx trial (PrEP), trunk fat declined through 48 weeks in those with detectable plasma TDF while increasing in those on placebo or without detectable plasma TDF.[42] Importantly, lipoatrophy from exposure to older ART persists even after changing off the offending agent.[66] These data indicate that weight gain after ART initiation or on long-term therapy is primarily through fat mass increase and occurs preferentially at visceral sites, which are linked to the development of metabolic diseases.

Metabolic Effects of Antiretroviral Therapy

Greater weight has been linked to deleterious changes in lipid and glucose homeostasis. Several studies have examined changes in lipid and/or glucose homeostasis in PWH on ART. In the TANGO switch study described earlier, the DTG/3TC arm compared with TAF-based regimen had lower total cholesterol, low-density lipoprotein

(LDL), and triglycerides (TG).[53] However, the improvement in lipids in the DTG/3TC arm was only observed in those who switched off a regimen containing a boosting agent, suggesting the boosting agent may have affected the TAF component of the regimen as well, potentially by raising plasma levels. There were no differences in insulin resistance, development of metabolic syndrome, cardiac risk, or hepatic fibrosis.[53] In the 96-week follow-up from the GEMINI-1 and GEMINI-2 trials, ART-naive PWH randomized to DTG/3TC versus TDF/FTC + DTG (not TAF) had significantly higher total cholesterol, high-density lipoprotein (HDL), LDL, and TG.[39] Switching from TAF-based to TDF-based regimens had the opposite effect. In the PWH switched from TAF-based to TDF-based regimens, total cholesterol, TG, LDL, and HDL decreased in the switch group but not the control group.[67]

In the CHARACTERISE study, a follow-up of the ADVANCE trial in which participants were changed to the standard public treatment regimen TDF/3TC/DTG, individuals on TAF/FTC + DTG at baseline had a significant decrease in total cholesterol, LDL, TG, glucose, and hemoglobin A1c (HbA1c) and those on EFV/TDF/FTC at baseline had significant decrease in total cholesterol, LDL, HDL, and HbA1c.[68] Thus, switching from TAF to TDF or changing from EVF to DTG appears to improve lipid profiles. Similar results were found in other large cohorts.[50,69] In the iPrEx trial comparing placebo versus TDF/FTC for PrEP, individuals with detectable plasma TDF had significantly reduced total cholesterol, LDL, and HDL.[42] In the DISCOVER trial, lipids were significantly lower in the TDF/FTC arm compared to the TAF/FTC arm[70]

In comparison to TDF and EVF, INSTIs have less influence on lipids. In the HPTN 077 trial randomizing HIV-negative individuals to either CAB + RPV or placebo, there were no differences in lipid or glucose measures between the groups.[43] However, individuals on DTG + TAF/FTC in the ADVANCE trial had a significantly increased 10-year CVD risk by QRISK equation compared with EFV/TDF/FTC.[10] The 10-year diabetes risk using the QDiabetes equation was significantly greater after 96 weeks in the TAF/FTC + DTG compared with the TDF/FTC + DTG group (6 extra cases per 1000 people treated over 10 years) and was greater in women than men. In the NA-ACCORD analysis of ART-naïve PWH, INSTI-based versus NNRTI-based regimens had an incident diabetes risk of 1.17 [0.92, 1.48] with the highest risk with RAL-based regimens.[11] In mediation analysis accounting for 12-month weight gain, the hazard ratio was attenuated suggesting the majority of increased risk for diabetes on INSTI-based regimens was mediated by weight gain. A recent study evaluating ART-experienced PWH from the Modena HIV Metabolic Clinic switched to either INSTI or non-INSTI regimens, accounting for baseline homeostatic model assessment of insulin resistance (HOMA-IR), switching to INSTI-based regimen was associated with a lower risk of HOMA-IR $\geq$ 2 with similar incidence of overall diabetes.[71] However, a weight gain of $\geq$5% would offset this risk reduction. Other studies have found a relationship between INSTIs and glucose intolerance.[72] Thus, INSTIs are likely associated with insulin resistance, most likely mediated through weight gain though further studies are necessary to elucidate the specific mechanism. In the RESPOND cohort, INSTI-based versus non-INSTI-based regimens were associated with a higher incidence of CVD, but further studies are needed to understand the mechanisms or whether confounders could contribute to this observation.[73] Taken together, changes in lipid and glucose homeostasis with ART are small, but at a population level, may influence the incidence of cardiometabolic diseases.

Weight Gain Reversal with Antiretroviral Therapy Switches

Whether weight changes occurring on INSTI-based and/or TAF-based regimens are reversible is an important clinical question. In CHARACTERISE, women changed from TAF/FTC + DTG to DTG/TDF/3TC lost 1.6 kg whereas in men, there was no significant difference.[68] In contrast, PWH who changed from EFV/TDF/FTC gained weight with absolute weight change similar among men and women. In a retrospective observation cohort of PWH switched from TAF-based to TDF-based regimens, weight remained stable in those changed to TDF but increased in those who remained on TAF.[67] The DEFINE trial evaluated switching to boosted darunavir + TAF/FTC versus continuing INSTI + TAF/FTC in PWH who had at least a 10% increase in weight on an INSTI-based regimen and found no difference in weight change after 24 weeks.[74] Similarly, NCT04223791 randomized individuals to either continue BIC/TAF/FTC or switch to DOR/islatravir and found no difference in weight or body fat distribution after 48 weeks.[75] Several trials including TANGO and SOLAR that removed TAF but continued an INSTI did not result in substantially changed weight trajectories. In summary, switching from TAF- or TAF-sparing regimens to TDF-based regimens is associated with weight reduction, though the changes overall are quite modest for most individuals and the durability of these reversals warrants further investigation.

Counseling and Choice of Antiretroviral Therapies

At the authors' center, the authors adhere to the recommendations in the IAS and HHS guidelines when determining ART regimens.[37,38] The authors do not deviate from recommended first-line therapies solely due to concern about weight gain as there is limited data on whether this is an effective and safe strategy. For ART-naïve patients, the authors counsel patients that weight gain is expected with ART regardless of the ART-regimen choice and closely monitor for excess weight gain and metabolic complications. Though all patients should be counseled about the importance of healthy diet and regular exercise, it is unknown whether concurrent interventions in individuals at risk for excessive weight gain (lifestyle changes ± weight loss medications) would be effective in preventing the emergence of metabolic complications after ART initiation. The authors suggest that in addition to BMI, other measures including waist circumference are collected since BMI is a poor indicator of adiposity. Additionally, the authors screen at baseline and follow-up for dyslipidemia and glucose intolerance (oral glucose tolerance test or fasting glucose preferred over hemoglobin A1c) and treat if indicated.[76,77] For ART-experienced individuals, they do not use second-line therapies that include EFV or TDF solely for weight suppressive effects nor are they routinely changing patients with weight gain on TAF and/or INSTIs back to TDF-based or non-INSTI-based regimens outside of clinical trials due to limited data on long-term effectiveness and durability of weight loss.

Management of Excessive Weight Gain on Antiretroviral Therapy

In the authors' clinical practice, the authors take a multifaceted approach. Individuals should be offered a visit with a dietician to optimize nutrition. Additionally, patients should be counseled about physical exercise, which has been shown to improve weight,[78] though with variable effects on metabolic measures.[79] Recent data in the general population have shown dramatic and durable weight changes and improvement in weight-associated comorbid conditions with glucagon-like peptide-1 receptor agonists (GLP-1) and dual acting glucose-dependent insulinotropic polypeptide (GIP) and GLP-1 receptor agonist.[80,81] Several studies of GLP-1 agonists in PWH are currently ongoing including the ACTG A5371 (Slim Liver) and NCT04019197, though preliminary study data suggest they are effective strategies to address weight gain in PWH.[82,83]

Bariatric surgery is a well-established procedure that promotes durable weight loss and results in reversal of weight-associated comorbidities.[84,85] A recent large retrospective analysis in the AIDS Therapy evaluation in the Netherlands (ATHENA) cohort

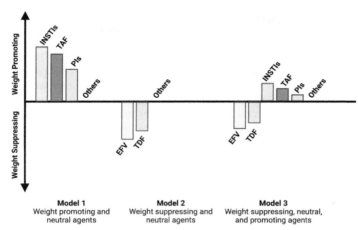

Fig. 3. Potential models of antiretroviral therapy (ART) agents and relationship with weight gain. In model 1, all excess weight gain is due to their weight-promoting effects. Model 1 is not compatible with the most recent data. In model 2, ART agents are only weight suppressing or weight neutral. In model 3, ART agents can be weight suppressing, neutral, or promoting. It is not clear whether model 2 or model 3 is correct. *Abbreviation:* EFV, efavirenz; INSTIs, integrase strand transfer inhibitors; PIs, protease inhibitors; TAF, tenofovir alafenamide; TDF, tenofovir disoproxil fumarate.

including 51 PWH who underwent bariatric surgery showed significant weight loss at 18 months, improvement in weight-associated comorbidities, therapeutic levels of DTG, EVG, FTC, and TDF, and only 1 participant with virologic failure post-surgery (resistance testing not performed).[86] In summary, changing ART regimen is unlikely to promote significant weight loss and multiple interventions addressing the complex pathogenesis of obesity are needed.

Current Controversies

Despite considerable progress in understanding ART-associated weight gain, several issues remain unresolved.

- While some studies suggest changing to TDF might promote weight loss, TDF is associated with adverse renal and bone mineral density, which may limit its use.
- PWH accumulate fat mass mainly at ectopic sites, including VAT. While some studies have implicated SAT injury and inflammation,[87] the mechanisms that underlie these observations remain poorly understood.
- GLP-1 and other weight loss medications are highly effective, but are known to cause sarcopenia through loss of lean mass.[81] PWH are already at higher risk for sarcopenia than HIV-negative persons,[88] so further studies are needed to investigate whether the benefits of weight loss outweigh the risks of worsening sarcopenia.
- Weight gain directly attributable to ART does not seem to increase cardiometabolic risk in most individuals, and identifying individuals who might respond to ART-switches is not known at this time.

SUMMARY

Effective ART has dramatically changed the landscape of HIV care and contemporary first-line ART is characterized by few off-target effects and increased tolerability.

However, PWH have an increasing burden of obesity and weight-associated comorbidities, which mirrors long-standing trends in the general population. Whereas it was previously thought that TAF and INSTI-related weight gain was solely due to their weight-promoting effects, data from high-quality clinical trials in PWH and HIV-negative persons on PrEP demonstrate that EFV and TDF have weight-suppressing properties. The loss of this effect may account for the vast majority of weight gain after ART regimen switches (**Fig. 3**). While switch studies to reverse weight gain are ongoing, management of excess weight gain and weight-associated comorbidities with lifestyle interventions, bariatric surgery, or weight loss drugs are likely to have a larger impact in reducing cardiometabolic disease in PWH on long-term ART.

CLINICS CARE POINTS

- The authors adhere to the ART guideline recommendations from IAS and HHS and do not routinely deviate from first-line therapies for weight gain concerns.
- All ART-naïve PWH should be counseled about expected weight gain after starting ART.
- The authors suggest obtaining measures aside from BMI, including waist circumference or waist-to-hip ratio at baseline and regular follow- up appointments.
- Patients should be counseled to eat a balanced diet and incorporate regular physical activity.
- For patients who develop excess weight gain and/or weight-associated comorbidities, a multi-disciplinary approach that includes the primary care physician, dietician, and weight loss specialist may be needed to address the complex pathophysiology of obesity.
- Bariatric surgery is safe and effective in PWH. More data are needed on the use of newer weight loss medications and ART changes.

DISCLOSURE

J.R. Koethe has served as a consultant to Gilead Sciences, Merck, ViiV Healthcare, Theratechnologies, and Janssen, and has received research support from Gilead Sciences, United States and Merck, United States.

FUNDING

Grant number: NIDDK K23DK135414 and CFAR P30AI110527.

REFERENCES

1. Marcus JL, Leyden WA, Alexeeff SE, et al. Comparison of overall and comorbidity-free life expectancy between insured adults with and without HIV Infection, 2000-2016. JAMA Netw Open 2020;3(6):e207954.
2. Marcus JL, Chao CR, Leyden WA, et al. Narrowing the gap in life expectancy between HIV-infected and HIV-uninfected individuals with access to care. J Acquir Immune Defic Syndr 2016;73(1):39–46.
3. Shah ASV, Stelzle D, Lee KK, et al. Global burden of atherosclerotic cardiovascular disease in people living with HIV: systematic review and meta-analysis. Circulation 2018;138(11):1100–12.
4. Bischoff J, Gu W, Schwarze-Zander C, et al. Stratifying the risk of NAFLD in patients with HIV under combination antiretroviral therapy (cART). EClinicalMedicine 2021;40:101116.

5. Nansseu JR, Bigna JJ, Kaze AD, et al. Incidence and risk factors for prediabetes and diabetes mellitus among HIV-infected Adults on antiretroviral therapy: a systematic review and meta-analysis. Epidemiology 2018;29(3):431–41.
6. Croxford S, Kitching A, Desai S, et al. Mortality and causes of death in people diagnosed with HIV in the era of highly active antiretroviral therapy compared with the general population: an analysis of a national observational cohort. Lancet Public Health 2017;2(1):e35–46.
7. Koethe JR, Jenkins CA, Lau B, et al. Rising obesity prevalence and weight gain among adults starting antiretroviral therapy in the United States and Canada. AIDS Res Hum Retroviruses 2016;32(1):50–8.
8. Sax PE, Erlandson KM, Lake JE, et al. Weight gain following initiation of antiretroviral therapy: risk factors in randomized comparative clinical trials. Clin Infect Dis 2020;71(6):1379–89.
9. Erlandson KM, Carter CC, Melbourne K, et al. Weight change following antiretroviral therapy switch in people with viral suppression: pooled data from randomized clinical trials. Clin Infect Dis 2021;73(8):1440–51.
10. McCann K, Shah S, Hindley L, et al. Implications of weight gain with newer antiretrovirals: 10-year predictions of cardiovascular disease and diabetes. AIDS 2021;35(10):1657–65.
11. Rebeiro PF, Jenkins CA, Bian A, et al. Risk of incident diabetes mellitus, weight gain, and their relationships with integrase inhibitor-based initial antiretroviral therapy among persons with human immunodeficiency virus in the United States and Canada. Clin Infect Dis 2021;73(7):e2234–42.
12. Fan JX, Brown BB, Hanson H, et al. Moderate to vigorous physical activity and weight outcomes: does every minute count? Am J Health Promot 2013;28(1):41–9.
13. Rao S, Pandey A, Garg S, et al. Effect of exercise and pharmacological interventions on visceral adiposity: a systematic review and meta-analysis of long-term randomized controlled trials. Mayo Clin Proc 2019;94(2):211–24.
14. Graff M, Scott RA, Justice AE, et al. Genome-wide physical activity interactions in adiposity - A meta-analysis of 200,452 adults. PLoS Genet 2017;13(4):e1006528.
15. Loos RJF, Yeo GSH. The genetics of obesity: from discovery to biology. Nat Rev Genet 2022;23(2):120–33.
16. Bell CN, Kerr J, Young JL. Associations between obesity, obesogenic environments, and structural racism vary by county-level racial composition. Int J Environ Res Publ Health 2019;16(5).
17. Cuevas AG, Chen R, Slopen N, et al. Assessing the role of health behaviors, socioeconomic status, and cumulative stress for racial/ethnic disparities in obesity. Obesity 2020;28(1):161–70.
18. Collaboration NCDRF. Trends in adult body-mass index in 200 countries from 1975 to 2014: a pooled analysis of 1698 population-based measurement studies with 19.2 million participants. Lancet 2016;387(10026):1377–96.
19. Fryar CD, Caroll MD, Afful J. Prevalence of overweight, obesity, and severe obesity among adults aged 20 and over: United States, 1960-1962 through 2017 — 2018. MD, USA: NCHS Health E-Stats; 2020.
20. Collaborators GBDO, Afshin A, Forouzanfar MH, et al. Health effects of overweight and obesity in 195 countries over 25 years. N Engl J Med 2017;377(1):13–27.
21. Venter WDF, Sokhela S, Simmons B, et al. Dolutegravir with emtricitabine and tenofovir alafenamide or tenofovir disoproxil fumarate versus efavirenz, emtricitabine, and tenofovir disoproxil fumarate for initial treatment of HIV-1 infection (ADVANCE): week 96 results from a randomised, phase 3, non-inferiority trial. Lancet HIV 2020;7(10):e666–76.

22. Nuttall FQ. Body Mass Index: Obesity, BMI, and Health: A Critical Review. Nutr Today 2015;50(3):117–28.

23. Powell-Wiley TM, Poirier P, Burke LE, et al. Obesity and cardiovascular disease: a scientific statement from the American Heart Association. Circulation 2021; 143(21):e984–1010.

24. Fabbrini E, Sullivan S, Klein S. Obesity and nonalcoholic fatty liver disease: biochemical, metabolic, and clinical implications. Hepatology 2010;51(2):679–89.

25. Achhra AC, Sabin C, Ryom L, et al. Body mass index and the risk of serious non-AIDS Events and all-cause mortality in treated HIV-Positive Individuals: D: A: D Cohort Analysis. J Acquir Immune Defic Syndr 2018;78(5):579–88.

26. Fox CS, Massaro JM, Hoffmann U, et al. Abdominal visceral and subcutaneous adipose tissue compartments: association with metabolic risk factors in the Framingham Heart Study. Circulation 2007;116(1):39–48.

27. Deurenberg P, Yap M, van Staveren WA. Body mass index and percent body fat: a meta analysis among different ethnic groups. Int J Obes Relat Metab Disord 1998;22(12):1164–71.

28. Bhagwat P, Ofotokun I, McComsey GA, et al. Changes in abdominal fat following antiretroviral therapy initiation in HIV-infected individuals correlate with waist circumference and self-reported changes. Antivir Ther 2017;22(7):577–86.

29. Mohammad A, De Lucia Rolfe E, Sleigh A, et al. Validity of visceral adiposity estimates from DXA against MRI in Kuwaiti men and women. Nutr Diabetes 2017; 7(1):e238.

30. Fourman LT, Kileel EM, Hubbard J, et al. Comparison of visceral fat measurement by dual-energy X-ray absorptiometry to computed tomography in HIV and non-HIV. Nutr Diabetes 2019;9(1):6.

31. Zhang YN, Fowler KJ, Hamilton G, et al. Liver fat imaging-a clinical overview of ultrasound, CT, and MR imaging. Br J Radiol 2018;91(1089):20170959.

32. Macallan DC, McNurlan MA, Milne E, et al. Whole-body protein turnover from leucine kinetics and the response to nutrition in human immunodeficiency virus infection. Am J Clin Nutr 1995;61(4):818–26.

33. Yuh B, Tate J, Butt AA, et al. Weight change after antiretroviral therapy and mortality. Clin Infect Dis 2015;60(12):1852–9.

34. Koethe JR, Lukusa A, Giganti MJ, et al. Association between weight gain and clinical outcomes among malnourished adults initiating antiretroviral therapy in Lusaka, Zambia. J Acquir Immune Defic Syndr 2010;53(4):507–13.

35. Bourgi K, Jenkins CA, Rebeiro PF, et al. Weight gain among treatment-naive persons with HIV starting integrase inhibitors compared to non-nucleoside reverse transcriptase inhibitors or protease inhibitors in a large observational cohort in the United States and Canada. J Int AIDS Soc 2020;23(4):e25484.

36. Bansi-Matharu L, Phillips A, Oprea C, et al. Contemporary antiretrovirals and body-mass index: a prospective study of the RESPOND cohort consortium. Lancet HIV 2021;8(11):e711–22.

37. Panel on Antiretroviral Guidelines for Adults and Adolescents. Guidelines for the Use of Antiretroviral Agents in Adults and Adolescents with HIV. In: Department of Health and Human Services: Available at: https://clinicalinfo.hiv.gov/en/guidelines/hiv-clinical-guidelines-adult-and-adolescent-arv/whats-new. Accessed October 4, 2023.

38. Gandhi RT, Bedimo R, Hoy JF, et al. Antiretroviral drugs for treatment and prevention of HIV infection in adults: 2022 recommendations of the International Antiviral Society-USA Panel. JAMA 2023;329(1):63–84.

39. Cahn P, Madero JS, Arribas JR, et al. Durable Efficacy of Dolutegravir Plus Lamivudine in Antiretroviral Treatment-Naive Adults With HIV-1 Infection: 96-Week Results From the GEMINI-1 and GEMINI-2 Randomized Clinical Trials. J Acquir Immune Defic Syndr 2020;83(3):310–8.

40. Orkin C, Squires KE, Molina JM, et al. Doravirine/Lamivudine/Tenofovir Disoproxil Fumarate (TDF) Versus Efavirenz/Emtricitabine/TDF in Treatment-naive Adults With Human Immunodeficiency Virus Type 1 Infection: Week 96 Results of the Randomized, Double-blind, Phase 3 DRIVE-AHEAD Noninferiority Trial. Clin Infect Dis 2021;73(1):33–42.

41. Delany-Moretlwe S, Hughes JP, Bock P, et al. Cabotegravir for the prevention of HIV-1 in women: results from HPTN 084, a phase 3, randomised clinical trial. Lancet 2022;399(10337):1779–89.

42. Glidden DV, Mulligan K, McMahan V, et al. Metabolic effects of preexposure prophylaxis with coformulated tenofovir disoproxil fumarate and emtricitabine. Clin Infect Dis 2018;67(3):411–9.

43. Landovitz RJ, Zangeneh SZ, Chau G, et al. Cabotegravir is not associated with weight gain in human immunodeficiency virus-uninfected individuals in HPTN 077. Clin Infect Dis 2020;70(2):319–22.

44. Leonard MA, Cindi Z, Bradford Y, et al. Efavirenz pharmacogenetics and weight gain following switch to integrase inhibitor-containing regimens. Clin Infect Dis 2021;73(7):e2153–63.

45. Lake JE, Wu K, Bares SH, et al. Risk factors for weight gain following switch to integrase inhibitor-based antiretroviral therapy. Clin Infect Dis 2020;71(9):e471–7.

46. Esber AL, Chang D, Iroezindu M, et al. Weight gain during the dolutegravir transition in the African Cohort Study. J Int AIDS Soc 2022;25(4):e25899.

47. Hickey MD, Wafula E, Ogachi SM, et al. Weight change following switch to Dolutegravir for HIV treatment in rural Kenya during country roll-out. J Acquir Immune Defic Syndr 2023;93(2):154–61.

48. Consolidated Guidelines on the Use of Antiretroviral Drugs for Treating and Preventing HIV Infection: Recommendations for a Public Health Approach. Geneva: World Health Organization; 2013. Available at: https://www.ncbi.nlm.nih.gov/books/NBK374294/.

49. Taramasso L, Berruti M, Briano F, et al. The switch from tenofovir disoproxil fumarate to tenofovir alafenamide determines weight gain in patients on rilpivirine-based regimen. AIDS 2020;34(6):877–81.

50. Surial B, Mugglin C, Calmy A, et al. Weight and Metabolic Changes After Switching From Tenofovir Disoproxil Fumarate to Tenofovir Alafenamide in People Living With HIV : A Cohort Study. Ann Intern Med 2021;174(6):758–67.

51. Mallon PW, Brunet L, Hsu RK, et al. Weight gain before and after switch from TDF to TAF in a U.S. cohort study. J Int AIDS Soc 2021;24(4):e25702.

52. Palella FJ, Hou Q, Li J, et al. Weight gain and metabolic effects in persons with hiv who switch to art regimens containing integrase inhibitors or tenofovir alafenamide. J Acquir Immune Defic Syndr 2023;92(1):67–75.

53. Batterham RL, Espinosa N, Katlama C, et al. Cardiometabolic parameters 3 years after switch to dolutegravir/lamivudine vs maintenance of tenofovir alafenamide-based regimens. Open Forum Infect Dis 2023;10(7):ofad359.

54. Llibre JM, Brites C, Cheng CY, et al. Efficacy and Safety of Switching to the 2-Drug Regimen Dolutegravir/Lamivudine Versus Continuing a 3- or 4-Drug Regimen for Maintaining Virologic Suppression in Adults Living With Human Immunodeficiency Virus 1 (HIV-1): Week 48 Results From the Phase 3, Noninferiority SALSA Randomized Trial. Clin Infect Dis 2023;76(4):720–9.

55. Tan DHS, Antinori A, Eu B, et al. Weight and metabolic changes with cabotegravir + rilpivirine long-acting or bictegravir. Seattle: Paper presented at: Conference on Retroviruses and Opportunistic Infections; 2023.

56. Ward BA, Gorski JC, Jones DR, et al. The cytochrome P450 2B6 (CYP2B6) is the main catalyst of efavirenz primary and secondary metabolism: implication for HIV/AIDS therapy and utility of efavirenz as a substrate marker of CYP2B6 catalytic activity. J Pharmacol Exp Therapeut 2003;306(1):287–300.

57. Desta Z, Gammal RS, Gong L, et al. Clinical Pharmacogenetics Implementation Consortium (CPIC) Guideline for CYP2B6 and Efavirenz-Containing Antiretroviral Therapy. Clin Pharmacol Ther 2019;106(4):726–33.

58. Griesel R, Maartens G, Chirehwa M, et al. CYP2B6 genotype and weight gain differences between dolutegravir and efavirenz. Clin Infect Dis 2021;73(11):e3902–9.

59. Shah S, Pilkington V, Hill A. Is tenofovir disoproxil fumarate associated with weight loss? AIDS 2021;35(Suppl 2):S189–95.

60. Ogbuagu O, Ruane PJ, Podzamczer D, et al. Long-term safety and efficacy of emtricitabine and tenofovir alafenamide vs emtricitabine and tenofovir disoproxil fumarate for HIV-1 pre-exposure prophylaxis: week 96 results from a randomised, double-blind, placebo-controlled, phase 3 trial. Lancet HIV 2021;8(7):e397–407.

61. Landovitz RJ, Donnell D, Clement ME, et al. Cabotegravir for HIV Prevention in Cisgender Men and Transgender Women. N Engl J Med 2021;385(7):595–608.

62. Calza L, Borderi M, Colangeli V, et al. Weight gain in treatment-naive HIV-1 infected patients starting abacavir/lamivudine/dolutegravir or tenofovir alafenamide/emtricitabine/bictegravir. AIDS 2022;36(1):153–5.

63. McComsey GA, Moser C, Currier J, et al. Body composition changes after initiation of raltegravir or protease inhibitors: ACTG A5260s. Clin Infect Dis 2016;62(7):853–62.

64. Kerchberger AM, Sheth AN, Angert CD, et al. Weight gain associated with integrase stand transfer inhibitor use in women. Clin Infect Dis 2020;71(3):593–600.

65. Debroy P, Sim M, Erlandson KM, et al. Progressive increases in fat mass occur in adults living with HIV on antiretroviral therapy, but patterns differ by sex and anatomic depot. J Antimicrob Chemother 2019;74(4):1028–34.

66. Grunfeld C, Saag M, Cofrancesco J Jr, et al. Regional adipose tissue measured by MRI over 5 years in HIV-infected and control participants indicates persistence of HIV-associated lipoatrophy. AIDS 2010;24(11):1717–26.

67. Kauppinen KJ, Aho I, Sutinen J. Switching from tenofovir alafenamide to tenofovir disoproxil fumarate improves lipid profile and protects from weight gain. AIDS 2022;36(10):1337–44.

68. Bosch B, Akpomiemie G, Chandiwana N, et al. Weight and metabolic changes after switching from Tenofovir Alafenamide/Emtricitabine (FTC)+Dolutegravir (DTG), Tenofovir Disoproxil Fumarate (TDF)/FTC + DTG, and TDF/FTC/Efavirenz to TDF/Lamivudine/DTG. Clin Infect Dis 2023;76(8):1492–5.

69. Martinez-Sanz J, Serrano-Villar S, Muriel A, et al. Metabolic-related outcomes after switching from tenofovir disoproxil fumarate to tenofovir alafenamide in adults with human immunodeficiency virus (HIV): a multicenter prospective cohort study. Clin Infect Dis 2023;76(3):e652–60.

70. Mayer KH, Molina JM, Thompson MA, et al. Emtricitabine and tenofovir alafenamide vs emtricitabine and tenofovir disoproxil fumarate for HIV pre-exposure prophylaxis (DISCOVER): primary results from a randomised, double-blind, multicentre, active-controlled, phase 3, non-inferiority trial. Lancet 2020;396(10246):239–54.

71. Milic J, Renzetti S, Ferrari D, et al. Relationship between weight gain and insulin resistance in people living with HIV switching to integrase strand transfer inhibitors-based regimens. AIDS 2022;36(12):1643–53.

72. Summers NA, Lahiri CD, Angert CD, et al. Metabolic changes associated with the use of integrase strand transfer inhibitors among virally controlled women. J Acquir Immune Defic Syndr 2020;85(3):355–62.

73. Neesgaard B, Greenberg L, Miro JM, et al. Associations between integrase strand-transfer inhibitors and cardiovascular disease in people living with HIV: a multicentre prospective study from the RESPOND cohort consortium. Lancet HIV 2022;9(7):e474–85.

74. Short WR, Ramgopal M, Hagins DP, et al. A prospective, randomized trial to assess a protease inhibitor–based regimen switch strategy to manage integrase inhibitor–related weight gain. Open Forum Infect Dis 2023;10(Suppl 2). ofad500.112.

75. McComsey GA, Molina J-M, Mills A, et al. Weight and body composition after switch to doravirine/islatravir (DOR/ISL) 100/0.75mg once daily: week 48 results from 2 randomized active-controlled phase 3 trials, MK8591A-017 (P017) and MK8591A-018 (P018). Brisbane: Paper presented at: IAS; 2023.

76. Monroe AK, Glesby MJ, Brown TT. Diagnosing and managing diabetes in HIV-infected patients: current concepts. Clin Infect Dis 2015;60(3):453–62.

77. American Diabetes Association Professional Practice C. 2. Classification and diagnosis of diabetes: standards of medical care in diabetes-2022. Diabetes Care 2022;45(Suppl 1):S17–38.

78. Becofsky K, Wing EJ, McCaffery J, et al. A randomized controlled trial of a behavioral weight loss program for human immunodeficiency virus-infected patients. Clin Infect Dis 2017;65(1):154–7.

79. Engelson ES, Agin D, Kenya S, et al. Body composition and metabolic effects of a diet and exercise weight loss regimen on obese, HIV-infected women. Metabolism 2006;55(10):1327–36.

80. Jastreboff AM, Aronne LJ, Ahmad NN, et al. Tirzepatide once weekly for the treatment of obesity. N Engl J Med 2022;387(3):205–16.

81. Wilding JPH, Batterham RL, Calanna S, et al. Once-weekly semaglutide in adults with overweight or obesity. N Engl J Med 2021;384(11):989–1002.

82. Nguyen QP, Wooten D, Duren K, et al. GLP-1 receptor agonists promote weight loss among people with HIV. Open Forum Infect Dis 2023;10(Suppl 2). ofad500.109.

83. McComsey GA, Sattar A, Albar Z, et al. Effects of semaglutide on adipose tissue in HIV-associated lipohypertrophy. Open Forum Infect Dis 2023;10(Suppl 2). ofad500.111.

84. Buchwald H, Avidor Y, Braunwald E, et al. Bariatric surgery: a systematic review and meta-analysis. JAMA 2004;292(14):1724–37.

85. Mingrone G, Panunzi S, De Gaetano A, et al. Bariatric-metabolic surgery versus conventional medical treatment in obese patients with type 2 diabetes: 5 year follow-up of an open-label, single-centre, randomised controlled trial. Lancet 2015;386(9997):964–73.

86. Zino L, Wit F, Rokx C, et al. Outcomes of bariatric surgery in people with HIV: a retrospective analysis from ATHENA cohort. Clin Infect Dis 2023;77(11):1561–8.

87. Leroyer S, Vatier C, Kadiri S, et al. Glyceroneogenesis is inhibited through HIV protease inhibitor-induced inflammation in human subcutaneous but not visceral adipose tissue. J Lipid Res 2011;52(2):207–20.

88. Oliveira VHF, Borsari AL, Webel AR, et al. Sarcopenia in people living with the Human Immunodeficiency Virus: a systematic review and meta-analysis. Eur J Clin Nutr 2020;74(7):1009–21.

Advances in the Management of Cardiovascular Disease in the Setting of Human Immunodeficiency Virus

Matthew S. Durstenfeld, MD, MAS[a,b,*], Priscilla Y. Hsue, MD[a,b]

KEYWORDS

- HIV • Cardiovascular diseases • Cardiovascular risk • Antiretroviral therapy

KEY POINTS

- Human immunodeficiency virus (HIV) is associated with increased cardiovascular risk including risk of atherosclerotic cardiovascular disease such as myocardial infarction and stroke, heart failure (HF), and arrhythmias.
- Mechanisms of increased cardiovascular risk are related in part due to worse cardiovascular health, but also to HIV-specific mechanisms and antiretroviral therapy-specific mechanisms.
- Statins have the strongest evidence as a safe and effective strategy for mitigating the risk of cardiovascular disease among people with HIV.
- Management of coronary artery disease, HF, and arrhythmias in the setting of HIV is largely consistent with management of these conditions among people without HIV.

INTRODUCTION

Increasing global access to human immunodeficiency virus (HIV) testing and treatment has transformed HIV into a chronic disease for many of the over 40 million people with HIV (PWH) worldwide. HIV is associated with increased risk of cardiovascular disease (CVD) including atherosclerotic CVD (ASCVD) resulting in myocardial infarction (MI) and stroke, heart failure (HF), and arrhythmias.

Funding: Dr P.Y. Hsue is funded by NIH/NIAID grant 2K24AI112393-06. Dr M.S. Durstenfeld is funded by NIH grant NIH/NHLBI (K12 HL143961). Its contents are solely the responsibility of the authors and do not necessarily represent the official views of the NIH.
[a] Department of Medicine, University of California, San Francisco, CA, USA; [b] Division of Cardiology, Zuckerberg San Francisco General, San Francisco, CA, USA
* Corresponding author. Division of Cardiology, UCSF at Zuckerberg San Francisco General Hospital, 1001 Potrero Avenue, 5G8, San Francisco, CA 94110.
E-mail address: matthew.durstenfeld@ucsf.edu
Twitter: @durstenfeld (M.S.D.)

Infect Dis Clin N Am 38 (2024) 517–530
https://doi.org/10.1016/j.idc.2024.04.006
0891-5520/24/© 2024 Elsevier Inc. All rights reserved.

id.theclinics.com

This state-of-the art review will discuss the underlying mechanisms that contribute to CVD among PWH, risk prediction and prevention of ASCVD, management, and key outstanding research questions. It highlights new research published in the last 5 years (2018 to 2024) focused on ASCVD, HF, and arrhythmias. HIV also increases the risk of cerebrovascular disease including stroke, peripheral vascular disease, venous thromboembolism, pulmonary hypertension, and aortic aneurysms but due to space limitations these conditions will not be covered.

EPIDEMIOLOGY OF CARDIOVASCULAR DISEASE AMONG PEOPLE WITH HUMAN IMMUNODEFICIENCY VIRUS

HIV is associated with more than twice the incidence of CVD (62 per 100,000 person-years; risk ratio 2.16, 95% Confidence Interval CI 1.68 to 2.77) compared to people without HIV.[1] The prevalence of CVD among PWH has tripled in the last 2 decades.[1] Modeling studies predict that the prevalence of CVD will increase with 78% of PWH in western countries with CVD by 2030.[2,3] The burden of CVD among PWH accounts for 2.6 million disability-adjusted life years per year, with the greatest burden in the Africa and Asia Pacific regions.[1] Among PWH in care, CVD is the second leading cause of death.[4] In the US, differences in HIV and CVD prevalence by race, ethnicity, and region are such that those who identify as Black/African American and Hispanic/Latino, and those who live in the Southern US are at the highest risk.[5]

ATHEROSCLEROTIC CARDIOVASCULAR DISEASE AMONG PEOPLE WITH HUMAN IMMUNODEFICIENCY VIRUS

ASCVD is a systemic vascular process that is initially asymptomatic and results in chronic vascular disease including chronic coronary syndromes (angina), carotid artery stenosis, peripheral arterial disease, and acute events such as (myocardial infarction [MI], orheart attack), cerebrovascular disease (stroke), and critical limb ischemia. Mechanisms of increased ASCVD among PWH include a higher prevalence of traditional risk factors, effects of antiretroviral therapy, and effects of HIV infection leading to chronic immune activation and inflammation, even among those who are treated and virally suppressed (**Fig. 1**).[6]

Cardiovascular health is operationalized by the American Heart Association (AHA) as "Life's Essential 8," which includes 4 health behaviors (eat better, be more active, quit tobacco, get healthy sleep) and 4 health factors (manage weight, control cholesterol, manage blood sugar, and manage blood pressure).[7] PWH have worse cardiovascular health.[8] This is partly due to a high burden of "traditional" ASCVD risk factors including smoking, dyslipidemia, and hypertension.[9] HIV infection and antiretroviral therapy (ART) can adversely affect lipid levels, including triglyceride levels. HIV infection and ART can also affect body composition, and contribute to lipodystrophy, insulin resistance, and obesity, with differences by ART classes. Newer ART including integrase strand transfer inhibitors (INSTI) have more favorable effects on lipids, but greater weight gain. Physical inactivity is common among PWH,[10] and PWH have lower cardiorespiratory fitness compared to people without HIV.[11] Hypertension is a major contributor to CVD, including among PWH, but whether HIV impacts hypertension remains unclear.[12]

HIV viremia, lower CD4 counts, and lower CD4/CD8 ratios are consistently associated with higher risk of ASCVD and MI. Early ART initiation is associated with reduced AIDS-related and non-AIDS-related events; however, in the strategic timing of antiretroviral therapy (START) trial, early ART initiation was not statistically significant for

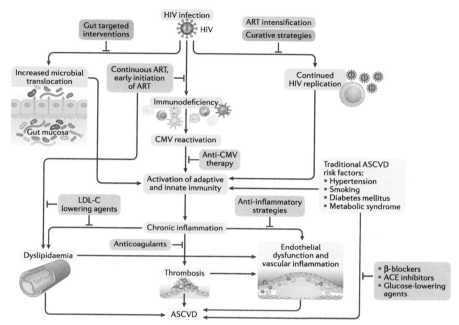

Fig. 1. Mechanisms of ASCVD and possible management strategies among PWH. HIV infection is associated with increased ASCVD risk due to an increased burden of traditional ASCVD risk factors, direct viral effects, ART effects. HIV increases immune activation and chronic inflammation via direct effects as well as via gut microbial translocation, reactivation of latent viruses. Statin therapy has the strongest evidence of benefit among PWH from the REPRIEVE Study. Further research is needed to develop anti-inflammatory strategies that are effective at reducing cardiovascular risk among PWH including efforts at HIV cure. (Hsue PY, Waters DD. HIV infection and coronary heart disease: mechanisms and management. Nature Reviews Cardiology. 2019;16(12):745–759. (13).)

cardiovascular events (likely due to young age and few events), and early initiation is associated with an increase in total cholesterol and low-density lipoprotein (LDL).

Consistent with this finding, older protease inhibitor (PI) based ART regimens, non-nucleoside reverse transcriptase inhibitors (NNRTIs), and nucleoside reverse transcriptase inhibitors (NRTIs), worsen lipid parameters especially triglycerides, and often LDL-C. Older PIs also have adverse effects on insulin resistance and cause lipodystrophy, resulting in higher risk of MI. Abacavir (NRTI) use is associated with increased risk of MI in some but not all studies and International AIDS Society (IAS) guidelines suggest avoiding abacavir in individuals with known or at high risk for ASCVD. NNRTIs also generally increase LDL-C and triglycerides, with efavirenz worse compared to rilpivirine. INSTIs, such as dolutegravir, raltegravir, elvitegravir, and CCR5 based regimens (maraviroc) are associated with more favorable lipid parameters but are associated with weight gain.[13] The cardiometabolic effects of ART must be weighed against selecting the most effective antiviral with high genetic barrier to resistance. In most cases, lipid abnormalities should be managed directly with statins rather than switching ART regimens.[14]

Concerns that INSTIs may be associated with increased cardiovascular risk were raised by an observational study within the RESPOND registry which includes 32,000 PWH in clinical care.[15] However, people at elevated ASCVD risk were more likely to be switched to INSTIs. A subsequent study of 5362 PWH within the Swiss HIV Cohort Study found that INSTIs were not associated with increased cardiovascular risk over a median 4.9 years.[16]

PWH, even those treated with ART, have higher immune activation leading to chronic inflammation that accelerates atherogenesis leading to cardiovascular events and mortality.[6] HIV-specific contributors to chronic inflammation may include direct effects of HIV proteins, co-infection with other viruses including Hepatitis C and cytomegalovirus, increased gut microbial translocation, immune responses to the viral reservoir, and clonal hematopoiesis of indeterminate potential.

Even among those virologically suppressed on ART, PWH have elevated inflammatory markers compared to the population without HIV, and inflammatory markers are strongly predictive of CVD events and mortality. Inflammation accelerates atherosclerosis and can precipitate acute plaque rupture leading to MI and stroke. Proteins encoded by HIV such as transactivator of transcription, negative factor, and gp120 induce inflammation and endothelial dysfunction. Markers of the viral reservoir among PWH without detectable viral loads are associated with ASCVD.[17] HIV-related immune dysfunction and immunosenescence (assessed crudely with CD4 count and CD4:CD8 ratio) are associated with CVD but the mechanistic links remain unclear. Co-infection with other viruses such as cytomegalovirus may impact the HIV viral reservoir, but its link to CVD remains uncertain.[18,19] The gastrointestinal microbiome and increased gut permeability play key roles in HIV disease pathogenesis and contribute to systemic inflammation[20]; interventional studies to probe this potential mechanism, however, have been largely negative.[21]

More recently, clonal hematopoiesis of indeterminate potential has been shown to be prevalent among PWH[22,23] and associated with subclinical ASCVD[24] and cardiovascular events, but requires further validation before it can be considered a CVD biomarker.[25]

Another potential contributor to CVD among PWH may be excess activation of the renin-angiotensin-aldosterone system related to hypertension and chronic kidney disease. Chronic kidney disease in the setting of HIV is associated with cardiovascular risk[26] and diastolic dysfunction.[27]

PREVENTION OF ATHEROSCLEROTIC CARDIOVASCULAR DISEASE

Prevention of CVD among people with HIV starts with effective ART and promoting cardiovascular health, and among people at risk for HIV this includes HIV prevention strategies including PrEP (**Fig. 2**). The EXTRA-CVD trial demonstrated that a nurse-led care coordination intervention that incorporated home blood pressure monitoring, treatment algorithms, and electronic health record tools to promote cardiovascular health among PWH resulted in better blood pressure and lipid control.[28]

Strong evidence supports the use of statins to prevent ASCVD among PWH. The Randomized Trial to Prevent Vascular Events in HIV (REPRIEVE) randomized 7769 individuals with treated HIV at low-to intermediate risk to pitavastatin 4 mg/day or placebo. In those treated with pitavastatin, the composite outcome of major adverse cardiovascular events was reduced compared to placebo by 35% (hazard ratio 0.65; 95% CI, 0.48–0.90; $P = .002$) from 7.32 to 4.81 per 1000 person-years among a population over a median follow-up of 5.1 years.[29] The median age was 50 and the median estimated 10-year ASCVD risk was 4.5%, below standard thresholds for recommendation of statin therapy, underscoring that statin therapy was effective for PWH with low risk. Importantly, muscle side effects were rare (2.3% vs 1.4%), and incident diabetes was only slightly more common (5.3% vs 4.0%).

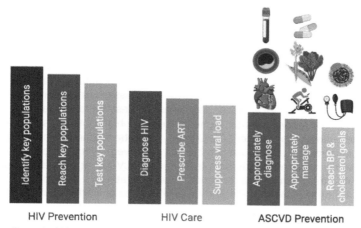

HIV Prevention HIV Care ASCVD Prevention

Fig. 2. The Extended HIV treatment Cascade for ASCVD Prevention. Because HIV is associated with increased cardiovascular risk, ASCVD prevention for people starts with HIV prevention and treatment. The care cascade including appropriately diagnosing and managing cardiovascular risk factors to reach optimal targets for cardiovascular health. (As published in McLaughlin et al. Cardiovascular health among persons with HIV without existing atherosclerotic cardiovascular disease. *AIDS* 2023; 37(14): p 2179-2183. Adapted with permission from: Okeke NL et al. Rationale and design of a nurse-led intervention to extend the HIV treatment cascade for cardiovascular disease prevention trial (EXTRA-CVD). *Am Heart J.* 2019;216:91-101.)

Based on the risk-based paradigm endorsed by the US Preventive Services Task Force (USPSTF) and cardiology societies, pharmacologic risk reduction is encouraged when absolute risk reduction exceeds potential risk of harm and societal costs. A major challenge to implementing this paradigm for PWH is poor calibration and discrimination of risk prediction models for PWH.[30] The pooled cohort equations endorsed by the AHA was used in REPRIEVE and is used in clinical practice in the US. However, it performs poorly among PWH, especially among women and those who are Black/African American. Unfortunately, HIV-specific calculators such as the D:A:D calculator[31] do not perform better[32] and have yet to be validated. The AHA recently developed a new risk calculator called "PREVENT" that incorporates cardiovascular-kidney-metabolic health, but it has not yet been evaluated among PWH.[33] Pre-REPRIEVE AHA guidelines considered HIV as a risk-enhancing factor that may be considered to recommend a statin at borderline elevated estimated risk (5%-7.5% 100 year risk).[34] Using prior guidelines, awareness of cardiovascular risk, and prescription of statins to those at elevated risk are quite low among clinicians caring for PWH.[8]

How will REPRIEVE inform clinical practice? The biggest immediate impacts are that it (1) raises awareness of cardiovascular risk and consideration of statins for PWH and (2) demonstrates that statins have a clinically meaningful benefit among lower risk PWH with low rates of adverse events. REPRIEVE raises several important questions for clinical consideration.

First, should pitavastatin be the preferred statin for people with HIV? As the statin studied in REPRIEVE, pitavastatin has the strongest evidence for efficacy and had a low rate of adverse effects including incident diabetes. A major advantage of pitavastatin is a lack of drug-drug interactions with older ART regimens, similar to pravastatin and fluvastatin, and unlike simvastatin and lovastatin. However, drug-drug interactions are no longer a major limitation with first line INSTI-based ART regimens.

Pitavastatin (along with pravastatin and fluvastatin), however, is a moderate intensity statin. Lower LDL is associated with improved cardiovascular benefit, so high intensity statins or non-statin alternatives such as PCSK9 inhibitors may be even more effective among high-risk PWH. Among people without HIV, earlier PCSK9 inhibition was associated with fewer CVD events in FOURIER-OLE, suggesting that earlier and longer LDL reductions are beneficial.[35] Furthermore, the mechanism-oriented imaging study of REPRIEVE demonstrated plaque regression among those treated with pitavastatin for 2 years[36] to a similar degree as atorvastatin for 1 year.[37]

Rosuvastatin or atorvastatin (at higher doses) are high-potency statins with anti-inflammatory effects. They lower LDL-C more than pitavastatin at a cost of increased drug-drug interactions and possibly more adverse events versus moderate-intensity statins. They are preferred for those with existing ASCVD or at high risk despite maximally tolerated treatment with a moderate-potency statin. For PWH on ART regimens that include ritonavir-boosted PIs, the dose should be limited to rosuvastatin 10 mg and atorvastatin 40 mg daily.

Cost is another important consideration as pitavastatin remains branded in the US. Pitavastatin is not cost-effective compared to pravastatin for primary prevention of ASCVD among PWH in the U.S. under a wide range of assumptions.[38]

A second question REPRIEVE raises is whether statins should be started on everyone with HIV without known ASCVD. The prespecified subgroup analysis did not suggest of heterogeneity of treatment effect by predicted risk. The REPRIEVE imaging sub study revealed that despite the low estimated risk, 49% had plaque; even among those with lowest predicted risk (<2.5% over 10 years), 30% had coronary plaque.[39] According to standard thresholds, the number needed to treat for 5 years to prevent 1 major adverse cardiovascular event meets even USPSTF thresholds for those with predicted risk greater than 5% and AHA/ACC thresholds for those predicted to have 2.5% to 5.0% 10-year risk.

For individuals without HIV at "borderline" risk, guidelines suggest imaging including coronary artery calcium scores may be considered. However, PWH predominantly have non-calcified plaque (particularly those not previously treated with a statin) which is invisible on a non-contrast, non-gated coronary artery calcium (CAC) computed tomographic scan. Within the REPRIEVE imaging sub study, only 35% had CAC even though 49% had plaque at baseline.[39] Non-calcified plaques are more inflammatory and exhibit features associated with increased risk of MI. A meta-analysis found that PWH had 3 times higher prevalence of non-calcified plaque compared to people without HIV.[40] There is a lack of evidence to support an imaging-based risk refinement strategy in HIV.[32]

In response to REPRIEVE, the British HIV Association recommended that all PWH over age 40 should be offered statins, and the United States Department of Health and Human Services Guidelines Panel for the Use of Antiretroviral Therapy in Adults and Adolescents with HIV recommended at least moderate intensity statin for all PWH age 40 to 75 with estimated risk of 5% to 20% with pitavastatin 4 mg, rosuvastatin 10 mg, or atorvastatin 20 mg daily and favors initiation in those with predicted risk less than 5%. For those with predicted risk less than 5%, an individualized approach of risk estimation and incorporation of patient preference may be the preferred strategy.

For those intolerant of statins or at high risk despite statins, lipid lowering therapies such as PCSK9 inhibitors, ezetimibe, and bempedoic acid may be considered. Evolocumab, a PCSK9 inhibitor, safely lowered LDL-C by 57% over 24 weeks among PWH.[41] Bempedoic acid is effective in the general population, lowering LDL-C by 21% and MACE by 13%, with favorable pleotropic effects, but has not been studied in HIV.[42]

Given associations between inflammation and ASCVD among PWH, there is a strong rationale to consider anti-inflammatory approaches. An important new paradigm within cardiology is the idea of residual cholesterol risk and residual inflammatory risk.[43] Residual inflammation predicts cardiovascular events among people without HIV.[43] The most common "anti-inflammatory" therapy in CVD, aspirin, had no effect on inflammatory markers among PWH,[44] but the net benefit or harm among PWH for primary prevention remains unknown. Therefore, there is an urgent need for identification of safe and effective anti-inflammatory strategies to reduce cardiovascular risk among PWH which may also have a beneficial impact on other comorbidities such as renal disease, neurologic disease, liver disease, pulmonary disease, and aging.

There have been several major trials of anti-inflammatory strategies to prevent CVD in the general population, with smaller proof-of-concept studies using similar agents among PWH. The CANTOS trial found that canakinumab, a monoclonal antibody targeting IL-1β reduced cardiovascular events among those with a reduction in hsCRP.[45] A small pilot study found that canakinumab reduced inflammatory markers among PWH.[46] Similarly, tocilizumab, an anti-IL-6 inhibitor, reduced inflammatory markers but increased lipid levels among PWH.[47] Based on observations in rheumatoid arthritis, the CIRT trial tested low-dose methotrexate in the general population, but it neither lowered inflammatory markers nor prevented cardiovascular events.[48] Similarly, methotrexate did not improve inflammatory markers or endothelial function among PWH.[49] In contrast, colchicine has strong evidence of efficacy and safety among people without HIV including those with chronic coronary artery disease[50] and recent MI,[51] and recently the Food and Drug Association approved for this indication. Its effect on clinical outcomes has not been studied specifically among PWH, and a small study suggested colchicine does not improve inflammatory markers or endothelial function among PWH.[52]

There have been 2 clinical trials of renin-angiotensin aldosterone system inhibitors to prevent CVD among PWH. Telmisartan, an angiotensin receptor blocker, was studied among PWH without hypertension; it did not improve insulin resistance, lipids, or adipokines.[53] In contrast, in the MIRACLE HIV study (n = 40), eplerenone 50 mg twice daily improved cardiac perfusion and strain compared to placebo.

Among PWH who are overweight or obese, there is enthusiasm regarding glucagon-like peptide-1 (GLP-1) agonists, in particular for semaglutide, which now has evidence of a cardiovascular benefit among the general population.[54] Tirzepatide, a novel glucose-dependent insulinotropic polypeptide and GLP-1 receptor agonist, is also effective for weight loss, but does not yet have evidence that it prevents cardiovascular events.[55]

TREATMENT OF ATHEROSCLEROTIC CARDIOVASCULAR DISEASE INCLUDING MYOCARDIAL INFARCTION

PWH who present with acute coronary syndromes (ACS) are on average a decade younger, have lower predicted ASCVD risk, and are more likely to present with single-vessel obstructive disease. Among those with Type 1 MI (plaque-rupture including ST-elevation and Non-ST elevation MI), treatment follows recommendations for people without HIV. In 1 study, the proportion of Type 2 MI (due to supply-demand mismatch) was 50% among PWH and was associated with higher mortality.[56] There is a lack of evidence regarding optimal treatment of Type 2 MI.

Recent data from 2009 to 2019 within the Veterans Affairs did not find differences in management of ACS by HIV status.[57] PWH who undergo percutaneous revascularization have similar short-term outcomes but increased risk of long-term mortality, even among those with treated HIV.[57] Short-term outcomes after coronary artery bypass graft surgery are similar but long-term outcomes have not been reported.

Drug-drug interactions are relevant for anti-platelet therapy, particularly among those on boosted ART regimens that include potent CYP3A inhibitors such as ritonavir and cobicistat, which decreases efficacy of clopidogrel and increases bleeding risk with ticagrelor.[58] INSTIs and maraviroc do not have drug-drug interactions with P2Y12 inhibitors. Among PWH, clopidogrel may be more effective than aspirin as monotherapy, for patients with chronic coronary syndromes or those without a recent stent placed.[59]

Management of chronic coronary syndromes, as well as vascular disease in other territories including stroke and peripheral arterial disease, is driven primarily by symptoms and does not vary by HIV status.

HEART FAILURE IN HUMAN IMMUNODEFICIENCY VIRUS

The risk of HF among PWH is approximately 1.5 to 2-fold greater than the population without HIV.[60] The phenotypes of HF with preserved ejection fraction (HFpEF) and HF with reduced ejection fraction (HFrEF) are both increased among PWH.[60] Among those with advanced HIV disease and viremia, the non-ischemic HFrEF phenotype is more common,[61] whereas among people with treated HIV the HFpEF phenotype may be more common.[62]

Imaging and autopsy studies have shed light on underlying mechanisms of HIV-associated HF. PWH, especially among those with greater immunodeficiency, have increased left ventricular mass. Cardiac MRI studies have demonstrated abnormalities suggestive of inflammation or fibrosis.[63] Circulating sCD163 and monocyte phenotypes are associated with fibrosis on cardiac MRI, suggesting this may be related to chronic systemic inflammation. Cardiac fibrosis is associated with diastolic dysfunction, which is common and occurs earlier among PWH.[64] On autopsy of PWH who died suddenly, there was cardiac interstitial fibrosis in contrast to the replacement fibrosis that occurs after an MI.[65] Abnormal cardiac perfusion from microvascular dysfunction may also contribute, although a recent study using the gold-standard, rubidium PET, did not find a difference in myocardial flow reserve among PWH compared to controls without HIV.[66]

In the general population, the greatest advances in HF care are in guideline directed medical therapy, which are not specific to PWH, and there are not major drug-drug interactions between standard HF medications and ART.

Among patients with advanced HF, outcomes after placement of ventricular assist devices and heart transplant are similar among people with and without HIV.[67,68]

ARRHYTHMIAS IN HUMAN IMMUNODEFICIENCY VIRUS

PWH are at increased risk of atrial fibrillation (AF) approximately 1.5 times that of the population without HIV, especially among those with viremia or low CD4 counts.[69] AF is more common among PWH who are older or have cardiopulmonary comorbidities.[70] Contributors to AF include obesity, alcohol, stress, and inflammation. The 2 main management decisions are regarding anticoagulation to reduce risk of thromboembolism and the choice of rate or rhythm control. Scores to assess embolic risk and bleeding have poor calibration and discrimination when applied to PWH, with CHA_2DS_2-VASC underestimating risk.[71] Apixaban and rivaroxaban are metabolized by the CYP3A4 system resulting in interactions with older ART regimens; dabigatran has the fewest drug-drug interactions. There is no HIV-specific evidence regarding rate versus rhythm control, but emerging evidence in the general population suggests that early rhythm control may be favorable over rate control. Beta-blockers are safe for rate control, whereas, diltiazem and verapamil (calcium channel blockers) have drug-drug interactions with older ART regimens.

PWH also have double the risk of sudden cardiac death (SCD) compared to the general population.[65,72,73] On autopsy, PWH have a higher burden of myocardial interstitial fibrosis.[65] In the general population, myocardial fibrosis by MRI is predictive of SCD, which raises the question of use of implantable cardiac defibrillators among PWH. PWH with defibrillators receive more appropriate shocks than people without HIV, suggestive of increased arrhythmia burden.[74] There are no risk stratification tools to predict SCD risk among PWH without HF.

SUMMARY

PWH remain at heightened risk for CVD, even among people with suppressed viral loads on ART. In the years since the first clinical features of HIV-associated atherosclerosis were described, there have been significant advances in the prevention and treatment of CVD among PWH, most notably the REPRIEVE study which is likely to increase statin utilization. Nonetheless, given the high-risk and the CVD burden that exists among PWH, urgent research priorities are needed including methods to optimize primary prevention and investigation of novel therapeutic strategies to reduce inflammation.

CLINICS CARE POINTS

- PWH are at increased risk of CVD including myocardial infarction, heart failure, and arrhythmias.
- Consider statins to prevent CVD among PWH, especially those over age 40 with predicted 10-year risk of ASCVD events greater than 5%.

DISCLOSURES

M.S. Durstenfeld has no disclosures. P.Y. Hsue has received modest honoraria from Gilead and Merck and a research grant from Novartis.

REFERENCES

1. Shah ASV, Stelzle D, Lee KK, et al. Global Burden of Atherosclerotic Cardiovascular Disease in People Living With HIV: Systematic Review and Meta-Analysis. Circulation 2018;138(11):1100–12.
2. Smit M, Brinkman K, Geerlings S, et al. Future challenges for clinical care of an ageing population infected with HIV: a modelling study. Lancet Infect Dis 2015; 15(7):810–8.
3. Smit M, van Zoest RA, Nichols BE, et al. Cardiovascular Disease Prevention Policy in Human Immunodeficiency Virus: Recommendations From a Modeling Study. Clin Infect Dis 2018;66(5):743–50.
4. Weber MSR, Duran Ramirez JJ, Hentzien M, et al. Time trends in causes of death in people with HIV: insights from the swiss HIV cohort study. Clin Infect Dis 2024;ciae014.
5. Bloomfield GS, Hill CL, Chiswell K, et al. Cardiology Encounters for Underrepresented Racial and Ethnic Groups with Human Immunodeficiency Virus and

Borderline Cardiovascular Disease Risk. J Racial Ethn Health Disparities 2023. https://doi.org/10.1007/s40615-023-01627-0.

6. Durstenfeld MS, Hsue PY. Mechanisms and primary prevention of atherosclerotic cardiovascular disease among people living with HIV. Curr Opin HIV AIDS 2021; 16(3):177–85.

7. Lloyd-Jones DM, Allen NB, Anderson CAM, et al. Life's Essential 8: Updating and Enhancing the American Heart Association's Construct of Cardiovascular Health: A Presidential Advisory From the American Heart Association. Circulation 2022; 146(5):e18–43.

8. McLaughlin MM, Durstenfeld MS, Gandhi M, et al. Cardiovascular health among persons with HIV without existing atherosclerotic cardiovascular disease. AIDS 2023;37(14):2179–83.

9. Grand M, Bia D, Diaz A. Cardiovascular Risk Assessment in People Living With HIV: A Systematic Review and Meta-Analysis of Real-Life Data. Curr HIV Res 2020;18(1):5–18.

10. Willig AL, Webel AR, Westfall AO, et al. Physical activity trends and metabolic health outcomes in people living with HIV in the US, 2008-2015. Prog Cardiovasc Dis 2020;63(2):170–7.

11. Durstenfeld MS, Peluso MJ, Spinelli MA, et al. Association of SARS-CoV-2 Infection and Cardiopulmonary Long COVID With Exercise Capacity and Chronotropic Incompetence Among People With HIV. J Am Heart Assoc 2023;12(20):e030896.

12. Davis K, Perez-Guzman P, Hoyer A, et al. Association between HIV infection and hypertension: a global systematic review and meta-analysis of cross-sectional studies. BMC Med 2021;19(1):105.

13. Eckard AR, McComsey GA. Weight gain and integrase inhibitors. Curr Opin Infect Dis 2020;33(1):10–9.

14. Lee FJ, Monteiro P, Baker D, et al. Rosuvastatin vs. protease inhibitor switching for hypercholesterolaemia: a randomized trial. HIV Med 2016;17(8):605–14.

15. Neesgaard B, Greenberg L, Miro JM, et al. Associations between integrase strand-transfer inhibitors and cardiovascular disease in people living with HIV: a multicentre prospective study from the RESPOND cohort consortium. Lancet HIV 2022;9(7):e474–85.

16. Surial B, Chammartin F, Damas J, et al. Impact of Integrase Inhibitors on Cardiovascular Disease Events in People With Human Immunodeficiency Virus Starting Antiretroviral Therapy. Clin Infect Dis 2023;77(5):729–37.

17. McLaughlin MM, Ma Y, Scherzer R, et al. Association of Viral Persistence and Atherosclerosis in Adults With Treated HIV Infection. JAMA Netw Open 2020; 3(10):e2018099.

18. Knudsen A, Kristoffersen US, Panum I, et al. Coronary artery calcium and intima-media thickness are associated with level of cytomegalovirus immunoglobulin G in HIV-infected patients. HIV Med 2019;20(1):60–2.

19. Schnittman SR, Lu MT, Mayrhofer T, et al. Cytomegalovirus Immunoglobulin G (IgG) Titer and Coronary Artery Disease in People With Human Immunodeficiency Virus (HIV). Clin Infect Dis 2023;76(3):e613–21.

20. Peters BA, Burk RD, Kaplan RC, et al. The Gut Microbiome, Microbial Metabolites, and Cardiovascular Disease in People Living with HIV. Curr HIV AIDS Rep 2023;20(2):86–99.

21. Hsue PY, Waters DD. HIV infection and coronary heart disease: mechanisms and management. Nat Rev Cardiol 2019;16(12):745–59.

22. Dharan NJ, Yeh P, Bloch M, et al. HIV is associated with an increased risk of age-related clonal hematopoiesis among older adults. Nat Med 2021;27(6):1006–11.

23. Bick AG, Popadin K, Thorball CW, et al. Increased prevalence of clonal hematopoiesis of indeterminate potential amongst people living with HIV. Sci Rep 2022; 12(1):577.
24. Wang S, Pasca S, Post WS, et al. Clonal hematopoiesis in men living with HIV and association with subclinical atherosclerosis. AIDS 2022;36(11):1521–31.
25. Wiley B, Parsons TM, Burkart S, et al. Effect of Clonal Hematopoiesis on Cardiovascular Disease in People Living with HIV. Exp Hematol 2022;114:18–21.
26. Ryom L, Lundgren JD, Ross M, et al. Renal Impairment and Cardiovascular Disease in HIV-Positive Individuals: The D:A:D Study. J Infect Dis 2016;214(8): 1212–20.
27. Peters M, Margevicius S, Kityo C, et al. Association of Kidney Disease With Abnormal Cardiac Structure and Function Among Ugandans With HIV Infection. J Acquir Immune Defic Syndr 2021;86(1):104–9.
28. Longenecker CT, Jones KA, Hileman CO, et al. Nurse-Led Strategy to Improve Blood Pressure and Cholesterol Level Among People With HIV: A Randomized Clinical Trial. JAMA Netw Open 2024;7(3):e2356445.
29. Grinspoon SK, Fitch KV, Zanni MV, et al. Pitavastatin to Prevent Cardiovascular Disease in HIV Infection. N Engl J Med 2023;389(8):687–99.
30. Triant VA, Perez J, Regan S, et al. Cardiovascular Risk Prediction Functions Underestimate Risk in HIV Infection. Circulation 2018;137(21):2203–14.
31. Friis-Moller N, Ryom L, Smith C, et al. An updated prediction model of the global risk of cardiovascular disease in HIV-positive persons: The Data-collection on Adverse Effects of Anti-HIV Drugs (D:A:D) study. Eur J Prev Cardiol 2016; 23(2):214–23.
32. Feinstein MJ, Hsue PY, Benjamin LA, et al. Characteristics, Prevention, and Management of Cardiovascular Disease in People Living With HIV: A Scientific Statement From the American Heart Association. Circulation 2019;140(2):e98–124.
33. Khan SS, Coresh J, Pencina MJ, et al. Novel Prediction Equations for Absolute Risk Assessment of Total Cardiovascular Disease Incorporating Cardiovascular-Kidney-Metabolic Health: A Scientific Statement From the American Heart Association. Circulation 2023;148(24):1982–2004.
34. Grundy SM, Stone NJ, Bailey AL, et al. 2018 AHA/ACC/AACVPR/AAPA/ABC/ ACPM/ADA/AGS/APhA/ASPC/NLA/PCNA Guideline on the Management of Blood Cholesterol: A Report of the American College of Cardiology/American Heart Association Task Force on Clinical Practice Guidelines. Circulation 2019;139(25): e1082–143.
35. O'Donoghue ML, Giugliano RP, Wiviott SD, et al. Long-Term Evolocumab in Patients With Established Atherosclerotic Cardiovascular Disease. Circulation 2022;146(15):1109–19.
36. Lu MT, Ribaudo H, Foldyna B, et al. Effects of Pitavastatin on Coronary Artery Disease and Inflammatory Biomarkers in HIV: Mechanistic Substudy of the REPRIEVE Randomized Clinical Trial. JAMA Cardiol 2024;9(4):323–34.
37. Lo J, Lu MT, Ihenachor EJ, et al. Effects of statin therapy on coronary artery plaque volume and high-risk plaque morphology in HIV-infected patients with subclinical atherosclerosis: a randomised, double-blind, placebo-controlled trial. Lancet HIV 2015;2(2):e52–63.
38. Boettiger DC, Newall AT, Phillips A, et al. Cost-effectiveness of statins for primary prevention of atherosclerotic cardiovascular disease among people living with HIV in the United States. J Int AIDS Soc 2021;24(3):e25690.
39. Hoffmann U, Lu MT, Foldyna B, et al. Assessment of Coronary Artery Disease With Computed Tomography Angiography and Inflammatory and Immune

Activation Biomarkers Among Adults With HIV Eligible for Primary Cardiovascular Prevention. JAMA Netw Open 2021;4(6):e2114923.

40. D'Ascenzo F, Cerrato E, Calcagno A, et al. High prevalence at computed coronary tomography of non-calcified plaques in asymptomatic HIV patients treated with HAART: a meta-analysis. Atherosclerosis 2015;240(1):197–204.

41. Boccara F, Kumar PN, Caramelli B, et al. Evolocumab in HIV-Infected Patients With Dyslipidemia: Primary Results of the Randomized, Double-Blind BEIJER-INCK Study. J Am Coll Cardiol 2020;75(20):2570–84.

42. Nissen SE, Lincoff AM, Brennan D, et al. Bempedoic Acid and Cardiovascular Outcomes in Statin-Intolerant Patients. N Engl J Med 2023;388(15):1353–64.

43. Ridker PM, Bhatt DL, Pradhan AD, et al. Inflammation and cholesterol as predictors of cardiovascular events among patients receiving statin therapy: a collaborative analysis of three randomised trials. Lancet 2023;401(10384):1293–301.

44. O'Brien MP, Hunt PW, Kitch DW, et al. A Randomized Placebo Controlled Trial of Aspirin Effects on Immune Activation in Chronically Human Immunodeficiency Virus-Infected Adults on Virologically Suppressive Antiretroviral Therapy. Open Forum Infect Dis 2017;4(1):ofw278.

45. Ridker PM, MacFadyen JG, Everett BM, et al. Relationship of C-reactive protein reduction to cardiovascular event reduction following treatment with canakinumab: a secondary analysis from the CANTOS randomised controlled trial. Lancet 2018;391(10118):319–28.

46. Hsue PY, Li D, Ma Y, et al. IL-1beta Inhibition Reduces Atherosclerotic Inflammation in HIV Infection. J Am Coll Cardiol 2018;72(22):2809–11.

47. Funderburg NT, Shive CL, Chen Z, et al. Interleukin 6 Blockade With Tocilizumab Diminishes Indices of Inflammation That Are Linked to Mortality in Treated Human Immunodeficiency Virus Infection. Clin Infect Dis 2023;77(2):272–9.

48. Ridker PM, Everett BM, Pradhan A, et al. Low-Dose Methotrexate for the Prevention of Atherosclerotic Events. N Engl J Med 2019;380(8):752–62.

49. Hsue PY, Ribaudo HJ, Deeks SG, et al. Safety and Impact of Low-dose Methotrexate on Endothelial Function and Inflammation in Individuals With Treated Human Immunodeficiency Virus: AIDS Clinical Trials Group Study A5314. Clin Infect Dis 2019;68(11):1877–86.

50. Nidorf SM, Fiolet ATL, Mosterd A, et al. Colchicine in Patients with Chronic Coronary Disease. N Engl J Med 2020;383(19):1838–47.

51. Tardif JC, Kouz S, Waters DD, et al. Efficacy and Safety of Low-Dose Colchicine after Myocardial Infarction. N Engl J Med 2019;381(26):2497–505.

52. Hays AG, Schar M, Barditch-Crovo P, et al. A randomized, placebo-controlled, double-blinded clinical trial of colchicine to improve vascular health in people living with HIV. AIDS 2021;35(7):1041–50.

53. Pushpakom S, Kolamunnage-Dona R, Taylor C, et al. TAILoR (TelmisArtan and InsuLin Resistance in Human Immunodeficiency Virus [HIV]): An Adaptive-design, Dose-ranging Phase IIb Randomized Trial of Telmisartan for the Reduction of Insulin Resistance in HIV-positive Individuals on Combination Antiretroviral Therapy. Clin Infect Dis 2020;70(10):2062–72.

54. Lincoff AM, Brown-Frandsen K, Colhoun HM, et al. Semaglutide and Cardiovascular Outcomes in Obesity without Diabetes. N Engl J Med 2023;389(24):2221–32.

55. Jastreboff AM, Aronne LJ, Ahmad NN, et al. Tirzepatide Once Weekly for the Treatment of Obesity. N Engl J Med 2022;387(3):205–16.

56. Feinstein MJ, Nance RM, Delaney JAC, et al. Mortality following myocardial infarction among HIV-infected persons: the Center for AIDS Research Network Of Integrated Clinical Systems (CNICS). BMC Med 2019;17(1):149.

57. Parikh RV, Hebbe A, Baron AE, et al. Clinical Characteristics and Outcomes Among People Living With HIV Undergoing Percutaneous Coronary Intervention: Insights From the Veterans Affairs Clinical Assessment, Reporting, and Tracking Program. J Am Heart Assoc 2023;12(4):e028082.

58. Marsousi N, Daali Y, Fontana P, et al. Impact of Boosted Antiretroviral Therapy on the Pharmacokinetics and Efficacy of Clopidogrel and Prasugrel Active Metabolites. Clin Pharm 2018;57(10):1347–54.

59. Marcantoni E, Garshick MS, Schwartz T, et al. Antiplatelet Effects of Clopidogrel Vs Aspirin in Virologically Controlled HIV: A Randomized Controlled Trial. JACC Basic Transl Sci 2022;7(11):1086–97.

60. Freiberg MS, Chang CH, Skanderson M, et al. Association Between HIV Infection and the Risk of Heart Failure With Reduced Ejection Fraction and Preserved Ejection Fraction in the Antiretroviral Therapy Era: Results From the Veterans Aging Cohort Study. JAMA Cardiol 2017;2(5):536–46.

61. Erqou S, Lodebo BT, Masri A, et al. Cardiac Dysfunction Among People Living With HIV: A Systematic Review and Meta-Analysis. JACC Heart Fail 2019;7(2): 98–108.

62. Ntsekhe M, Baker JV. Cardiovascular Disease Among Persons Living With HIV: New Insights Into Pathogenesis and Clinical Manifestations in a Global Context. Circulation 2023;147(1):83–100.

63. Ntusi N, O'Dwyer E, Dorrell L, et al. HIV-1-Related Cardiovascular Disease Is Associated With Chronic Inflammation, Frequent Pericardial Effusions, and Probable Myocardial Edema. Circulation Cardiovascular imaging 2016;9(3):e004430.

64. Butler J, Greene SJ, Shah SH, et al. Diastolic Dysfunction in Patients With Human Immunodeficiency Virus Receiving Antiretroviral Therapy: Results From the CHART Study. J Card Fail 2020;26(5):371–80.

65. Tseng ZH, Moffatt E, Kim A, et al. Sudden Cardiac Death and Myocardial Fibrosis, Determined by Autopsy, in Persons with HIV. N Engl J Med 2021;384(24): 2306–16.

66. Knudsen A, Christensen TE, Ghotbi AA, et al. Normal Myocardial Flow Reserve in HIV-Infected Patients on Stable Antiretroviral Therapy: A Cross-Sectional Study Using Rubidium-82 PET/CT. Medicine (Baltim) 2015;94(43):e1886.

67. Birk SE, Baran DA, Campbell R, et al. Clinical outcomes of ventricular assist device support by HIV infection status: An STS-INTERMACS analysis. J Heart Lung Transplant 2023;42(9):1185–93.

68. Osobamiro O, Stempein-Otero A, Ssinabulya I, et al. Cardiac transplantation in people living with HIV: the global context. Heart 2022;108(7):573–4.

69. Sardana M, Hsue PY, Tseng ZH, et al. Human Immunodeficiency Virus Infection and Incident Atrial Fibrillation. J Am Coll Cardiol 2019;74(11):1512–4.

70. Nance RM, Delaney JAC, Floyd JS, et al. Risk factors for atrial fibrillation in a multicenter United States clinical cohort of people with HIV infection. AIDS 2022;36(6):903–5.

71. Jung H, Yang PS, Jang E, et al. Prevalence and Associated Stroke Risk of Human Immunodeficiency Virus-Infected Patients With Atrial Fibrillation - A Nationwide Cohort Study. Circ J 2019;83(12):2547–54.

72. Sardana M, Nah G, Hsue PY, et al. Human Immunodeficiency Virus Infection and Out-of-Hospital Cardiac Arrest. Am J Cardiol 2022;163:124–9.

73. Garcia R, Warming PE, Hansen CJ, et al. Out-of-Hospital Cardiac Arrest in individuals with Human Immunodeficiency Virus infection - A nationwide population-based cohort study. Clin Infect Dis 2023;77(11):1578–84.

74. Alvi RM, Neilan AM, Tariq N, et al. Incidence, Predictors, and Outcomes of Implantable Cardioverter-Defibrillator Discharge Among People Living With HIV. J Am Heart Assoc 2018;7(18):e009857.

Cancer in People with HIV

Thomas A. Odeny, MD, MPH, PhD[a], Valeria Fink, MD[b],
Mazvita Muchengeti, PhD, MSc (Epidemiology & Biostatistics)[c,d],
Satish Gopal, MD, MPH[e,*]

KEYWORDS

- Human immunodeficiency virus-associated cancers
- Human immunodeficiency virus malignancies
- Cancer in people with human immunodeficiency virus
- Acquired immunodeficiency disease defining cancers

KEY POINTS

- Many factors contribute to a continued increased cancer risk among people with HIV (PWH) globally, despite advancements in antiretroviral therapy (ART).
- Behavioral, vaccination, and screening interventions are currently available to reduce cancer risk and should be integrated into routine healthcare, alongside continued research and tailoring to meet the diverse needs of PWH globally.
- PWH diagnosed with cancer can often be treated similarly to people without HIV in the ART era – including with novel cancer therapies and in clinical trials – but unique treatment challenges and opportunities remain among PWH.
- Collaborative multidisciplinary efforts, leveraging implementation science, are critical for continued progress against cancer in PWH, especially in parts of the world with the greatest burden of HIV.

INTRODUCTION

In this review, we provide an overview of the intersection between human immunodeficiency virus (HIV) and cancer. Addressing cancer in the context of HIV requires consideration not only of the specific cancer type but also the broader context. We therefore consider throughout disparities in access to care for people with HIV (PWH), including in low- and middle-income countries (LMICs) where most PWH

[a] Division of Oncology, Department of Medicine, Washington University School of Medicine, 660 S. Euclid Ave., CB 8056, St. Louis, MO 63110-1093, USA; [b] Research Department, Fundación Huésped, Av. Forest 345 (C1427CEA) Buenos Aires, Argentina; [c] School of Public Health, University of the Witwatersrand, Johannesburg, South Africa; [d] South African DSI-NRF Centre of Excellence in Epidemiological Modelling and Analysis (SACEMA), Stellenbosch University, South Africa; [e] Center for Global Health, National Cancer Institute, 9609 Medical Center Drive, Rockville MD 20850, USA
* Corresponding author. 9609 Medical Center Drive Rockville MD 20850
E-mail address: satish.gopal@nih.gov

Infect Dis Clin N Am 38 (2024) 531–557
https://doi.org/10.1016/j.idc.2024.06.007
0891-5520/24/Published by Elsevier Inc.

live. We analyze existing evidence to shed light on current clinical management strategies, complications, controversies, and emerging opportunities.

EPIDEMIOLOGY
The Global Human Immunodeficiency Virus Epidemic

In some world regions, the HIV epidemic is largely generalized, while in others the HIV epidemic is more concentrated among specific key populations.[1] These key populations include men who have sex with men (MSM), transgender people, male and female sex workers and their sexual partners, people who inject drugs, incarcerated persons, migrants or refugees, and people of African ancestry. Even within a largely generalized HIV epidemic in sub-Saharan Africa, there are key populations requiring specific attention. These include highly mobile populations (eg, seasonal farm workers, construction workers, long-distance truck drivers, and uniformed forces), people with disabilities, young women (15–24 years), and fishing communities.[2–4] Recognizing these key populations is critical in identifying individuals at higher risk of HIV, and consequently, HIV-associated malignancies. Social, behavioral, and structural factors often act to increase cancer risk for such key populations independent of HIV infection, while also increasing risk for HIV infection, which itself potentiates cancer risk.[5] PWH may also be socially and structurally disadvantaged relative to individuals without HIV, making them susceptible to health disparities across the cancer control continuum. Finally, cancer is now a leading cause of death in PWH as they live longer on antiretroviral therapy (ART).[6,7]

Cancer Risk and Antiretroviral Therapy Among People with Human Immunodeficiency Virus

Early in the global HIV epidemic, it became clear that PWH had a higher risk of developing cancer. By 1993, Kaposi sarcoma (KS), non-Hodgkin lymphoma (NHL), and cervical cancer were included in the surveillance case definition of acquired immunodeficiency syndrome (AIDS).[8] Subsequently, additional cancers were recognized as associated with HIV, including Hodgkin lymphoma, cancers associated with human papillomavirus (HPV), lung cancer, liver cancer, and, in sub-Saharan Africa, conjunctival cancer and squamous cell carcinoma of the skin.[9–11] As noted in **Table 1**, the introduction of ART ushered in a marked decline in some HIV-associated cancers, particularly those most strongly associated with immunodeficiency.[21] Many of these declines have been replicated as ART has been progressively introduced and expanded worldwide, although there are important differences observed across world regions. In particular, high-quality epidemiologic data are often not as readily available to assess trends in LMICs. Finally, risk for some HIV-associated cancers has not been reduced by the introduction of ART, leading to changes in the distribution of specific cancer types among PWH.

Social, Demographic, and Behavioral Risk Transitions Worldwide

In addition to global trends with respect to the HIV epidemic and ART scale-up, and as reflected in **Table 1**, HIV-associated cancer burden is also influenced by broader demographic and socioeconomic changes within and across populations over time.[22] Countries characterized by a low Human Development Index (HDI) have a higher prevalence of infection-related cancers such as cervical, KS, stomach, and liver cancers. Conversely, countries with a high HDI have increased prevalence of cancers associated with reproductive, dietary, and hormonal factors such as female breast, colorectal, and prostate cancers.[23] Therefore, as populations' age and human

Table 1
Illustrative population-based epidemiologic studies detailing human immunodeficiency virus-associated cancer risk worldwide and across antiretroviral therapy scale-up periods

Study	Pre-ART			Range	Early ART Scale-up			Range	Late ART Scale-up						Range
	Dal Maso et al,[12] 2009	Mbulaiteye et al,[13] 2006	Stein et al,[14] 2008		Clifford et al,[15] 2005	Godbole et[16] 2016	Muchengeti et al,[10] 2023		Dal Maso et al,[12] 2009	Dhokotera et al,[17] 2019	Akarolo-Anthony et al,[18] 2014	Hernandez Ramirez et al,[19] 2017	Tanon et al,[11] 2012	Jaquet et al,[20] 2015	
Countries	Italy	Uganda	South Africa		Switzerland	India	South Africa		Italy	South Africa	Nigeria	USA	Cote d'Ivoire, Benin	Benin, Cote d'Ivoire, Nigeria, Togo	
Study period	1986–1996	1998–2002	1995–2004		1985–2002	1996–2008	1995–2016		1997–2004	2004–2014	2005–2012	1996–2012	2009–2011	2009–2012	
Measure	SIR	SIR	OR		SIR	SIR	OR		SIR	OR	SIR	SIR	OR	OR	
Infection-related Cancers															
Kaposi sarcoma	1792 (1640–1956)	6.4 (4.8–8.4)	47.1 (31.9–69.8)	6.4–1792	192 (170–217)		99.1 (72.6–135.1)	99.1–192	572 (508–641)	134 (111–161)	5.7 (4.1–7.2)	498 (478–519)	62.2 (22.1–175.5)	34.6 (17.3–69.0)	5.7–572
Non-Hodgkin lymphoma	497 (450–546)	6.7 (1.8–17)	5.9 (4.3–8.1)	5.9–479	76.4 (66.5–87.4)	10.6 (5.9–17.5)	11.3 (9.3–13.6)	11.3–76.4	93.4 (83.9–104)	2.7 (2.6–2.9)		11.5 (11.1–11.9)	4.0 (2.0–8.0)	3.6 (1.9–6.8)	2.7–93.4
Cervix	51.0 (23.1–97.3)	2.4 (1.1–4.4)	1.6 (1.3–2.0)	1.6–51.0	8.0 (2.9–17.4)	15.7 (11–22)	2.7 (2.4–3.0)	2.7–15.7	41.5 (28.0–59.3)	1.7 (1.6–1.8)	2.0 (0.4–3.5)	3.24 (2.94–3.56)	7.9 (3.8–16.7)	4.3 (2.2–8.3)	1.7–41.5
Hodgkin lymphoma		5.7 (1.2–17)	1.6 (1.0–2.7)	1.6–5.7	17.3 (10.2–27.4)	7.7 (2.1–19.7)	3.1 (2.4–4.2)	3.1–17.3		1.2 (1.1–1.4)		7.70 (7.20–8.23)	3.0 (0.7–13.3)	3.4 (0.9–13.5)	1.2–7.7
Anogenital (other than cervix)			2.2 (1.4–3.3)	2.2								11.6 (2.9–46.3)	17.7 (6.9–45.2)		11.6–17.7
Vulva and vagina	24.6 (2.3–90.6)			24.6					24.3 (4.6–71.8)						24.3
Vulva						4.8 (3.5–6.4)		4.8		1.9 (1.7–2.2)		9.35 (7.91–11.0)			1.9–9.35
Vagina						25.2 (3.1–91.1)	5.5 (3.0–10.2)	5.5–25.2		0.8 (0.7–1.0)		3.55 (2.30–5.24)			3.55
Penis							5.4 (2.7–10.5)	5.4	12.0 (2.3–35.5)	2.3 (1.8–3.0)		5.33 (4.39–6.40)			2.3–12.0
Anus	35.5 (12.8–77.7)			35.5	33.4 (10.5–78.6)		2.1 (1.4–3.2)	2.1–33.4	44.0 (21.8–78.9)	1.6 (1.3–2.0)	0.3 (0–17.8)	19.1 (18.1–20.0)			1.6–44.0
Merkel cell carcinoma												2.58 (1.24–4.74)			2.58

(continued on next page)

Table 1
(continued)

Liver	2.1 (0.4–6.4)		2.1	7.0 (2.2–16.5)	8.1 (3.5–15.9)	0.8 (0.5–1.3)	7.0–8.1	6.4 (3.7–10.5)	0.4 (0.4–0.5)	0.5 (0–5.1)	3.21 (3.02–3.41)	2.7 (1.1–7.7)	2.2 (1.0–5.8)	2.2–6.4
Oral cavity and pharynx				4.1 (2.1–7.4)		1.6 (1.3–1.9)	1.6–4.1		0.5 (0.5–0.6)		1.64 (1.46–1.84)	1.0 (0.2–4.9)	1.6 (0.6–4.4)	0.5–1.64
Other cancer types where role of infection is unknown but for which HIV association is known or postulated														
Squamous cell carcinoma of skin		2.6 (1.4–4.9)	2.6			3.5 (2.5–4.9)	3.5		1.8 (1.6–2.0)			3.4 (0.6–18.3)	5.2 (2.0–14.4)	1.8–5.2
Non-epithelial skin										4.0 (0–8.5)				
Eye Cancer					157 (32–458.2)	18.7 (10.1–34.7)	18.7–157		5.9 (5.1–6.8)	1.5 (0–18.1)				5.9
Conjunctiva	4 (1.5–8.7)		4						21.5 (16.3–28.4)			5.56 (3.44–8.50)		5.6–21.5
Lip						-			2.7 (1.7–4.3)			2.35 (1.43–3.62)		2.35–2.7
Non-melanoma skin	2.1 (1.2–3.3)		2.1	3.2 (2.2–4.5)					1.8 (1.2–2.6)					1.8
Basal cell carcinoma									1.3 (1.1–1.5)					1.3
Melanoma	0.9 (0.2–2.6)			1.1 (0.3–2.8)	6.0 (1.2–17.4)	2.0 (1.2–3.5)	2.0–6.0	0.6 (0.1–1.7)	0.8 (0.6–0.9)		0.86 (0.75–0.98)			0.8–0.86
Lung	2.1 (1.2–3.3)		2.1	3.2 (1.7–5.4)	8.8 (4.8–14.7)	1.2 (0.9–1.4)	3.2–8.8	4.1 (2.9–5.5)	0.5 (0.5–0.6)		1.97 (1.89–2.05)		2.0 (0.4–8.9)	0.5–4.1
Larynx						1.7 (1.3–2.4)	1.7		0.6 (0.5–0.6)		2.11 (1.89–2.05)			0.6–2.11
Myeloma	5.5 (1.0–16.4)			5.5 (0.5–20.4)		1.1 (0.7–1.5)		3.9 (1.0–10.0)	0.6 (0.6–0.7)		0.89 (0.78–1.02)			0.6
Leukemia	4.9 (2.4–8.8)		4.9	1.8 (0.2–6.7)	23.9 (7.8–55.9)	0.7 (0.4–1.3)	23.9	1.1 (0.2–3.3)	0.2 (0.2–0.3)		1.18 (1.00–1.37)	0.8 (0.2–2.4)	0.7 (0.2–2.4)	0.2

Abbreviations: ART, antiretroviral therapy; OR, odds ratio; SIR, standardized incidence ratio. Please see Refs.[10–20]

development improves worldwide, cancer burden among PWH will increasingly include malignancies that are not infection-associated, like breast, colorectal, prostate, and lung cancers, especially in parts of the world with more generalized HIV epidemics.[24,25]

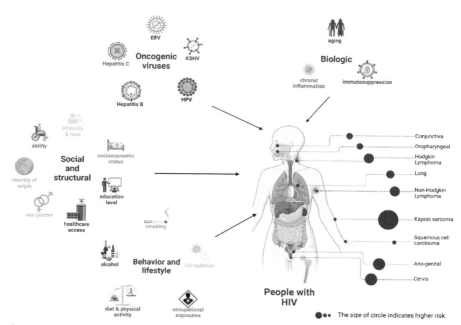

Fig. 1. The complex and intersecting social, structural, behavioral, and lifestyle factors that affect cancer risk for people with HIV. EBV, Epstein-Barr virus; HPV, human papillomavirus; KSHV, Kaposi sarcoma-associated herpesvirus.

PATHOBIOLOGY

The interplay between cancer and HIV is complex and multifactorial as illustrated in **Fig. 1**, reflecting elements that are unique or related to HIV and others that are related to cancer in the general population and may be exacerbated among PWH.

Oncogenic Infections

Many cancers associated with HIV have an underlying viral infectious cause such as Kaposi sarcoma herpesvirus (KSHV), Epstein-Barr virus (EBV), HPV, and hepatitis B viruses (HBVs) and hepatitis C viruses (HCVs).[26] HIV infection primarily contributes to increased cancer risk by inducing immunosuppression, potentiating oncogenic viruses, and other indirect mechanisms. However, more recent evidence has suggested that HIV-1 itself may be directly carcinogenic, for example, via expression of specific HIV proteins, which induce oxidative stress thereby promoting malignant transformation.[27]

In **Table 2**, we show a brief timeline of HIV and viral infections associated with cancer. With each subsequent discovery of the association between cancer and oncogenic viral infections, the importance of immunosuppression in viral oncogenesis was confirmed.

Epstein-Barr virus and non-Hodgkin lymphoma

EBV, a gamma-herpesvirus, was the first virus to be causally associated with cancer in humans in 1964. It was initially identified as the causative agent for Burkitt lymphoma, and later as the cause of undifferentiated nasopharyngeal carcinoma and other lymphoma subtypes.[37] EBV is ubiquitous, with approximately 90% of the world's

Table 2	
A brief timeline of human immunodeficiency virus and cancer	
1981	Clusters of KS and *Pneumocystis carinii* Pneumonia are identified Among Homosexual Male Residents of California.[28]
1982	HPV is identified as the necessary cause of cervical cancer.[29]
1983	HIV is identified as the cause of AIDS[30]
1984	Baruch Blumberg and Irving Millman develop the HBV vaccine, which reduces risk of liver cancer associated with chronic HBV infection.[31]
1987	The first antiretroviral drug, zidovudine is developed and approved by the US FDA for the treatment of HIV.[32]
1988	Michael Houghton and colleagues discover HCV, which is an important cause of HCC.[33]
1993	Inclusion of KS, NHL, and ICC in the case definition of AIDS by the Centers for Disease Control.[8]
1994	KSHV is discovered.[34]
1996	Highly active ART, typically with three complementary antiviral medicines, is introduced to treat HIV in the US and Europe. HIV-1 is classified as a human carcinogen by the International Agency for Research on Cancer.[26]
1997	EBV is classified as a human carcinogen by the International Agency for Research on Cancer.[26]
1998+	HIV-cancer record linkage studies shed light on the spectrum and risk of cancers in HIV.
1999+	KS and NHL incidence decline in the US and Europe after the introduction of ART. Cancers not classically associated with AIDS emerge and eventually predominate among people with HIV in the US and Europe.
2002	HPV is recognized as a cause of anal, vulvar and oropharyngeal cancers.[35]
2004	ART is introduced into national public health programs in sub-Saharan Africa.
2005+	Cancer becomes a leading cause of death in HIV-infected people in the US and Europe.
2008	Researchers discover Merkel Cell Polyomavirus associated with Merkel cell carcinoma, a rare and aggressive skin cancer.[36]

Abbreviations: ART, antiretroviral therapy; EBV, Epstein-Barr virus; HBV, hepatitis B virus; HCV, hepatitis C virus; HPV, human papillomavirus; ICC, invasive cervical carcinoma; KS, kaposi sarcoma; KSHV, Kaposi sarcoma-associated herpesvirus; NHL, non-Hodgkin lymphoma.

population having latent infection. In PWH, EBV can undergo reactivation, leading to the B-cell proliferation, which can contribute to lymphomagenesis. In part reflecting this, PWH have significantly elevated NHL and Hodgkin lymphoma (HL) risk as shown in **Table 1**.

Kaposi sarcoma herpesvirus and Kaposi sarcoma, primary effusion lymphoma, and multicentric Castleman disease

KSHV is another gamma-herpesvirus also referred to as human herpesvirus 8, first identified in 1994 and found to be causally associated with cancer. Chang and colleagues identified that patients with HIV-associated KS all had KSHV infection.[38] KSHV virus was later identified as the cause of other cancers in PWH, including primary effusion lymphoma,[39] and a form of the lymphoproliferative disorder multicentric Castleman disease.[40]

Human papillomavirus and cervical, anal, vulvar, vaginal, penile, and head and neck cancer

HPV constitutes the most common sexually transmitted disease, with around 80% of sexually active people being infected sometime in their life.[41] HPV infections are more prevalent and more likely to persist in PWH compared to the general population,[8,42,43] leading to a higher prevalence and incidence of HPV-related cancers among PWH. Cervical cancer was included in the surveillance case definition of AIDS in 1993.[8] A recent metanalysis showed that the risk of cervical cancer is 6 times higher among women with HIV, with most cases occurring in LMICs, especially Sub-Saharan Africa.[44] Despite the advent of ART, nearly all HPV-related cancers are still observed at higher frequency among PWH.[43] In particular, PWH have greater than 20 times increased risk of anal cancer, and HIV-infected MSM have even greater risk (60–80 times greater).[45]

Hepatitis B virus, Hepatitis C virus, and hepatocellular carcinoma

Given common routes of transmission, PWH experience higher incidence of coinfection with HBV and HCV compared to the general population. In the United States (US), estimates indicate chronic HCV prevalence of 26% among PWH versus 0.9% in the general adult population. Similarly, for HBV infection, the prevalence is 5% among PWH versus 0.3% in the general population.[42] That prevalence may vary between 2% and 30% in LMICs.[46] PWH further have increased risk of chronic hepatitis due to compromised immunity, which further elevates the risk of hepatocellular carcinoma (HCC). Data from various cohorts demonstrate recent increases in HCC incidence among PWH in recent years.[47]

Contributing Factors Other than Oncogenic Viruses

Chronic inflammation

Chronic inflammation from HIV infection persistently activates the immune system, leading to cytokine dysregulation that creates a microenvironment that favors oncogenesis.[48] This inflammatory milieu amplifies production of inflammatory mediators such as IL-6 and TNF-alpha, which facilitate angiogenesis and cancer cell survival.[49] In PWH, chronic immune activation is further worsened by infections and toxins (eg, from smoking), which are much more prevalent than in people without HIV (see **Fig. 1**).

Immunosuppression

HIV infection compromises immune surveillance by targeting CD4 cells, allowing cancer cells to evade detection and elimination. This mechanism is likely important even for cancers not clearly associated with oncogenic viruses. An example is squamous cell carcinoma of the skin, for which HIV-related immune suppression might impair immune surveillance of precancerous mutational events triggered by exposure to ultraviolet (UV) light. Reflecting this, the lowest historic CD4 cell count, known as the nadir CD4 cell count, and more prolonged periods of severe immunosuppression correlate with a higher likelihood of developing cancer in PWH.[49] As noted earlier, immunodeficiency also induces reactivation and replication of latent viral infections (eg, cytomegalovirus [CMV], EBV), which can be directly carcinogenic (eg, EBV) or indirectly through chronic activation of the immune system (eg, CMV).[50]

Accelerated aging

Although ART has dramatically increased life expectancy for PWH, HIV infection may also be associated with accelerated aging relative to populations without HIV. This premature aging is driven by persistent immune activation, shortening of telomeres, and mitochondrial dysfunction,[48] and potentially contributes to increased risk of age-related cancers.

Direct human immunodeficiency virus effects

There is recent evidence indicating that HIV itself may have direct pro-oncogenic effects through multiple potential mechanisms, involving synergism with other pro-oncogenic viruses, disruption of cell cycle regulation, blockage of tumor suppressor gene function, promotion of chromosome instability through inhibition of telomerase activity, impairment of DNA repair function, induction of tumor angiogenesis, and enhancement of the effects of exogenous carcinogens.[51] Some HIV proteins, including envelope protein gp120, accessory protein negative factor Nef, matrix protein p17, transactivator of transcription Tat, and reverse transcriptase RT may promote malignant transformation, providing increasing support to potential direct carcinogenic effects of HIV.[51]

Effect of antiretroviral therapy

Some studies suggest a potential association between certain ART medicines and increased risk of specific cancers,[52] but such associations are generally not confirmed. ART exposure was not associated with increased risk of non-AIDS defining cancers, except for long-term use of protease inhibitors (PIs), which might be associated with increased anal cancer risk.[52] Interestingly, PIs have anti-angiogenic effect and induce regression of KS in animal models. In clinical practice both non-nucleoside reverse transcriptase inhibitor-based and PI-based regimens are equally effective in reducing incidence of KS.[53] Ongoing studies within the AIDS Malignancy Consortium (AMC) are evaluating the role of PIs for treating KS.

Behavioral and Lifestyle Factors

Tobacco, alcohol, obesity, lack of physical activity, and an unhealthy diet are all known cancer risk factors. Tobacco is responsible for one-fifth of the cancer burden of PWH in the US.[54] Tobacco use is consistently more common among PWH than in the general population worldwide.[42] The synergistic effect of HIV infection and tobacco accentuates the risk of cancer and contributes to the observed higher incidence of lung cancer in PWH. Smoking cessation interventions, therefore, are crucial in cancer prevention among PWH.[55]

Alcohol use disorder and increased alcohol use has been reported among PWH. Alcohol has been related to an increased risk of cancers such as liver and head and neck cancers. It also leads to worse cancer-related outcomes.[56]

Obesity has been reported to be less frequent among PWH in the US.[42] On the contrary, a study in women with HIV in South Africa showed a prevalence of 67.5% of obesity and overweight status.[57] Such regional variations likely reflect not only HIV-related issues, but also dietary and physical activity patterns worldwide. Overweight status and obesity have been increasing across multiple world regions since the advent of ART, in particular with greater use of integrase inhibitors and tenofovir alafenamide (TAF).

Finally, unprotected sexual practices and a higher number of sexual partners contribute to increased risk of oncogenic viral infections, emphasizing the importance of safe sex practices and regular screenings in PWH.

Health Care Disparities

While a comprehensive review of multilevel health care disparities globally is outside the scope of this review, it is important to note that disparities in access to health care services play a role in risk of cancer among PWH. For example, due to complex social, economic, and structural factors, PWH may have limited access to cancer screening (eg, cervical, anal) leading to delayed diagnoses and increased cancer morbidity and mortality. Access to timely HIV diagnosis and treatment and vaccines also play a role. Moreover, disparities significantly influence the complex and intersecting social, structural, behavioral, and lifestyle factors that affect cancer risk and outcomes for PWH as shown in **Fig. 1**.

SCREENING AND PREVENTION

Given the increasing lifespan of PWH along with increased cancer risk and burden, optimized cancer screening and prevention for this population has become critical. Considering that the highest burden of HIV is in LMICs, these settings present additional challenges in developing appropriate and cost-effective cancer prevention and screening strategies.

Vaccination and Treatment for Oncogenic Viruses

Vaccination is effective against HBV and HPV infection, and treatment is effective for HBV and HCV even after infection to reduce complications, including liver cirrhosis and cancer. Despite the wide availability of vaccines, there are 300 million people with chronic HBV infection worldwide. The World Health Organization (WHO) hepatitis elimination strategy includes 90% of infants vaccinated for HBV by 2030, 90% of viral hepatitis infections diagnosed, and 80% of viral hepatitis infections treated.[58] Because PWH have higher rates of HBV and HCV infection than individuals without HIV, several guidelines recommend testing of all PWH for HBV and HCV.[59,60] All PWH co-infected with HCV are candidates for curative treatment.[59,60] Direct-acting antiviral HCV regimens in PWH have shown the same efficacy and adverse events profile as in people without HIV. PWH with active HBV should receive an ART regimen that includes emtricitabine (follicular thyroid carcinoma) or lamivudine (3 TC), and tenofovir disoproxil fumarate (TDF) or TAF that are active against HIV and HBV.[59,60] Currently, the fixed dose combination of dolutegravir/TDF/3TC is the most frequent first line regimen used globally. In many LMICs, therefore, routine testing for HBV among PWH is not done since commonly prescribed ART regimens are effective for both HIV and HBV.

Many guidelines, especially from high- and upper-middle income countries, recommend HBV vaccination for PWH.[47,60] WHO recommends HBV vaccination of persons at high risk of HBV infection in older age groups including PWH.[61] Where HBV testing is available, it is recommended in order to identify those who are already immune and therefore, may not need vaccination. Although earlier studies showed a reduced response to HBV vaccination among PWH (35%–70%),[62] longer-term follow-up shows no difference between standard and booster doses.[61] There are currently no clear recommendations for routine booster vaccination among PWH and no information is available regarding lifelong protection in HIV-infected or HIV-exposed infants receiving HBV vaccination.[61]

The high burden of HPV, its persistence, and the elevated risk of HPV-related precancer and cancer among PWH,[42] support the need for targeted vaccination and screening against HPV-associated cancers in this population. Guidelines in high- and upper-middle income countries recommend HPV vaccination before the onset of sexual activity, and it is currently recommended to start vaccination at 11 to 12 years and extending through age 26 years. Catch-up vaccination is advised for all individuals aged 13 to 26 years who have not been vaccinated, and may be offered to older people in selected cases. Despite evidence supporting abbreviated 1-dose and 2-dose vaccination schedules,[63] the current recommendation for PWH is still a 3-dose schedule.[64] While the HPV vaccine is generally safe and well-tolerated by PWH,[65] those with lower CD4 counts (<200 cells/ml) and unsuppressed HIV may have lower seropositivity rates compared to those with well-controlled HIV.[66]

Global HPV vaccine uptake varies. Less than 25% to 30% of most LMICs have introduced the vaccine into national immunization schedules, compared to greater than 85% in high-income countries. Notably, there is no specific vaccine recommendation for women with HIV in the global strategy to accelerate the elimination of cervical cancer as a public health problem.[67] Additional challenges in LMIC include HPV vaccination programs being school-based, with HPV vaccination not being routinely offered for PWH outside childhood immunization programs.

Behavioral Risk Reduction

As noted previously, several behavioral cancer risk factors are more frequent among PWH. A systematic review evaluating smoking cessation interventions in PWH showed that the most successful approaches were tailored to the needs of PWH, including assessment of and intervention for polysubstance abuse and mental health issues, and use of cell phone-based strategies.[68] WHO recommends healthy lifestyle counseling, smoking cessation advice, healthy diet, and exercise among other modifiable factors for PWH to prevent non-communicable diseases.[69] Other factors such as exposure to UV radiation, or occupational hazards must also be considered (see **Fig. 1**).

Timely Human Immunodeficiency Virus Diagnosis and Treatment

The Strategic Timing of Antiretroviral Therapy study led to universal treatment recommendations for PWH, in part by demonstrating that the risk of cancer was higher among those who started ART with CD4 less than 350 cells per ml than for those starting with CD4 greater than 500 cells per ml.[70] PWH starting immediate ART reduced cancer risk by 64% compared to the deferred arm.[71] Current guidelines recommend that all PWH should start ART as soon as possible.[59,64,72]

Screening for Specific Cancer Sites

Cancer screening practices for PWH should address cancers with higher prevalence among PWH (cervical, anal, and liver cancer) but also cancers for which screening is recommended in the general population (breast, colon, and prostate). In **Table 3**, we have summarized current recommendations from various representative international guidelines regarding cancer screening among PWH, including recommendations extrapolated from the general population.

To provide a global perspective, we have included current guidelines and recommendations from the WHO, the United States Department of Health and Human Services, the European AIDS Clinical Society, along with representative countries from Africa, Latin America, and Asia.

As illustrated in **Table 3**, all guidelines recommend regular cervical cancer screening, with cytology still the most frequently recommended technique. Although WHO has recommended the transition to HPV DNA testing as the primary screening test for cervical cancer screening, visual inspection with acetic acid or cytology continue to be the primary screening tests in most LMIC settings,[87] although these are likely suboptimal.[88] Lack of access to cryotherapy, excision, or thermal ablation for preneoplastic lesions identified via screening is another major challenge in the control of cervical cancer in LMIC, as screening programs will have limited value if follow-up care for screen-positive women is not assured. Single-visit screen and treat approaches have, therefore, been recommended for low-resource settings.[89]

Table 3
Representative contemporary cancer screening guidelines for people with human immunodeficiency virus across different world regions

		DHHS[64] and USPSTF[79]	EACS[59]	WHO[72,74–76]	South Africa[77–79]	Kenya[80]	Thailand[81–83]	Brazil[84,85]
Cervix	Target populations	Women >21 y	Women >21 y	Women ≥ 25 y Children and adolescents after sexual debut	All women Children and adolescents after sexual debut	Women 18–65 y	Women	Women
	Method	21–29 y: Cytology >30 y: Cytology or Cytology + HPV DNA	Cytology HPV DNA	HPV DNA Alternative: Cytology or VIA	Cytology	HPV test VIA-VILI	Cytology	Cytology
	Frequency	1–3 y	1–3 y	3–5 y	At diagnosis and every 3 y	1–2 y	During the first y and once a y	Every 6 mo during first y; yearly afterwards, if normal
Anus	Target populations	People with HIV	MSM and persons with HPV-associated dysplasia	MSM, trans and gender diverse people and other people who are more likely to engage in anal sex			Anal sex	Receptive anal intercourse, prior HPV or abnormal vulvar or cervical histology
	Method	DRE Cytology (only if HRA is available) HRA (specialists recommendation)	DRE Cytology HRA	Cytology Skin anal and genital examination	Not stated	Not stated	Cytology	DRE Cytology Anoscopy if abnormal
	Frequency	1 y	1–3 y	Not mentioned			In the first y and once a y afterwards	1 y
Liver	Target populations	HIV/HBV > 40 y HIV/HCV, in particular if cirrhosis	HBV or HCV with cirrhosis if treatment available for HCC HBV- non-cirrhotics, consider risk factors	People with cirrhosis			People with cirrhosis, Men> 40 y or Female > 50 y or family history of liver cancer	Cirrhosis and HBV
	Method	Ultrasound	Ultrasound (and alphafetoprotein)	Not stated	Not stated	Not stated	Ultrasound and alphafetoprotein (HBV) Ultrasound (HCV + cirrhosis)	Ultrasound and alphafetoprotein
	Frequency	6 mo	6 mo	Not stated			6–12 mo	6 mo
Lung	Target populations	50–80 y with history of ≥ 20 pack-ye smoking and currently smoke or have quit within the past 15 y	50–80 y with history of ≥ 20 pack-y smoking, and are current smokers or former smokers that quit within the past 15 y	Not stated	Symptom-based work-up	Not stated	Not stated	No recommendations to screen for lung cancer. However, services should have a harm reduction policy and promote tobacco cessation.
	Method	Low-dose CT	Low-dose helical CT (where local screening programs are available)	Low dose helical CT WHO supports but no guidelines.[86]	Chest x-ray			
	Frequency	1 y (stop if > 15 y	1 y	Not stated	Not			

(continued on next page)

Table 3
(continued)

		after quitting or limited life expectancy)			applicable			
Breast	Target populations	Women (40) 50–74	Women 50–74 y	Not stated	Women >40 y	40–74 y	Women 30–70 y	Women 50–69 y
	Method	Mammography	Mammography	Mammography wherever available. Early detection programs prioritized	CBE	Mammography CBE if not available	30–70 y: BSE 40–70 y: CBE >45 y mammography	Mammography
	Frequency	2 y	1–3 y	2 y	2 y	1–2 y	2 y	2 y
Colorectal	Target populations	50–75 y (45–49 y moderate benefit)	Persons 50–75 y or with a life expectancy > 10 y	Not stated	Symptom-based work-up	40–75 y	50–70 y	50–70 y
	Method	Stool-based tests or Direct visualization tests	According to local screening program Colonoscopy FIT for occult blood, or MT-sDNA or CT colonography	Stool-based tests	Colonoscopy	FIT FOBT Colonoscopy	FIT	Stool based test or colonoscopy or sigmoidoscopy
	Frequency	Depending on method 1–10 y	Depending on method 1–10 y	Not stated	Not applicable	1 y (10 y if colonoscopy)	2 y	Not stated
Prostate	Target populations	55–69 y	Men > 50 y with a life expectancy >10 y		Symptom-based work-up	Men > 40 y		
	Method	PSA (to be discussed on a individual basis)	Use of PSA controversial	Not mentioned	DRE	PSA DRE if not available	Not mentioned	Not recommended
	Frequency	Periodic	1–2 y		Not applicable	1 y		

Guidelines or recommendations specific for PWH.   Guidelines or recommendations for the general population.

Abbreviations: BSE, breast self-examination; CBE, clinical breast examination; CT, computed tomography; DHHS, United States Department of Health and Human Services; DRE, digital rectal exam; EACS, European Academy of Cancer Sciences; FIT, fecal immunochemistry test; FOBT, fecal occult blood test; HBV, hepatitis B Virus; HCV, hepatitis C Virus; HPV, Human Papilomavirus; HRA, high-resolution anoscopy; MT-sDNA, multitarget stool DNA; PSA, prostate specific antigen; USPSTF, United States Preventive Services Task Force; Via, visual inspection with acetic acid; VILI, visual inspection with Lugol's iodine; WHO, World Health Organization.
Please see Refs.[59,64,72–86]

Timely detection and treatment of anal precancerous lesions was recently shown to reduce the risk of anal cancer for PWH.[90] Recently published consensus guidelines recommend anal cancer screening for populations at high risk of anal cancer.[91]

Despite PWH experiencing a lower risk of breast, prostate, and colorectal cancers in the US, and increased mortality after cancer diagnosis for PWH, recommended screening interventions for these cancers in the general population are generally extrapolated to PWH.[92]

Additionally, some as yet unproven cancer screening interventions might have value for PWH in certain settings. For example, skin cancer screening is not routinely recommended for the general population.[93] However, for PWH in endemic areas for KSHV or with very low CD4 counts, comprehensive skin examination for KS lesions integrated into routine HIV care might be a relatively simple and inexpensive method of reducing KS morbidity and mortality in settings with high burden. While rare in other settings, conjunctival cancer is particularly frequent in Africa with a risk 21 times higher in PWH.[94] Early-stage conjunctival lesions might be identified through routine external inspection in high-incidence settings despite not having been formally studied as a cancer screening intervention.

TREATMENT

Treatment of HIV-associated cancers is multifaceted. ART is an essential component, restoring immune function and reducing risk of infectious complications during cancer treatment. ART has enabled treatment of cancer in PWH to be similar in most instances to treatment of cancer in people without HIV, including with intensive curative-intent regimens. However, there are a few special considerations in PWH, including co-infections, drug-drug interactions (DDI), and diagnostic challenges.

Special Considerations or Departures from General Standards-of-Care

Co-management of human immunodeficiency virus and cancer

Co-management of HIV and cancer may result in better outcomes,[95] but management of HIV and cancer is often verticalized.[96,97] Greater integration of HIV and cancer care for PWH and cancer, including through physical co-location of services, can improve outcomes for PWH across the cancer prevention and treatment continuum.[55,98] For example, ART-naïve PWH whose first clinical presentation results from a new diagnosis of cancer may experience delays in initiating ART,[99] yet these delays can be successfully reduced using HIV and cancer co-management models. This is important because initiation or continuation of ART among PWH who have cancer improves cancer treatment outcomes. For example, PWH in LMIC with locally advanced cervical cancer receiving ART experience similar 5-year overall survival[100] and adverse effect rates[101] as those without HIV after curative-intent chemoradiation therapy. Similarly, PWH with lymphoma in LMICs experience significantly improved overall survival when ART is initiated soon after lymphoma diagnosis.

Supportive care

PWH receiving cancer therapies have a higher risk of opportunistic infections than HIV-negative cancer patients due to immunosuppression from both HIV and cancer therapies. As such, supportive care during cancer treatment for PWH requires careful consideration. As with PWH without cancer, prophylaxis against Pneumocystic jiroveci pneumonia and toxoplasmosis is recommended with CD4 counts less than 200 cells per uL and *Mycobacterium avium* complex prophylaxis for CD4 less than 50 cells per uL. Routine growth factor supports with granulocyte-colony stimulating factor may be indicated in some instances for PWH receiving chemotherapy even if not indicated for HIV-negative individuals, for example, with curative-intent ABVD chemotherapy for HL.[102]

Drug interactions

Older ART regimens have significant DDI, overlapping toxicities with cancer therapies, and adverse effects that precluded combination with chemotherapy. Fortunately, current ART regimens, such as those that include HIV integrase inhibitors, are well-tolerated and do not have significant DDI with common cancer therapies.[103] ART regimens boosted with cobicistat or ritonavir, as well as antifungals such as fluconazole, by strongly inhibiting CYP3A4, may increase toxicity of cancer chemotherapeutic agents that are metabolized by CYP3A4. This is especially well-documented with vinca alkaloid-containing treatment regimens such as ABVD for HL where neurotoxicity is worse when combined with ritonavir-based ART.[104,105] Some chemotherapeutic agents used for treatment of lung cancer (eg, platinum agents) may need to be used with caution, with close monitoring of renal function, in PWH due to potential for additive renal toxicity when combined with ART containing tenofovir. Notably, newer cancer therapies may be associated with increased risk of opportunistic infections. For example, use of the Bruton tyrosine kinase inhibitor (TKI) ibrutinib in cancer treatment has been associated with increased risk of serious infections, including invasive fungal infections such as aspergillosis.[106] This risk is higher in patients already predisposed to invasive fungal infections such as PWH.[107] Finally, for PWH receiving hematopoietic stem-cell transplants, teams will need to include experts in HIV care for close monitoring of pharmacologic interactions between post-transplant immunosuppression and ART. Important DDI between cancer therapies and ART are summarized in **Table 4** as follows.

Specific Cancers for Which Management May Depart from General Standards-of-Care

Kaposi sarcoma
ART alone may be sufficient for limited KS. In PWH with advanced stage KS, addition of chemotherapy to ART improves survival and is considered the standard-of-care.[108] Liposomal doxorubicin is commonly used as the first-line chemotherapy option and has shown efficacy in treating KS in PWH while minimizing toxicity. Paclitaxel has also shown efficacy in treating advanced KS and is also an option, although with more toxicity that liposomal doxorubicin.[109] Importantly, in the ART era, single-agent paclitaxel showed superiority to oral etoposide and bleomycin or vincristine regimens in resource-limited settings,[110] and may be preferred to liposomal doxorubicin due to lower cost.[111] Pomalidomide, an oral immunomodulatory drug, is also now approved by the US Food and Drug Administration (FDA) for KS treatment,[112] and may be particularly attractive for use in LMICs as it does not require visits to a

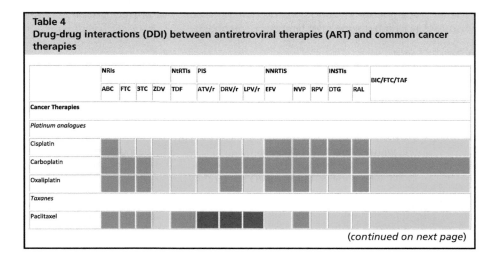

Table 4
Drug-drug interactions (DDI) between antiretroviral therapies (ART) and common cancer therapies

	NRIs				NtRTIs	PIS			NNRTIS			INSTIs		BIC/FTC/TAF
	ABC	FTC	3TC	ZDV	TDF	ATV/r	DRV/r	LPV/r	EFV	NVP	RPV	DTG	RAL	
Cancer Therapies														
Platinum analogues														
Cisplatin														
Carboplatin														
Oxaliplatin														
Taxanes														
Paclitaxel														

(continued on next page)

Table 4
(continued)

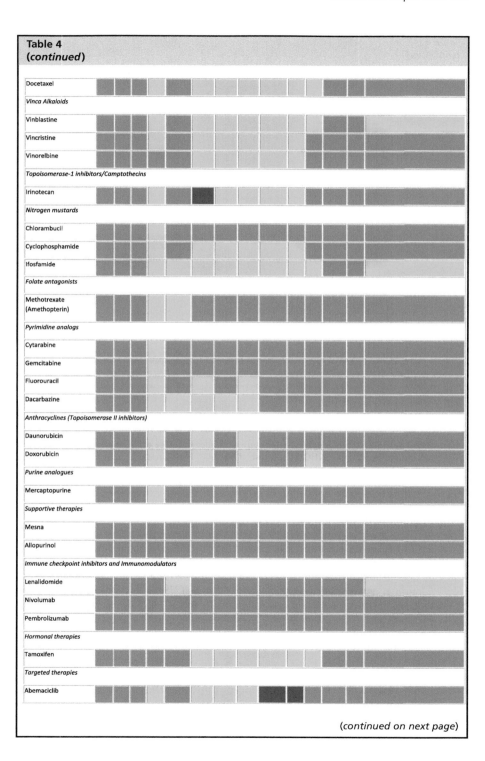

(continued on next page)

Table 4
(continued)

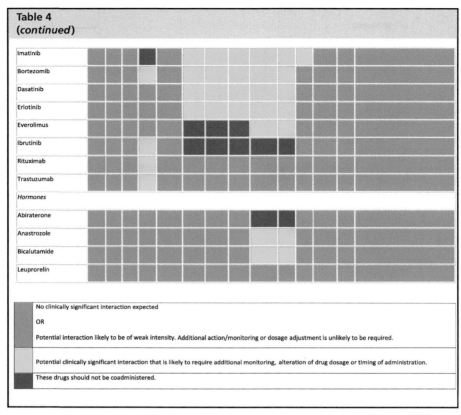

	No clinically significant interaction expected
	OR
	Potential interaction likely to be of weak intensity. Additional action/monitoring or dosage adjustment is unlikely to be required.
	Potential clinically significant interaction that is likely to require additional monitoring, alteration of drug dosage or timing of administration.
	These drugs should not be coadministered.

Adapted and modified from WHO HIV treatment guidelines, Rudek et al., University of Liverpool hiv-druginteractions.org tool, WHO Model List of Essential Medicines.

chemotherapy clinic for intravenous infusion. Recently, immune checkpoint inhibitors (ICI) (eg, pembrolizumab) have shown promise in treating advanced KS.[113]

Hodgkin lymphoma and non-Hodgkin lymphoma
While ART has lowered the incidence of some virus-associated cancers (KS, NHL),[19] in the era of ART scale-up there has been a significant increase in the fraction of HL among all lymphomas in Africa.[114] There has also been increased incidence of HL observed in the first 3 months of ART, likely triggered by immune reconstitution.[115] HL in general is associated with declines in CD4-cell,[116] likely due to sequestration of these cells in the tumor microenvironment. In PWH, HL risk increases with low CD4 cell counts less than 100 cells per μL.[115] Therefore, consideration should be given for routine growth factor support when treating HL among PWH with regimens such as ABVD, although not typically considered for people without HIV. In addition, dose reductions may be necessary for PWH with HL who experience prolonged neutropenia with ABVD. In cases of relapsed or refractory HL, both autologous and allogeneic stem cell transplants are safe in PWH, as in people without HIV. There is an emerging role for use of immunotherapy for HL in the first and subsequent lines, although research specifically for PWH is ongoing.[117]

NHLs that occur in PWH tend to be aggressive and are often associated with EBV or KSHV, including diffuse large B-cell lymphoma, Burkitt lymphoma, primary central nervous system lymphoma, primary effusion lymphoma, and plasmablastic lymphoma.[118] The infusional dose-adjusted EPOCH chemotherapy regimen has demonstrated particularly good results for most aggressive systemic NHL subtypes among PWH and is the typical backbone used in clinical trials conducted by the AMC. Pembrolizumab, an ICI, has shown particular promise in treating HIV-associated NHL caused by oncogenic viruses, despite general lack of efficacy for NHL in the general population.[119] Chimeric antigen receptor T-cells (CAR-Ts) have been successfully used to treat lymphoma in PWH similar to the general population.[120]

Non-small cell lung cancer

People with HIV have higher risk of lung-cancer specific mortality and all-cause mortality than those without HIV, even adjusting for cancer stage, treatment, and health care-related factors such as treating cancer facility and type of health insurance.[121,122] The underlying mechanisms for this elevated risk are unclear.

Targeted therapies (eg, TKIs against EGFR, ALK, ROS1) have greatly improved outcomes for patients with lung cancer harboring targetable genetic alterations. Data about DDI between targeted TKI therapies for lung cancer and ART are sparse, but in general support avoidance of concomitant CYP3A4 inhibiting ARTs (eg, PIs) and the need for multidisciplinary care.[123–125]

ICI have revolutionized the treatment of lung cancer and are as safe and efficacious in PWH who are on suppressive ART as in people without HIV.[126–128]

Application of Novel Therapies

Immunotherapy, cellular therapy, and immunomodulatory drugs

Classical cancer treatments such as chemotherapy and radiotherapy are often more difficult to apply in PWH due to worsening CD4 counts, myelosuppression, and infectious risks that may result in increased treatment-related morbidity and mortality.[129] Conversely, immunotherapy shows promise in harnessing the immune system to combat both HIV and cancer without worsening immunosuppression. PWH have disproportionately higher risk of many cancers for which ICIs are currently approved. Immune checkpoints such as PD-1 and CTLA4 are upregulated in PWH as a result of persistent immune stimulation by chronic HIV infection and, in those with virus-associated cancers (eg, KS, NHL, cervical cancer, HCC), chronic viral stimulation, both of which lead to T-cell exhaustion and impairment of their killing function. ICIs are safe in PWH receiving ART with CD4 counts above 100 cells per uL.[113,128,130] In fact, among patients with advanced cancer enrolled into trials of ICIs, PWH have similar baseline CD4 counts as HIV-negative patients, and these low CD4 counts neither increase the risk of treatment-related adverse events nor lower survival after receiving immunotherapy.[127] Pembrolizumab, an ICI, has shown particular promise in treating HIV-associated NHL,[119] and KS.[113]

The immunomodulatory drug, pomalidomide, is associated with reduced downregulation or increased cell surface expression of MHC-1 in cells infected by the oncogenic viruses KSHV, HTLV-1, and EBV.[131] Pomalidomide has been shown to be particularly effective in treatment of KS, which is caused by KSHV, and is currently approved by the US FDA for this indication.[112] Ongoing studies show promise for the combination of pomalidomide with ICIs to treat virus-associated cancers in PWH.[119]

Implications and opportunities for cure of both human immunodeficiency virus and cancer

Allogeneic hematopoietic stem cell transplantation using suitable donor stem cells in PWH with hematological malignancies such as acute myeloid leukemia and HL can result in long-term remission with potential for cure of both conditions.[132,133] However, the logistical and cost implications make it likely unsuitable for large scale adoption. CAR-Ts have been successfully used to treat lymphoma in PWH,[120] and offer promise for targeting HIV cure.[134] Interestingly, even though CAR-Ts have revolutionized treatment of relapsed lymphoma, they were originally developed in search of HIV cure. More recently, the ICI pembrolizumab has been shown to reverse the latency of HIV and might provide insights and opportunities that are informative to ongoing HIV cure efforts.[135]

Clinical Trials

Clinical trials usually offer the best cancer treatment options.[102] However, PWH are often excluded from cancer clinical trials. The American Society of Clinical Oncology and the US National Institutes of Health (NIH) both support the inclusion of PWH in cancer clinical trials.[136,137] However, where PWH are included, there are usually arbitrary CD4 count thresholds for eligibility. Emerging research shows that among people with relapsed and refractory cancers, CD4 counts are similar between PWH and people without HIV.[138] Moreover, for those who are enrolled in clinical trials of immunotherapy, there is no significant association between low CD4 counts less than 350 cells per μL and either the proportion of adverse events or overall survival in both people with and without HIV.[127] Real-world data further show that the use of ICIs in PWH does not increase toxicity.[126] Therefore, PWH should be included in clinical trials of immunotherapy without regard to CD4 count thresholds. A recent assessment by the National Cancer Institute's Cancer Therapy Evaluation Program found that there is increasing intention to include PWH in cancer immunotherapy trials, but that actual inclusion in trial protocols remains unchanged.[139]

Reflecting this need for rigorous clinical trials to inform cancer treatment and prevention among PWH, including in LMICs where HIV-associated malignancies burden is high, it is important to note efforts like the AMC. AMC is an NIH-sponsored network to study cancer and precancer pathobiology and to evaluate new treatment and prevention approaches among PWH, first launched in 1995. Initially limited to the US, it has more recently expanded internationally to include Africa and Latin America. This consortium has contributed significantly to advancements in prevention and treatment of cancer in PWH.[140]

IMPLEMENTATION SCIENCE

Finally, as new cancer control interventions become available, implementation science enables contextual adaptation to ensure relevance and feasibility. Because different populations of PWH have cultural nuances, implementation science provides a framework for tailoring interventions in ways that respect their beliefs, attitudes, and practices. Implementation science methodologies also facilitate the systematic evaluation of barriers and facilitators to adoption of cancer control interventions, thereby enabling development of targeted strategies. Application of implementation science principles to cancer control in PWH also ensures that the perspectives and experiences of all stakeholders are considered in the design and execution of cancer control interventions. Particularly in LMICs, implementation science can allow comprehensive and coordinated cancer control efforts to effectively leverage the existing strong HIV infrastructure.

SUMMARY

The complex interplay between HIV and cancer requires a holistic approach that transcends traditional disease boundaries. Collaboration between infectious disease specialists, oncologists, and public health experts is paramount to comprehensively address the continued challenges posed by HIV-associated cancers even in the ART era, toward improving outcomes for PWH worldwide. (see **Table 2**)

CLINICS CARE POINTS

- Many factors contribute to a continued increased cancer risk among PWH globally, despite advancements in ART.
- Behavioral, vaccination, and screening interventions are currently available to reduce cancer risk and should be integrated into routine health care, alongside continued research and tailoring to meet the diverse needs of PWH globally.
- PWH diagnosed with cancer can often be treated similarly to people without HIV in the ART era – including with novel cancer therapies and in clinical trials – but unique treatment challenges and opportunities remain among PWH.
- Collaborative multidisciplinary efforts, leveraging implementation science, are critical for continued progress against cancer in PWH, especially in parts of the world with the greatest burden of HIV.

DISCLOSURE

T.A. Odeny received grant funding from Gilead Sciences. V. Fink participated as speaker and expert discussant for MSD. The opinions expressed in this article are the authors own and do not reflect the view of the NIH, the Department of Health and Human Services, or the United States Government.

REFERENCES

1. Beyrer C, Baral SD, Weir BW, et al. A call to action for concentrated HIV epidemics. Curr Opin HIV AIDS 2014;9(2):95–100.
2. Musumari PM, Techasrivichien T, Srithanaviboonchai K, et al. HIV epidemic in fishing communities in Uganda: A scoping review. PLoS One 2021;16(4): e0249465.
3. Key Populations - Eswatini National AIDS Program. 2023. Available at: http://swaziaidsprogram.org/key-populations/.
4. Simbayi LC, Zuma K, Zungu N, Moyo S, Marinda E, Jooste S, Mabaso M, Ramlagan S, North A, van Zyl J, Mohlabane N, Dietrich C, Team NlatSV. South African National HIV Prevalence, Incidence, Behaviour and Communication Survey, 2017. Cape Town: HSRC Press; 2019.
5. Suneja G, Coghill A. Cancer care disparities in people with HIV in the United States. Curr Opin HIV AIDS 2017;12(1):63–8.
6. Trickey A, McGinnis K, Gill MJ, et al. Longitudinal trends in causes of death among adults with HIV on antiretroviral therapy in Europe and North America from 1996 to 2020: a collaboration of cohort studies. Lancet HIV 2024;11(3): e176–85.
7. Weber MSR, Duran Ramirez JJ, Hentzien M, et al. Time trends in causes of death in people with human immunodeficiency virus: insights from the swiss HIV cohort study. Clin Infect Dis 2024. https://doi.org/10.1093/cid/ciae014.
8. 1993 revised classification system for HIV infection and expanded surveillance case definition for AIDS among adolescents and adults. MMWR Recomm Rep (Morb Mortal Wkly Rep) 1992;41(Rr-17):1–19.

9. Yarchoan R, Uldrick T, Polizzotto M. Cancers in people with HIV and AIDS. Springer; 2014.

10. Sengayi-Muchengeti M, Singh E, Chen WC, et al. Thirteen cancers associated with HIV infection in a Black South African cancer patient population (1995-2016). Int J Cancer 2023;152(2):183–94.

11. Tanon A, Jaquet A, Ekouevi DK, et al. The spectrum of cancers in West Africa: associations with human immunodeficiency virus. PLoS One 2012;7(10): e48108.

12. Dal Maso L, Polesel J, Serraino D, et al. Pattern of cancer risk in persons with AIDS in Italy in the HAART era. Br J Cancer 2009;100(5):840–7.

13. Mbulaiteye SM, Katabira ET, Wabinga H, et al. Spectrum of cancers among HIV-infected persons in Africa: the Uganda AIDS-Cancer Registry Match Study. Int J Cancer 2006;118(4):985–90.

14. Stein L, Urban MI, O'Connell D, et al. The spectrum of human immunodeficiency virus-associated cancers in a South African black population: results from a case-control study, 1995-2004. Int J Cancer 2008;122(10):2260–5.

15. Clifford GM, Polesel J, Rickenbach M, et al. Cancer risk in the Swiss HIV Cohort Study: associations with immunodeficiency, smoking, and highly active antiretroviral therapy. J Natl Cancer Inst 2005;97(6):425–32.

16. Godbole SV, Nandy K, Gauniyal M, et al. HIV and cancer registry linkage identifies a substantial burden of cancers in persons with HIV in India. Medicine (Baltim) 2016;95(37):e4850.

17. Dhokotera T, Bohlius J, Spoerri A, et al. The burden of cancers associated with HIV in the South African public health sector, 2004-2014: a record linkage study. Infect Agent Cancer 2019;14:12.

18. Akarolo-Anthony SN, Maso LD, Igbinoba F, et al. Cancer burden among HIV-positive persons in Nigeria: preliminary findings from the Nigerian AIDS-cancer match study. Infect Agent Cancer 2014;9(1):1.

19. Hernández-Ramírez RU, Shiels MS, Dubrow R, et al. Cancer risk in HIV-infected people in the USA from 1996 to 2012: a population-based, registry-linkage study. Lancet HIV 2017;4(11):e495–504.

20. Jaquet A, Odutola M, Ekouevi DK, et al. Cancer and HIV infection in referral hospitals from four West African countries. Cancer Epidemiol 2015;39(6):1060–5.

21. Ruffieux Y, Muchengeti M, Egger M, et al. Immunodeficiency and Cancer in 3.5 Million People Living With Human Immunodeficiency Virus (HIV): The South African HIV Cancer Match Study. Clin Infect Dis 2021;73(3):e735–44.

22. Greenberg L, Ryom L, Bakowska E, et al. Trends in cancer incidence in different antiretroviral treatment-eras amongst people with HIV. Cancers 2023;(14):15.

23. Bray F, Jemal A, Grey N, et al. Global cancer transitions according to the Human Development Index (2008-2030): a population-based study. Lancet Oncol 2012; 13(8):790–801.

24. Haas CB, Engels EA, Horner MJ, et al. Trends and risk of lung cancer among people living with HIV in the USA: a population-based registry linkage study. Lancet HIV 2022;9(10):e700–8.

25. Shiels MS, Islam JY, Rosenberg PS, et al. Projected cancer incidence rates and burden of incident cancer cases in hiv-infected adults in the United States Through 2030. Ann Intern Med 2018;168(12):866–73.

26. International Agency for Research on Cancer. IARC monographs on the identification of carcinogenic hazards to humans. IARC Monogr Meet 2019;124:1–4.

27. Isaguliants M, Bayurova E, Avdoshina D, et al. Oncogenic Effects of HIV-1 Proteins, Mechanisms Behind. Cancers 2021;13(2).

28. A cluster of Kaposi's sarcoma and Pneumocystis carinii pneumonia among homosexual male residents of Los Angeles and Orange Counties, California. MMWR Morb Mortal Wkly Rep 1982;31(23):305–7.

29. zur Hausen H. Papillomaviruses in the causation of human cancers - a brief historical account. Virology 2009;384(2):260–5.

30. Gallo RC, Montagnier L. The discovery of HIV as the cause of AIDS. N Engl J Med 2003;349(24):2283–5.

31. Blumberg BS. The discovery of the hepatitis B virus and the invention of the vaccine: a scientific memoir. J Gastroenterol Hepatol 2002;17(Suppl):S502–3.

32. Powderly WG. Zidovudine. Mo Med 1989;86(11):741–3.

33. Houghton M. Discovery of the hepatitis C virus. Liver Int 2009;29(Suppl 1):82–8.

34. Agut H, Calvez V, Fillet AM, et al. [The discovery of three novel human viruses, human herpesviruses 6, 7, and 8]. Bull Acad Natl Med Jun-Jul 1997;181(6): 1009–22. La découverte de trois nouveaux virus humains, les herpèsvirus humains 6, 7 et 8.

35. Muñoz N, Castellsagué X, Berrington de González A, et al. Chapter 1: HPV in the etiology of human cancer. Vaccine 2006;24(Suppl 3):S3/1–10.

36. Shuda M, Arora R, Kwun HJ, et al. Human Merkel cell polyomavirus infection I. MCV T antigen expression in Merkel cell carcinoma, lymphoid tissues and lymphoid tumors. Int J Cancer 2009;125(6):1243–9.

37. Yu H, Robertson ES. Epstein-Barr Virus History and Pathogenesis. Viruses 2023;15(3).

38. Chang Y, Cesarman E, Pessin MS, et al. Identification of herpesvirus-like DNA sequences in AIDS-associated Kaposi's sarcoma. Science 1994;266(5192): 1865–9.

39. Cesarman E, Chang Y, Moore PS, et al. Kaposi's Sarcoma–Associated Herpesvirus-Like DNA Sequences in AIDS-Related Body-Cavity–Based Lymphomas. N Engl J Med 1995;332(18):1186–91.

40. Soulier J, Grollet L, Oksenhendler E, et al. Kaposi's Sarcoma-Associated Herpesvirus-Like DNA Sequences in Multicentric Castleman's Disease. Blood 1995/08/15/1995;86(4):1276–80.

41. Workowski KA, Bachmann LH, Chan PA, et al. Sexually transmitted infections treatment guidelines, 2021. MMWR Recomm Rep (Morb Mortal Wkly Rep) 2021;70(4):1–187.

42. Park LS, Hernández-Ramírez RU, Silverberg MJ, et al. Prevalence of non-HIV cancer risk factors in persons living with HIV/AIDS: a meta-analysis. Aids 2016;30(2):273–91.

43. Patel P, Hanson DL, Sullivan PS, et al. Incidence of types of cancer among HIV-infected persons compared with the general population in the United States, 1992-2003. Ann Intern Med 2008;148(10):728–36.

44. Stelzle D, Tanaka LF, Lee KK, et al. Estimates of the global burden of cervical cancer associated with HIV. Lancet Glob Health 2021;9(2):e161–9.

45. Silverberg MJ, Lau B, Justice AC, et al. Risk of anal cancer in HIV-infected and HIV-uninfected individuals in North America. Clin Infect Dis 2012;54(7):1026–34.

46. Global progress report on HIV, viral hepatitis and sexually transmitted infections, 2021: Accountability for the global health sector strategies 2016–2021: actions for impact. Geneva: World Health Organization; 2021. ISBN: 978-92-4-002707-7.

47. Sherman KE, Peters MG, Thomas DL. HIV and the liver. Top Antivir Med 2019; 27(3):101–10.

48. Dubrow R, Silverberg MJ, Park LS, et al. HIV infection, aging, and immune function: implications for cancer risk and prevention. Curr Opin Oncol 2012;24(5): 506–16.

49. Goncalves PH, Montezuma-Rusca JM, Yarchoan R, et al. Cancer prevention in HIV-infected populations. Semin Oncol 2016;43(1):173–88.

50. Appay V, Sauce D. Immune activation and inflammation in HIV-1 infection: causes and consequences. J Pathol 2008;214(2):231–41.

51. Borges AH, Dubrow R, Silverberg MJ. Factors contributing to risk for cancer among HIV-infected individuals, and evidence that earlier combination antiretroviral therapy will alter this risk. Curr Opin HIV AIDS 2014;9(1):34–40.

52. Chao C, Leyden WA, Xu L, et al. Exposure to antiretroviral therapy and risk of cancer in HIV-infected persons. Aids 2012;26(17):2223–31.

53. Borges ÁH. Combination antiretroviral therapy and cancer risk. Curr Opin HIV AIDS 2017;12(1):12–9.

54. Altekruse SF, Shiels MS, Modur SP, et al. Cancer burden attributable to cigarette smoking among HIV-infected people in North America. Aids 2018;32(4):513–21.

55. Parascandola M, Neta G, Bloch M, et al. Colliding epidemics: research gaps and implementation science opportunities for tobacco use and HIV/AIDS in low- and middle-income Countries. J Smok Cessat 2022;2022:6835146.

56. Williams EC, Hahn JA, Saitz R, et al. Alcohol Use and Human Immunodeficiency Virus (HIV) Infection: Current Knowledge, Implications, and Future Directions. Alcohol Clin Exp Res 2016;40(10):2056–72.

57. Hanley S, Moodley D, Naidoo M. Obesity in young South African women living with HIV: A cross-sectional analysis of risk factors for cardiovascular disease. PLoS One 2021;16(11):e0255652.

58. Interim guidance for country validation of viral hepatitis elimination. Geneva: World Health Organization; 2021. ISBN: 978-92-4-002839-5.

59. Ambrosioni J, Levi L, Alagaratnam J, et al. Major revision version 12.0 of the European AIDS Clinical Society guidelines 2023. HIV Med 2023. https://doi.org/10.1111/hiv.13542.

60. Gandhi RT, Bedimo R, Hoy JF, et al. Antiretroviral drugs for treatment and prevention of HIV infection in adults: 2022 Recommendations of the International Antiviral Society–USA Panel. JAMA 2023;329(1):63–84.

61. World Health Organization. Hepatitis B vaccines: WHO position paper-July 2017. Wkly Epidemiol Rec 2017;92(27):369–92.

62. Farooq PD, Sherman KE. Hepatitis B Vaccination and Waning Hepatitis B Immunity in Persons Living with HIV. Curr HIV AIDS Rep 2019;16(5):395–403.

63. Palefsky JM. Human papillomavirus-associated anal and cervical cancers in HIV-infected individuals: incidence and prevention in the antiretroviral therapy era. Curr Opin HIV AIDS 2017;12(1):26–30.

64. Hepatitis B vaccines: WHO position paper – July 2017. Wkly Epidemiol Rec. 2017;92(27):369-92. Epub 20170707. PubMed PMID: 28685564.

65. Losada C, Samaha H, Scherer EM, et al. Efficacy and durability of immune response after receipt of HPV vaccines in people living with HIV. Vaccines (Basel) 2023;11(6).

66. Ghebre RG, Grover S, Xu MJ, et al. Cervical cancer control in HIV-infected women: Past, present and future. Gynecol Oncol Rep 2017;21:101–8.

67. Global strategy to accelerate the elimination of cervical cancer as a public health problem. Geneva: World Health Organization; 2020. ISBN: 978-92-4-001410-7.

68. Moscou-Jackson G, Commodore-Mensah Y, Farley J, et al. Smoking-cessation interventions in people living with HIV infection: a systematic review. J Assoc Nurses AIDS Care Jan-Feb 2014;25(1):32–45.

69. World Health Organization. Scoping consultation on noncommunicable diseases and mental health conditions in people living with HIV: meeting report. Geneva, Switzerland: Global Health Campus; 9-10 2019. 2021.

70. Lundgren JD, Babiker AG, Gordin F, et al. Initiation of antiretroviral therapy in early asymptomatic HIV infection. N Engl J Med 2015;373(9):795–807.

71. Borges ÁH, Neuhaus J, Babiker AG, et al. Immediate antiretroviral therapy reduces risk of infection-related cancer during early HIV infection. Clin Infect Dis 2016;63(12):1668–76.

72. Consolidated guidelines on HIV prevention, testing, treatment, service delivery and monitoring: recommendations for a public health approach. Geneva: World Health Organization; 2021. ISBN: 978-92-4-003159-3.

73. United States Preventive Services Task Force. 2024. Available at: https://www.uspreventiveservicestaskforce.org/uspstf/search_results?searchterm=cancerscreening.

74. Guidance for country validation of viral hepatitis elimination and path to elimination: technical report. Geneva: World Health Organization; 2023. ISBN: 978-92-4-007863-5.

75. World Health Organization. Global Breast Cancer Initiative Implementation Framework: assessing, strengthening and scaling-up of services for the early detection and management of breast cancer. Geneva: World Health Organization; 2023.

76. World Health Organization. Colorectal cancer. 2023. Available at: https://www.who.int/news-room/fact-sheets/detail/colorectal-cancer.

77. Republic of South Africa National Department of Health. 2023 ART Clinical Guidelines for the Management of HIV in Adults, Pregnancy and Breastfeeding, Adolescents, Children, Infants and Neonates. 2023. Available at: https://knowledgehub.health.gov.za/elibrary/2023-art-clinical-guidelines-management-hiv-adults-pregnancy-and-breastfeeding-adolescents.

78. Breast Cancer Prevention and Control Policy: Department of Health Republic of South Africa; 2017. Available at: https://knowledgehub.health.gov.za/system/files/elibdownloads/2023-04/Breast-Cancer-Policy-2017.pdf. Accessed July 11, 2024.

79. Symptom-based integrated approach to the adult in primary care.: Department of Health, Republic of South Africa; 2023. Available at: https://knowledgehub.health.gov.za/system/files/elibdownloads/2023-10/APC_2023_Clinical_tool-PRINT.pdf. Accessed July 11, 2024.

80. National AIDS & STI Control Program. Kenya HIV Prevention and Treatment Guidelines, 2022. Available at: https://www.differentiatedservicedelivery.org/wp-content/uploads/Kenya-ARV-Guidelines-2022-Final-1.pdf. Accessed July 10, 2024

81. Ruxrungtham KCK, Chetchotisakd P, Chariyalertsak S, et al. Thailand National Guidelines on HIV/AIDS Treatment and Prevention 2021/2022. Division of AIDS and STIs, Department of Disease Control. Available at: https://www.prepthai.net/Paper/HIVAIDS_Guidelines.pdf.

82. Insamran W, Sangrajrang S. National Cancer Control Program of Thailand. Asian Pac J Cancer Prev 2020;21(3):577–82.

83. Cancer screening tests provided to Thais. 2023. Available at: https://eng.nhso. go.th/view/1/DescriptionNews/Cancer-screening-tests-provided-to-Thais/415/ EN-US.

84. Protocolo clínico e diretrizes terapêuticas para manejo da infecção pelo hiv em adultos. Ministério da Saúde. Secretaria de Vigilância em Saúde. Departamento de Vigilância. Prevenção e Controle das Infecções Sexualmente. Transmissíveis. do HIV/Aids e das Hepatites Virais. Available at: https://www.gov.br/aids/ pt-br/central-de-conteudo/pcdts/2013/hiv-aids/pcdt_manejo_adulto_12_2018_ web.pdf/@@download/file. Accessed July 11, 2024.

85. Detecção precoce do câncer Instituto Nacional de Câncer José Alencar Gomes da Silva; 2021. Available at: https://www.inca.gov.br/sites/ufu.sti.inca.local/files/ media/document/deteccao-precoce-do-cancer.pdf. Accessed July 11, 2024.

86. World Health Organization. Lung Cancer. 2023. Available at: https://www.who. int/news-room/fact-sheets/detail/lung-cancer.

87. WHO guideline for screening and treatment of cervical pre-cancer lesions for cervical cancer prevention. Geneva: World Health Organization; 2021. ISBN: 978 92 4 003082 4.

88. Asangbeh-Kerman SL, Davidović M, Taghavi K, et al. Cervical cancer prevention in countries with the highest HIV prevalence: a review of policies. BMC Publ Health 2022;22(1):1530.

89. Shin MB, Liu G, Mugo N, et al. A framework for cervical cancer elimination in low-and-middle-income countries: a scoping review and roadmap for interventions and research priorities. Front Public Health 2021;9:670032.

90. Palefsky JM, Lee JY, Jay N, et al. Treatment of anal high-grade squamous intraepithelial lesions to prevent anal cancer. N Engl J Med 2022;386(24):2273–82.

91. Stier EA, Clarke MA, Deshmukh AA, et al. International Anal Neoplasia Society's consensus guidelines for anal cancer screening. Int J Cancer 2024;154(10): 1694–702.

92. Horner MJ, Gopal S. Opportunities to understand unique cancer risks in global HIV-infected populations. J Natl Cancer Inst 2018;110(9):923–4.

93. Henrikson NB, Ivlev I, Blasi PR, et al. Skin cancer screening: updated evidence report and systematic review for the US Preventive Services Task Force. JAMA 2023;329(15):1296–307.

94. Muchengeti M, Bohlius J, Dhokotera TG. Conjunctival cancer in people living with HIV. Curr Opin Infect Dis 2021;34(1):1–7.

95. Burger H, Ismail Z, Taljaard JJ. Establishing a multidisciplinary AIDS-associated Kaposi's sarcoma clinic: Patient characteristics, management and outcomes. S Afr Med J 2018;108(12):1059–65.

96. Ehrenkranz P, Grimsrud A, Holmes CB, et al. Expanding the Vision for Differentiated Service Delivery: A Call for More Inclusive and Truly Patient-Centered Care for People Living With HIV. J Acquir Immune Defic Syndr 2021;86(2): 147–52.

97. Marquez PV, Farrington JL. No more disease silos for sub-Saharan Africa. Bmj 2012;345:e5812.

98. Sivaram S, Sanchez MA, Rimer BK, et al. Implementation science in cancer prevention and control: a framework for research and programs in low- and middle-income countries. Cancer Epidemiol Biomarkers Prev 2014;23(11):2273–84.

99. Oseso LN, Chiao EY, Bender Ignacio RA. Evaluating Antiretroviral Therapy Initiation in HIV-Associated Malignancy: Is There Enough Evidence to Inform Clinical Guidelines? J Natl Compr Canc Netw 2018;16(8):927–32.

100. MacDuffie E, Bvochora-Nsingo M, Chiyapo S, et al. Five-year overall survival following chemoradiation therapy for locally advanced cervical carcinoma in women living with and without HIV infection in Botswana. Infect Agent Cancer 2021;16(1):55.

101. Grover S, Bvochora-Nsingo M, Yeager A, et al. Impact of human immunodeficiency virus infection on survival and acute toxicities from chemoradiation therapy for cervical cancer patients in a limited-resource setting. Int J Radiat Oncol Biol Phys 2018;101(1):201–10.

102. Reid E, Suneja G, Ambinder RF, et al. Cancer in People Living With HIV, Version 1.2018, NCCN Clinical Practice Guidelines in Oncology. J Natl Compr Canc Netw 2018;16(8):986–1017.

103. Yang J, Wei G, Gui F, et al. Safety and efficacy of pharmacotherapy containing INSTIs and chemotherapy drugs in people living with HIV and concomitant colorectal cancer. AIDS Res Ther 2022;19(1):45.

104. Rubinstein PG, Braik T, Jain S, et al. Ritonavir Based Highly Active Retroviral Therapy (HAART) Correlates with Early Neurotoxicity When Combined with ABVD Treated HIV Associated Hodgkin Lymphoma but Not Non-Hodgkin Lymphoma. A Retrospective Study. Blood 2010/11/19/2010;116(21):2807.

105. Ezzat HM, Cheung MC, Hicks LK, et al. Incidence, predictors and significance of severe toxicity in patients with human immunodeficiency virus-associated Hodgkin lymphoma. Leuk Lymphoma 2012;53(12):2390–6.

106. Varughese T, Taur Y, Cohen N, et al. Serious infections in patients receiving ibrutinib for treatment of lymphoid cancer. Clin Infect Dis 2018;67(5):687–92.

107. Ghez D, Calleja A, Protin C, et al. Early-onset invasive aspergillosis and other fungal infections in patients treated with ibrutinib. Blood 2018;131(17):1955–9.

108. Ramaswami R, Lurain K, Yarchoan R. Oncologic Treatment of HIV-Associated Kaposi Sarcoma 40 Years on. J Clin Oncol 2022;40(3):294–306.

109. Cianfrocca M, Lee S, Von Roenn J, et al. Randomized trial of paclitaxel versus pegylated liposomal doxorubicin for advanced human immunodeficiency virus-associated Kaposi sarcoma: evidence of symptom palliation from chemotherapy. Cancer 2010;116(16):3969–77.

110. Krown SE, Moser CB, MacPhail P, et al. Treatment of advanced AIDS-associated Kaposi sarcoma in resource-limited settings: a three-arm, open-label, randomised, non-inferiority trial. Lancet 2020;395(10231):1195–207.

111. Raimundo K, Biskupiak J, Goodman M, et al. Cost effectiveness of liposomal doxorubicin vs. paclitaxel for the treatment of advanced AIDS-Kaposi's sarcoma. J Med Econ 2013;16(5):606–13.

112. Ramaswami R, Polizzotto MN, Lurain K, et al. Safety, activity, and long-term outcomes of pomalidomide in the treatment of Kaposi sarcoma among individuals with or without HIV Infection. Clin Cancer Res 2022;28(5):840–50.

113. Uldrick TS, Gonçalves PH, Abdul-Hay M, et al. Assessment of the safety of pembrolizumab in patients with HIV and advanced cancer-a phase 1 study. JAMA Oncol 2019;5(9):1332–9.

114. Vaughan J, Perner Y, McAlpine E, et al. Brief Report: HIV-Associated Hodgkin Lymphoma Involving the Bone Marrow Identifies a Very High-Risk Subpopulation in the Era of Widescale Antiretroviral Therapy Use in Johannesburg, South Africa. J Acquir Immune Defic Syndr 2020;83(4):345–9.

115. Lanoy E, Rosenberg PS, Fily F, et al. HIV-associated Hodgkin lymphoma during the first months on combination antiretroviral therapy. Blood 2011;118(1):44–9.

116. Tullgren O, Grimfors G, Holm G, et al. Lymphocyte abnormalities predicting a poor prognosis in Hodgkin's disease. A long-term follow-up. Cancer 1991; 68(4):768–75.
117. Herrera AF, LeBlanc ML, Castellino SM, et al. SWOG S1826, a randomized study of nivolumab(N)-AVD versus brentuximab vedotin(BV)-AVD in advanced stage (AS) classic Hodgkin lymphoma (HL). J Clin Oncol 2023/06/10 2023; 41(17_suppl):LBA4.
118. Re A, Cattaneo C, Montoto S. Treatment management of haematological malignancies in people living with HIV. Lancet Haematol 2020;7(9):e679–89.
119. Lurain K, Ramaswami R, Mangusan R, et al. Use of pembrolizumab with or without pomalidomide in HIV-associated non-Hodgkin's lymphoma. J Immunother Cancer 2021;9(2).
120. Abramson JS, Irwin KE, Frigault MJ, et al. Successful anti-CD19 CAR T-cell therapy in HIV-infected patients with refractory high-grade B-cell lymphoma. Cancer 2019;125(21):3692–8.
121. Coghill AE, Shiels MS, Suneja G, et al. Elevated cancer-specific mortality among HIV-infected patients in the United States. J Clin Oncol 2015;33(21):2376–83.
122. Coghill AE, Han X, Suneja G, et al. Advanced stage at diagnosis and elevated mortality among US patients with cancer infected with HIV in the National Cancer Data Base. Cancer 2019;125(16):2868–76.
123. Okuma Y, Hosomi Y, Imamura A. Lung cancer patients harboring epidermal growth factor receptor mutation among those infected by human immunodeficiency virus. OncoTargets Ther 2015;8:111–5.
124. Pichardo R, Go RF, Qu L, et al. HIV-associated non-small-cell lung cancer with rearrangement of the anaplastic lymphoma kinase gene: a report of two patients. Cureus 2019;11(8):e5466.
125. Deeken JF, Beumer JH, Anders NM, et al. Preclinical assessment of the interactions between the antiretroviral drugs, ritonavir and efavirenz, and the tyrosine kinase inhibitor erlotinib. Cancer Chemother Pharmacol 2015;76(4):813–9.
126. El Zarif T, Nassar AH, Adib E, et al. Safety and activity of immune checkpoint inhibitors in people living with HIV and cancer: a real-world report from the cancer therapy using checkpoint inhibitors in people living with HIV-International (CATCH-IT) Consortium. J Clin Oncol 2023;41(21):3712–23.
127. Odeny TA, Lurain K, Strauss J, et al. Effect of CD4+ T cell count on treatment-emergent adverse events among patients with and without HIV receiving immunotherapy for advanced cancer. J Immunother Cancer 2022;10(9):e005128.
128. Gonzalez-Cao M, Morán T, Dalmau J, et al. Assessment of the Feasibility and Safety of Durvalumab for Treatment of Solid Tumors in Patients With HIV-1 Infection: The Phase 2 DURVAST Study. JAMA Oncol 2020;6(7):1063–7.
129. Calkins KL, Chander G, Joshu CE, et al. Immune status and associated mortality after cancer treatment among individuals with HIV in the antiretroviral therapy era. JAMA Oncol 2020;6(2):227–35.
130. Cook MR, Kim C. Safety and efficacy of immune checkpoint inhibitor therapy in patients with HIV infection and advanced-stage cancer: a systematic review. JAMA Oncol 2019;5(7):1049–54.
131. Davis DA, Shrestha P, Aisabor AI, et al. Pomalidomide increases immune surface marker expression and immune recognition of oncovirus-infected cells. OncoImmunology 2019;8(2):e1546544.
132. Hütter G, Nowak D, Mossner M, et al. Long-term control of HIV by CCR5 Delta32/Delta32 stem-cell transplantation. N Engl J Med 2009;360(7):692–8.

133. Gupta RK, Abdul-Jawad S, McCoy LE, et al. HIV-1 remission following CCR5Δ32/Δ32 haematopoietic stem-cell transplantation. Nature 2019; 568(7751):244–8.

134. Rust BJ, Kiem HP, Uldrick TS. CAR T-cell therapy for cancer and HIV through novel approaches to HIV-associated haematological malignancies. Lancet Haematol 2020;7(9):e690–6.

135. Uldrick TS, Adams SV, Fromentin R, et al. Pembrolizumab induces HIV latency reversal in people living with HIV and cancer on antiretroviral therapy. Sci Transl Med 2022;14(629):eabl3836.

136. Uldrick TS, Ison G, Rudek MA, et al. Modernizing clinical trial eligibility criteria: recommendations of the American Society of Clinical Oncology-Friends of Cancer Research HIV Working Group. J Clin Oncol 2017;35(33):3774–80.

137. Denicoff AM, Ivy SP, Tamashiro TT, et al. Implementing modernized eligibility criteria in US National Cancer Institute Clinical Trials. J Natl Cancer Inst 2022; 114(11):1437–40.

138. Odeny TA, Rosenthal MH, Lurain KA, et al. CD4+ T-cell count eligibility by HIV status among participants receiving immunotherapy for cancer diagnoses. J Clin Oncol 2021;39(15_suppl):12104.

139. Reuss JE, Stern D, Foster JC, et al. Assessment of cancer therapy evaluation program advocacy and inclusion rates of people living with hiv in anti-PD1/PDL1 clinical trials. JAMA Netw Open 2020;3(12):e2027110.

140. Lin LL, Lakomy DS, Chiao EY, et al. Clinical trials for treatment and prevention of HIV-associated malignancies in sub-saharan africa: building capacity and overcoming barriers. JCO Glob Oncol 2020;6:1134–46.

Sexually Transmitted Infections in People with Human Immunodeficiency Virus

Jessica Tuan, MD, MS[a], Morgan M. Goheen, MD, PhD[a],
William Trebelcock, MD[b], Dana Dunne, MD, MHS[a],*

KEYWORDS

- Sexually transmitted infections • Human immunodeficiency virus • Syphilis
- Gonorrhea • Chlamydia • Trichomonas • Mpox • Mycoplasma

KEY POINTS

- People with human immunodeficiency virus (HIV) have higher rates of sexually transmitted infections (STIs) compared to patients without HIV, especially among men who have sex with men (MSM).
- Many cases of chlamydia and gonorrhea are missed with urine-only diagnostic testing; routinely asking about sites exposed during sexual activity or adopting universal 3 site testing leads to increased rates of diagnosis and treatment.
- Syphilis rates continue to rise, and providers need to be expert in the signs and symptoms of this complex disease, including recognition of symptomatic early neurosyphilis, and ocular and otic disease.
- Vaccines can help prevent some STIs, including human papillomavirus, hepatitis B virus, and mpox, and are in development for gonorrhea. Prevention of chlamydia, gonorrhea, and syphilis using postexposure prophylaxis with doxycycline is showing promise in certain populations, such as MSM.

INTRODUCTION

Sexually transmitted infections (STIs) encompass a wide variety of pathogens including bacteria (*Neisseria gonorrhoeae*, *Chlamydia trachomatis* [CT], *Mycoplasma genitalium* [MG], and *Treponema pallidum*), viruses (human immunodeficiency virus [HIV], herpes simplex types 1 and 2, mpox, human papillomavirus [HPV], and hepatitis B and C viruses), parasites (*Trichomonas vaginalis* [TV]), and ectoparasites (scabies[1] and lice). The term "sexually transmitted disease" is used when an individual infected with one of these microorganisms is symptomatic.

[a] Department of Internal Medicine (Infectious Diseases), Yale School of Medicine, New Haven, CT, USA; [b] Yale New Haven Hospital, New Haven, CT, USA
* Corresponding author. Department of Internal Medicine, Section of Infectious Diseases, Yale School of Medicine, 20 York Street, LMP 1074, New Haven, CT 06511.
E-mail address: dana.dunne@yale.edu

Infect Dis Clin N Am 38 (2024) 559–579
https://doi.org/10.1016/j.idc.2024.04.007
0891-5520/24/© 2024 Elsevier Inc. All rights reserved.

Epidemiology and trends will be reviewed by pathogen in the following sections. Overall, incidence rates of bacterial STIs have been rising steadily for years.[1,2] Patients with HIV (PWH) have even higher incidence rates compared to patients without HIV (**Figs. 1** and **2**).[3] Additionally, infection with many STIs increases the risk of acquiring and/or transmitting HIV.[4–6] Therefore, preventing, diagnosing, and treating patients with STIs is an important component of HIV infection prevention strategies. This review will summarize the screening recommendations for STIs in PWH, as well as important epidemiologic, clinical, diagnostic, and treatment details for the major STIs, with emphasis on where these may differ compared to patients without HIV and will conclude with established and emerging strategies for STI prevention.

Screening Recommendations

Recommendations for STI screening in PWH (**Table 1**) are similar to those in patients without HIV, with a few notable exceptions: (1) In people who are receptive partners for vaginal intercourse, screening for TV is recommended, (2) screening for gonorrhea (GC), chlamydia, and syphilis is recommended for all.

Nucleic acid amplification testing (NAAT) is the test of choice for diagnosis of chlamydia and GC including from extragenital sites. For patients with vaginas, either vaginal swabs (provider-collected or patient-collected) or endocervical swabs are preferred, as urine testing can be less sensitive. First-void urine samples are preferred in patients with penile sexual exposure. NAAT performance for chlamydia and GC from these sites are 95% to 98% specific and 98% to 100% specific, respectively.[7,8] Chlamydia and GC screening should include genital and extragenital testing and should be based on current anatomy. It is extremely important to screen all sites of exposure (pharynx, rectum, and urine) in men who have sex with men (MSM) and/or transgender women, as urine-only testing can miss a significant portion of infections.[9,10] Serology-based screening recommendations (syphilis and viral hepatitis) for transgender patients are similar to cisgender screening guidelines.

While recommended by many guidelines and funding agencies, STI screening rates are often still low. A study examining STI screening in PWH found only approximately two-thirds had appropriate site-specific sexual screening. Test positivity was highest among MSM (3.1%, compared to a low of 0.2% in women). Of patients diagnosed with STI who had multisite testing, 96% were only positive at an extragenital site, indicating that without expanded screening, many infections would be missed.[11]

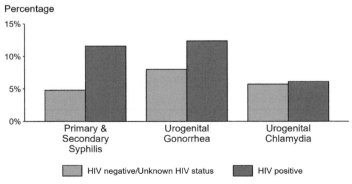

Fig. 1. Proportion of MSM with primary and secondary syphilis, urogenital GC, or urogenital chlamydia by HIV status, STD surveillance network, 2021. (Source and figure from CDC 2021 STI Surveillance Report.)

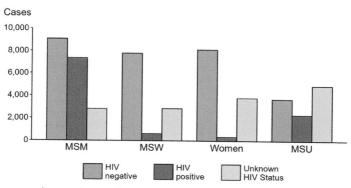

Fig. 2. Primary and secondary syphilis—reported cases by sex, sex of sex partners, and HIV status, 2021. (Source and figure from CDC 2021 STI Surveillance Report.).

Chlamydia

Epidemiology

CT (serovars D–K) remains the most prevalent bacterial STI in the United States, with 1,649,716 cases reported in 2022,[1] representing a steady increase over the past decades. Younger MSM populations have the highest rates of infection,[3] thus overlapping with many people with or at risk for HIV. In general, parsing out bacterial STI rates among PWH has involved relying on sentinel studies and surveillance networks. A 2011 systematic review reported overall mean point prevalence of STIs as 16.3% among PWH (from 33 studies with confirmed STI testing from both developed and developing countries), with 5% mean prevalence of chlamydia.[12] A 2018 Centers for Disease Control and Prevention (CDC) STI surveillance report noted in populations attending sentinel sexually transmitted disease (STD) surveillance clinics in 2018, urogenital chlamydia positivity was essentially the same in HIV-positive or HIV-negative MSM (6.1% and 6.7%, respectively).[13]

Lymphogranuloma venereum (LGV), caused by CT serovars L1 to L3, is rare, and prior to 2003, had been endemic primarily in Africa, India, and Southeast Asia. An outbreak of proctocolitis due to CT LGV serovars was reported in Amsterdam in 2003. Subsequently, large case reports were published describing hundreds of cases in Europe and the United States. HIV coinfection rates reported in these outbreaks were extremely high (upward of 90%). In Europe, where there has been more monitoring than in the United States, LGV rates have trended upwards and are higher among PWH. LGV diagnoses among MSM visiting STI clinics in the Netherlands increased from less than 100 in 2010 to greater than 250 in 2017, with LGV positivity rate of all positive CT samples also increasing to approximately 10% by 2017. The vast majority of these cases involved PWH.[14]

Clinical manifestations

Chlamydia can infect mucosal tissue of the urogenital tract, oropharynx, rectum, and eye. Infections are most commonly asymptomatic.[15] In PWH, there are no significant reports to suggest different manifestations of CT presentation.[6,16] Clinical syndromes caused by the common urogenital serovars (D–K) can include urethritis, epididymoorchitis, cervicitis, vaginal discharge, and pelvic inflammatory disease (PID).

LGV can present as an ulceroglandular syndrome occurring in stages: first with a small painless ulcer at the infection site, then a few weeks later with large, tender inguinal lymph nodes (with risk for perforation) and eventual scarring, lymphatic

Table 1
Sexually transmitted infection screening recommendations in PWH

	Recommendation Timing and Frequency	Notes
Chlamydia and GC	Screening at first visit and at least annually thereafter (more frequent screening if risk factors[a])	• Patient with vagina: vaginal or endocervical specimens favored over urine • Patient with penis: first-void urine recommended • Include all exposed sites for MSM (pharynx, rectum, and urethra)
Syphilis	At first visit and at least annually thereafter If pregnant, add first and last trimester screening (State policy-dependent)	Consider rescreening every 3–6 mo if new partners
MG	No screening recommendation	—
Trichomonas	All persons having vaginal sex at intake visit and annually (more frequent screening if risk factors[a])	• Vaginal or endocervical specimens favored over urine • No screening recommendation for patients without native vaginas
HSV	Type-specific serology for HSV-2 infection is not generally recommended in patients presenting for STI evaluation but may be considered in unique cases	—
Mpox virus	No screening recommendation	—
HBV	HBsAg, HBsAb, HBcAb at first visit If nonimmune, offer vaccination	If HBsAb positive, check HBV viral load Anti-HBs should be obtained 1–2 mo after completion of vaccine series to assess for vaccine response
Hepatitis C virus	HCV antibody all patients aged >18 y old once Annually if ongoing IDU; consider annually for MSM	If HCV antibody positive, check HCV RNA

Abbreviations: HBcAb, hepatitis B core antibody; HBsAb, hepatitis B surface antibody; HBsAg, hepatitis B surface antigen; IDU, injection drug users; MSM, men who have sex with men.
[a] Risk factors: New or multiple sexual partners, inconsistent use of barrier contraception, transactional sex work, partner with STI, and/or other partners.

fibrosis, and lymphedema. In outbreaks associated with unprotected anal receptive intercourse (primarily in MSM), the presentation is an acute and/or chronic proctitis/proctocolitis, and if untreated, can lead to rectal fissures and perforation. Infection with CT LGV serovars can also be asymptomatic.[17]

Diagnosis
Recommended diagnostics for chlamydia infection rely on NAAT technology and can be done from urogenital sampling (urine, vaginal, endocervical, and endourethral), or rectal or pharyngeal swab. The most recent 2021 CDC guidelines suggest that new point-of-care (POC) NAATs (eg, Cepheid - Sunnyvale, CA, USA, neisseria gonorrhea [NG]/CT Cepheid Xpert CT/NG) are performing well and can be used reliably, relative to conventional, more time-consuming NAATs.[18] Testing does not differ for PWH,

except for the emphasis on extragenital screening.[7] High rates of rectal CT have been reported in women who deny anal sex exposure, suggesting either contiguous spread, self-inoculation, or underreported anal receptive intercourse.[19] Self-testing has been demonstrated to be well-accepted and also have good performance compared to physician sample collection making it a useful tool that should be incorporated into care, particularly if it increases screening uptake and patient comfort.[20,21]

For LGV diagnosis, commercial chlamydia NAAT tests will be able to detect LGV serovars, though these tests do not distinguish between the LGV serovars and the classic urogenital serovars D to K. There are no Food and Drug Administration (FDA)-approved molecular tests to confirm LGV infection. Therefore, the diagnosis of LGV is often clinical and presumptive when a chlamydia NAAT is positive from the rectum in setting of proctitis or proctocolitis symptoms.[22] Serovar-specific serologic testing for chlamydia is not recommended as it is neither standardized nor performance validated for proctitis presentations. Serology may be useful as supportive evidence in patients presenting with inguinal adenopathy (inguinal syndrome) when no material is available for NAAT testing.[23]

Management

Treatment recommendations are summarized in **Table 2** and is not different in PWH. Treatment of CT infection with standard urogenital strains (serovars D–K) has shifted to now recommend doxycycline 100 mg bid × 7 days as first-line treatment, relegating azithromycin to an alternative therapy. This change was based on clinical trials that showed approximately 20% greater cure rates of rectal chlamydia with doxycycline than with azithromycin in MSM study populations.[24,25] This recommendation is also extended to women who test positive for CT (from genital sites) because of high rates of concomitant rectal infection. One-time azithromycin remains an alternative regimen, particularly if there is concern about treatment completion or in pregnant patients.

For LGV serovars, longer doxycycline treatment courses (of 21 days) are necessary.[26] However, given standard NAAT testing does not differentiate serovars and the prevalence of LGV in the United States is extremely low, the decision to extend treatment should be based on clinical symptoms. If rectal screening is positive without proctitis symptoms, it is reasonable to treat with only the standard 7 day course.[18]

Test-of-cure (TOC) is not recommended (except during pregnancy, in which TOC is recommended 4 weeks posttreatment) although rescreening should still be performed 3 to 4 months after treatment given high reinfection rates.

Gonorrhea

Epidemiology

GC (*Neisseria gonorrhoeae*) is the second most common bacterial STI reported in the United States, steadily increasing annually with 648,056 cases in 2022.[3] A 2011 systematic review reported an overall median point prevalence of GC of 9.5% among PWH.[12] In the HIV-positive MSM population, urogenital GC positivity was 12.7% compared to 7.6% among HIV-negative MSM,[13] highlighting especially high GC rates in some subpopulations of PWH.

Clinical manifestations

Uncomplicated GC infection may involve the urogenital tract, oropharynx, rectum, or eye, in both men and women. Like chlamydia, the majority of infections can be asymptomatic, with reports of ranges of approximately 50% to 90% of infections being asymptomatic at either urogenital or extragenital infection sites.[17] Diagnosis of GC should be suspected in patients presenting with urethritis, urethral discharge, acute

Table 2
Centers for Disease Control and Prevention-recommended treatments for selected sexually transmitted infections in human immunodeficiency virus-infected patients

Infection	Preferred Treatment	Alternative Treatment(s)	Notes
Chlamydia	Doxycycline 100 mg PO bid × 7 d	Azithromycin 1 g PO × 1	• Do not use doxycycline in pregnancy • TOC at 4 wk posttreatment in pregnancy
GC: uncomplicated (urogenital, rectal, and pharyngeal)	Ceftriaxone 500 mg IM × 1 (increase dose to 1 g for people >150 kg)	*Cefixime 800 mg PO × 1 Cephalosporin allergy: Gentamicin 240 mg IM × 1 plus azithromycin 2 g PO × 1	• If it has not been ruled out, add empiric treatment to cover chlamydia • All non-ceftriaxone regimens less efficacious for pharyngeal GC • TOC 7–14 d after treatment needed for pharyngeal infection
GC: complicated Disseminated	Ceftriaxone 1 g IV or IM q 24 h × 7 d	Cefotaxime 1 g IV q 8 h or Ceftizoxime 1 g IV q 8 h	Can change to enteral therapy when clinically stable guided by susceptibility results
Syphilis: early (primary, secondary, early latent)	Benzathine penicillin 2.4 million units IM × 1	Penicillin allergic: Doxycycline 100 mg PO bid × 14 d	• If allergic to penicillin and concern for med adherence, should be desensitized and receive penicillin • Pregnancy: should be treated per syphilis stage with penicillin. Desensitize if allergic
Syphilis: late latent and tertiary syphilis (with normal CSF examination)	Benzathine penicillin 2.4 million units IM weekly × 3 wk (7.2 mU total)	Penicillin allergic: Doxycycline 100 mg PO bid × 28 d	Pregnancy: weekly benzathine penicillin as per nonpregnant, but cannot go >9 d between injections, or else need to repeat entire antibiotic series

Neurosyphilis	Aqueous penicillin G 18–24 million units divided q 4 h × 10–14 d	Procaine penicillin G 2.4 million units IM once daily plus probenecid 500 mg PO qid both for 10–14 d	Can consider benzathine penicillin 2.4 million units IM × 1 dose at completion of IV therapy if infection thought to be present >1 y (eg, late)
Trichomoniasis	Metronidazole 500 mg PO bid × 7 d	Metronidazole 2 g PO × 1 Tinidazole 2 g PO × 1	Sexual partners with penile exposure can be treated with 2 g one-time dose regimen
MG	Doxycycline 100 mg PO bid × 7 d followed by moxifloxacin 400 mg PO QD × 7 d	If known to be macrolide-susceptible: Doxycycline 100 mg PO bid × 7 d followed by azithromycin 1 g PO initial dose, then 500 mg PO QD × 3 d (2.5 g total)	Macrolide susceptibility testing not widely available
HSV: First episode*	Acyclovir 400 mg PO tid × 7–10 d or famciclovir 250 mg PO tid × 7–10 d or valacyclovir 1 g PO bid × 7–10 d		*May need to extend course if healing incomplete at day 10
HSV: Episodic	Acyclovir 400 mg PO tid × 5–10 d or famciclovir 500 mg PO tid × 5–10 d or valacyclovir 1 g PO bid × 5–10 d		
HSV: Suppression	Acyclovir 400–800 mg PO 2–3 times daily or famciclovir 500 mg PO bid or valacyclovir 500 mg PO bid		• Risk of recurrence highest first 6 mo after starting ART—consider suppression during this time • Suppression associated with lower likelihood of acyclovir resistance compared to episodic
Mpox	No FDA-approved treatments. Treatment recommended for advanced or poorly controlled HIV or for severe disease	*Tecovirimat	*Not FDA-approved as of October 2021 for mpox Available through IND from CDC

Abbreviations: ART, antiretroviral therapy; CDC, Centers for Disease Control and Prevention; GC, gonorrhea; IM, intramuscular; IND, investigational new drug; IV, intravenous; PO, per os; TOC, test-of-cure.
The Symbol * indicates all non-ceftriaxone regimens less efficacious for pharyngeal GC

epididymo-orchitis, cervicitis, PID, or proctitis. Additionally, GC should be considered when evaluating pharyngitis in sexually active persons. Rare complications include gonococcal conjunctivitis in adults (frequently from autoinoculation) and disseminated gonococcal infection (DGI), which can lead to purulent arthritis or a classic triad of tenosynovitis, dermatitis, and polyarthralgia. There are reports of increased DGI in patients taking eculizumab,[27] but otherwise no data to suggest immunosuppression, such as that from HIV, contributes to an increased DGI risk. In fact, as with CT, no significant data exist to suggest different manifestations of GC infection in PLH.[6,16] A study in sub-Saharan Africa comparing HIV-positive patients with and without STIs noted GC urethritis was associated with an increased HIV viral load in semen, even when comparing patients with otherwise matched CD4 counts and plasma virus levels. Furthermore, semen virus levels decreased with STI treatment (whereas blood plasma virus levels stayed consistent with STI treatment), demonstrating specificity of the STI effect on semen viral load and highlighting implications for transmission dynamics in high-risk populations.[4]

Diagnosis

In evaluating symptomatic urethral discharge, Gram staining is highly sensitive and specific and can be used as a POC test, if available, though definitive testing for both GC and chlamydia should still be pursued (for state reporting, ruling out chlamydia coinfection). The preferred test for GC is NAAT. GC and chlamydia are cotested on most commercially available NAAT platforms, given the overlapping clinical syndromes caused by these organisms. With the continuous evolution of antimicrobial resistance, gonococcal cultures are necessary when susceptibility testing is desired.[28] The CDC supports sentinel sites across the United States to routinely perform N gonorrhoeae culture and susceptibility testing for the purpose of detecting emerging drug resistance.

Diagnosis of disseminated GC infection is more challenging, as yield of culturing the bacteria from sterile nonmucosal areas is often suboptimal. Recommendations for suspected DGI diagnosis include culturing from relevant dissemination sites (eg, skin, synovial fluid, blood, and central nervous system [CNS]) as well as simultaneously performing NAAT on any of these samples, and screening at all standard urogenital, pharyngeal, and rectal sites in order to increase the chance of diagnosis if present.[28]

Management

Drug resistance has been a long-standing concern for N gonorrhoeae, with resistance having developed to prior first-line treatment regimens including penicillins and fluoroquinolones. Ceftriaxone has remained the backbone of therapy for the past few decades, though also not without concern about developing resistance. As summarized in **Table 2**, there has been a recent major shift in the latest CDC treatment guidelines, which now recommend a larger dose of ceftriaxone (now a one-time 500 mg intramuscular [IM] dose) in order to try and combat resistance potential.[29] Despite concerns about possible emerging resistance, cases of ceftriaxone resistance in the United States are rare; there were less than 0.1% of isolates having concerning minimum inhibitory concentrations greater than 0.25 mcg/mL and no clinical treatment failures in the United States. CDC guidelines also note azithromycin resistance of ~5% in 2018; alternative treatment options are thus quite limited if a true beta-lactam allergy exists, and ceftriaxone remains the only recommended therapy for pharyngeal infection.[29]

TOC is only necessary for pharyngeal infection (where there are more concerns about persistence) and should be performed 7 to 14 days after initial treatment. Otherwise rescreening is recommended 3 months after treatment, particularly as partners can serve as a reservoir to reinfect patients.[29]

Mycoplasma

Epidemiology and clinical

MG has been an emerging STI since it was first isolated in 1981.[30] As sensitive NAAT testing has only recently become available, it is neither a reportable disease nor are there screening recommendations; thus, broad epidemiologic trends are less well known. It is responsible for up to 20% to 30% of symptomatic and asymptomatic nongonococcal urethritis in individuals with a penis,[31,32] and associated with a 2 fold increase in the risk for cervicitis, PID, spontaneous abortion, preterm birth, and infertility.[33] This bacterium has also been implicated as a cause of symptomatic proctitis among those engaging in receptive anal sex.[34] Like other STIs of the urogenital tract, MG causes local inflammation of the affected epithelium. This has been shown to increase transepithelial HIV transmission to deeper target cells, thereby serving as a significant route for HIV acquisition.[35] In cross-sectional analyses, there is a strong association between MG positivity and HIV infection.[36,37] A nested case–control study of women in Uganda and Zimbabwe demonstrated a 2 fold independent risk of HIV acquisition (adjusted odds ratio 2.45) if she had tested positive for MG in the visit prior to HIV acquisition.[38] It is noteworthy that although vaginal HIV shedding is higher in those with MG infection, it does not appear to cause increased vertical transmission from mother to child.[39,40]

Diagnosis

There are now commercially available NAAT tests to detect MG infection with preferred specimen types of first-void urine or endourethral swabs for penile exposure and vaginal or endocervical swabs. Test performance of the transcription-mediated assays is excellent (92%–98% sensitivity and specificity),[41,42] similar to NAAT performance for CT and GC. Currently, the 2021 CDC STI consensus guidelines recommend reserving testing for men with recurrent or persistent urethritis symptoms and women with recurrent cervicitis, and testing can be considered for women with PID.[8]

Treatment

The landscape of MG treatment and diagnosis has evolved significantly due to the emergence of macrolide resistance, initially observed in penile urethritis in 2006.[43] The predominant cause of macrolide resistance in MG is attributed to specific mutations, known as macrolide resistance-mediating mutations (MRMs).[44] These MRMs are responsible for resistance levels that vary by region, but a recent meta-analysis showed on average 35.5% of tested samples had drug resistance.[45] In contrast, MSM with HIV in Alabama had much higher rates of resistance at 70.6% and 80% of urogenital and rectal samples, respectively.[46]

Although the FDA-approved NAATs described earlier can successfully identify MG, further polymerase chain reaction (PCR)-based assays are used to ascertain macrolide resistance.[47] While there are several commercial NAATs available that interrogate these MRMs outside the United States, they are not FDA-approved at this time. Present guidelines recommend a 2 stage, therapeutic approach that utilizes doxycycline followed by moxifloxacin (or azithromycin if the isolate is confirmed to be macrolide susceptible; see **Table 2**).[8] Until macrolide resistance testing is more widely available, fluoroquinolone use in lieu of azithromycin is recommended.

Syphilis

Epidemiology

Syphilis (caused by *T pallidum*) incidence rates in the United States have been increasing since 2001 and, as of 2022, have reached rates not seen since 1950.[1] Syphilis has been disproportionately affecting MSM since the early 2000s, but since

2013, rates have also started to rise in women, and concurrently, rates of congenital syphilis have also risen (219% increase from 2017 to 2021). In 2021, in patients with primary or secondary syphilis, 44.8% of cases among MSM were in PWH, compared with 38.3% of cases among men with unknown sex of sex partners, indicating a high level of coinfection (see **Fig. 2**). This high coinfection underscores the interplay of enhanced HIV acquisition risk associated with syphilis infection and potential impacts of HIV infection on syphilis diagnosis and management. Syphilis is a complex, multistage infection with clinical stages, diagnostics, and management well summarized in several recent reviews.[48,49.]

Clinical

Clinical manifestations are largely similar in PWH with some potential exceptions. There have been case reports and series of PWH presenting with more than one primary chancre and increased rates (compared to historic case series) of necrotic ulcerative cutaneous lesions (lues maligna).[50,51] Higher than expected case numbers of PWH with neurosyphilis were described early in the acquired immunodeficiency syndrome epidemic preantiretroviral therapy (ART).[52] Early neurologic involvement is common in all patients with syphilis,[53,54] so it is posited that difficulty clearing the infection is responsible for this observed increase in cases in PWH.

Diagnosis

The diagnosis of syphilis can be made directly (using dark-field microscopy or immunostaining) or indirectly using sera. Given the availability of and proficiency in dark-field microscopy has greatly diminished over the past 20 years, serology is the mainstay of diagnosis. Serologic diagnosis relies on using a combination of both treponemal-specific and nontreponemal tests. Historically, screening started with the nontreponemal test (assaying antibodies to nonspecific lipoidal antigens) and, if positive, was confirmed with a treponemal-specific test. More recently, many commercial and hospital laboratories have adopted a reverse approach, taking advantage of automated treponemal-specific tests with a suggested algorithm shown in **Fig. 3**.[55] A positive treponemal and nontreponemal test confirms syphilis, but clinical staging relies on a history and physical examination (including a careful neurologic examination) evaluating for signs and symptoms of primary (ulcerative disease), secondary (systemic involvement including rash, alopecia, oral lesions, and possible deep organ involvement), early symptomatic neurosyphilis (ocular, otic, cranial nerve abnormalities, and aseptic meningitis), or late neurologic manifestations (tabes dorsalis, Argyll-Robertson pupils, and cognitive changes). Latent syphilis, defined as seropositivity but without signs or symptoms, is divided into early (likely infected within past 12 months based on history, serial testing, exposure) or late (likely infected >12 months ago or unknown) for treatment purposes. Testing algorithms and interpretation of syphilis serology is unchanged for PWH. Prozone phenomena, which can cause a false-negative nontreponemal test, can be seen in secondary syphilis and has been reported in PWH.

Management

Broadly speaking, syphilis treatment in the HIV-positive population does not differ from recommendations for HIV-negative patients. First-line treatment (for any stage) involves penicillin (see **Table 2**), with doxycycline as an alternative for true penicillin allergy (though less published experience in PWH).[8,56] All pregnant people allergic to penicillin should undergo evaluation and desensitization as penicillin is the best-studied regimen to prevent congenital syphilis.

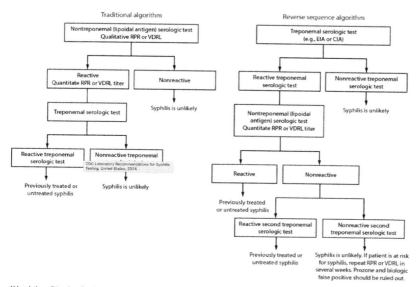

Abbreviations: CIA = chemiluminescence immunoassay; EIA = enzyme immunoassay; RPR = rapid plasma regain; TPPA = *Treponoma pallidum* particle agglutination; = Venereal Disease Research Laboratory.

Fig. 3. Algorithms that can be applied to screening for syphilis with serologic tests–CDC laboratory recommendations for syphilis testing in the United States, 2024 (From[55]).

Although treatment is the same, there are specific management aspects that should be emphasized in PWH. Given syphilis prevalence in PWH, particularly in MSM, emphasis on partner identification, notification, and treatment should be prioritized, as well as state department of public health reporting, in order to attempt to curb the syphilis epidemic. Furthermore, it is important to note that a syphilis diagnosis for someone not on ART should not preclude immediate initiation of ART, with relatively little risk of immune reconstitution inflammatory syndrome compared to other diseases.[57] Similarly, available data would not suggest an increased risk of Jarisch–Herxheimer reaction in PWH compared to that seen in HIV-negative individuals.

The data surrounding the risk of neurosyphilis in PWH are not definitive. Although some older studies suggested increased rates of neurosyphilis in PWH though others did not note a correlation (Rompalo, Karp).[55,58] While some continue to recommend cerebrospinal fluid (CSF) studies in patients with CD4 counts less than 350 cells/mm^3 or rapid plasma reagin (RPR) titer greater than 1:32 given reports these correlate with an increased neurosyphilis risk, data do not suggest improved clinical outcomes with this practice.[56,59] Furthermore, the effectiveness of standard early syphilis treatment even in the face of CNS abnormalities and concern for neurosyphilis risk is quite high.[60] Thus, current guidelines focus on only performing LPs in those with neurologic symptoms or inadequate treatment response. Lumbar puncture (LP) is no longer indicated for patients with isolated otic or ocular syphilis. If the diagnosis of neurosyphilis is made, follow-up CSF studies to monitor neurosyphilis treatment response are not recommended, as long as patients are clinically improved with decreasing serum nontreponemal titers.[56] Despite concerns about more prolonged time-to-treatment response in PWH, overall serologic response rates are still quite high in PWH (>90% regardless of stage[59]). While PWH may be at a slightly increased risk of treatment failure, available data suggest this risk is overall low.[57] Certainly, it was long ago established that enhanced or additional treatment of syphilis in PWH was not necessary.[58]

Follow-up

Several studies have documented delayed RPR response to treatment in PWH and more propensity to remain serologically nonresponsive (lack of at least 4 fold decrease in RPR titer after appropriate treatment).[61,62] This has led to recommendations for increased monitoring in HIV-positive patients with syphilis (at 3, 6, 9, 12, 24 month intervals) to ensure treatment has resulted in proper resolution of symptoms and appropriate RPR decline. Inadequate response requires initiation of further workup or treatment, with emphasis on concern for previously unappreciated neurosyphilis.[57]

Treatment failure and need for retreatment can be difficult to parse out, given high reinfection risk in many PWH. Re-evaluation should occur if signs or symptoms of syphilis persist, there is a sustained (>2 week) greater than 4 fold increase in RPR titer, or a lack of a 4 fold decrease in RPR titer over the appropriate monitoring period (12 months for early syphilis, 24 months for late latent syphilis). In many cases, this equates with CSF examination, especially if neurologic complaints are present. If CSF studies suggest a diagnosis of neurosyphilis, treatment of this should occur; otherwise, retreatment with 3 weekly penicillin IM injections is recommended. Finally, if detailed history raises concern for reinfection and early disease, proceeding with penicillin IM treatment is also appropriate.[57]

Trichomoniasis

TV is the most common nonviral STI globally. Data regarding TV rates in HIV-infected individuals, compared to non-HIV infected individuals, are sparse as it is not a reportable disease. However, most studies in the United States and Africa report rates of TV infection at 1.5 fold to 2 fold higher in HIV-infected women, when compared to HIV-negative women.[63] As summarized in a recent systematic review, and like the other STIs discussed earlier, trichomoniasis has important implications for HIV transmission and acquisition. Across a range of studies in Southern Africa, women with TV were 50% more likely to acquire HIV compared to women without TV.[64] In women with co-infection with *Trichomonas* who are not virally suppressed, successful treatment of TV was associated with a decrease in cervicovaginal fluid HIV viral load.[65]

Most people who are infected with TV will be asymptomatic, but when symptomatic, then prototypical vaginal discharge is profuse and malodorous and can be associated with vaginal irritation and dyspareunia. Men can experience urethritis symptoms. The preferred diagnostic test is a nucleic acid amplication test (NAAT) on patient-collected or provider-collected vaginal, endocervical swabs or female then urine, with a sensitivity and specificity of 95% to 100%. Two products are also approved for male urine testing—Max CTGCTV2 assay (Becton Dickinson) and GeneXpert TV (Cepheid), the latter of which can be performed in less than 1 hour.[66] If NAAT testing is not available, rapid antigen tests (OSOM, Sekisui Diagnostics - San Diego, CA, USA) perform better than wet mount microscopy (82%–95% sensitivity compared with culture and transcription-mediated assay), though this is not recommended for use on urine collected from male individuals, due to lower reported sensitivity (38%).[67]

Patients with trichomoniasis should be treated whether symptomatic or not and management should include the treatment of sexual partners. The preferred treatment is summarized in **Table 2**. The oral metronidazole 2 g single-dose regimen is not preferred for vaginal infection due to lower cure rates in both HIV-positive and HIV-negative patients.[68,69] Women who are diagnosed and treated for TV should be retested, preferably with a NAAT assay, 3 months after treatment to ensure no reinfection has occurred.

Herpes Simplex Virus

Epidemiology

Seroprevalence rates (estimated by using type-specific glycoprotein assays) for herpes simplex virus type 2 (HSV-2) infection in the United States is 11% in non-HIV-infected individuals,[70] but upward of 60% in PLH. Coinfected patients can experience increased rates of HSV recurrence, which can be associated with severe ulceration and higher amounts of HSV viral shedding. An association between HSV-2 seropositivity and increased HIV-1 acquisition risk has also been well described.[71,72]

Clinical

While HSV-1 (typically acquired through orogenital contact) and HSV-2 can cause both a clinically indistinguishable genital infection, most persistent infection in the genital area is caused by HSV-2. Most patients who acquire HSV-2 do so asymptomatically but can shed virus regardless of symptoms, with rates of shedding increased in PWH.[73] When symptoms do occur, first (primary) episodes typically appear 4 to 7 days after sexual contact with an infected partner. Patients experience multiple painful shallow ulcerations that can be bilateral, in contrast to the clinical symptoms of recurrence, which are marked by milder symptoms and fewer lesions that are typically unilateral. The risk of genital ulcerations caused by HSV is higher in those with HIV with CD4 count less than 200 cells/mm^3 and risk of ulceration increases within the first 3 months of starting ART.[74] Individuals with CD4 count less than 200 cells/mm^3 are at an increased risk of HSV complications, including disseminated HSV and nonhealing ulcers. The CNS is a target organ for HSV dissemination, with complications including vasculitis, meningitis, and optic neuritis.

Diagnosis

For symptomatic patients, direct testing of clinical specimens using NAAT is recommended, with 17 such assays approved by the FDA as of 2019. While these molecular diagnostics are highly sensitive and specific, sensitivity decreases as ulcers heal. Viral culture is less sensitive than NAAT but can be used on clinical specimens if NAAT testing is unavailable. In symptomatic patients, type-specific serology (HSV-1 and HSV-2 glycoprotein antibody assay) should not be relied upon for diagnostic purposes, as a positive result may not be related to the symptom and can be falsely negative if patients have been recently exposed.[75] Type-specific HSV serology can be a useful diagnostic adjunct for patients with repeatedly negative PCR or viral culture whose symptoms are otherwise compatible with genital HSV.[76]

Treatment

Treatment regimens are summarized in **Table 2**. Treatment is recommended in all patients for initial episodes. In general, initial episode treatment is similar in PWH compared to that of HIV-negative patients, except that time to healing may be protracted requiring a prolonged course. No short courses (less than 5 days) are recommended for episodic treatment. Doses for suppression are generally higher than those recommended for patients without HIV. As mentioned, rates of ulceration in patients infected with HSV-2 increase in the first 3 months of ART initiation, so suppression may be considered during this time (use for 6 months then re-evaluate).[74]

Mpox

The orthopoxvirus mpox (formerly monkeypox) was first noted in a human in 1970. This zoonotic disease, which has been endemic to Central and West Africa, had a global resurgence amid the 2022 to 2023 outbreak of mpox.[77] The incubation period of mpox can range from a few days to a couple of weeks. Mpox classically presents with a mucocutaneous vesiculopustular rash, associated with fever and lymphade-nopathy along with constitutional symptoms. In cases of mpox-associated proctitis, anorectal pain, tenesmus, rectal bleeding, and lesions can also be present. In dissem-inated disease, pulmonary, cardiac, gastrointestinal, or CNS involvement (including ocular involvement) have been reported. Those with HIV-related immunosuppression without virologic suppression (particularly if the CD4 count is <100 cells/mm^3) are at risk for severe manifestations and complications of mpox including prolonged or necrotizing skin lesions, lung involvement and secondary infections and sepsis, and death.[78] In addition, secondary infection of skin lesions is also possible.[79]

There are no FDA-approved medications for mpox. Mild cases can be treated with supportive care but for patients with late or poorly controlled HIV or with severe dis-ease, treatment is recommended. The antiviral tecovirimat can be acquired through an expanded investigational new drug (IND) application through the CDC and is dosed 2 to 3 times per day for 14 days (or longer, if needed based on lesion response). Other potentially effective antivirals include brincidofovir and cidofovir.[80] In addition, the JYNNEOS vaccine can also be given as postexposure prophylaxis (PEP), ideally within 4 days of exposure, using the same 2 dose interval recommended for primary preven-tion (see "Sexually transmitted infection Prevention" section for mpox vaccination pre-exposure strategy).

Sexually Transmitted Infection Prevention

Barrier protection
Condoms remain a highly effective method for decreasing transmission of many STIs including chlamydia, GC, and trichomonas, and Hepatitis B. For HSV, condoms differ-entially protected against HSV-2 transmission by sex, from men to women by 96% and from women to men by 65%.[81] Correct and consistent condom use should be reviewed at clinic visits, especially for patients with incident bacterial STIs. Risk-reduction counseling is recommended for all adolescents and adults at risk for STIs.

Preexposure and postexposure prophylaxis
The prophylactic use of antibiotics for the prevention of STIs is a concept with historical precedence, dating back to as early as the 1940s.[82] This was revisited in a 2015 study of MSM, which demonstrated a significant reduction in incidence of any STI at 48 weeks within the doxycycline arm of the study.[83] Given the alarming rise in STI rates, PEP with doxycycline (doxy-postexposure prophylaxis [PEP]) after unprotected sexual inter-course has been examined as an intervention to decrease rising STI numbers.

Prominent recent trials—DoxyPEP, DOXYVAC, and IPERGAY—have presented persuasive evidence supporting the use of doxycycline for the prevention of chla-mydia, syphilis, and to a lesser degree GC in MSM and transgender women (**Table 3**).[83–86] A similar study involving cisgender heterosexual women in Kenya did not yield comparable protective effects.[87] It remains unclear whether this discrepancy is mainly attributable to reduced drug levels in the vaginal mucosa, or if other factors such as medication adherence and social acceptability played a significant role. Within the DoxyPEP study, subgroup analyses showed that the cohort of PWH had a similar decrease in incidence as the preexposure prophylaxis (PrEP) cohort with a relative risk reduction of 62% versus 66%, respectively of any STI.[85]

Amid the increased utilization of doxycycline, concerns are emerging about poten-tial antibiotic resistance in STI-related pathogens. Within the DoxyPEP and DOXYVAC trials, no significant difference in GC resistance was found between baseline and study end time points; however, in DoxyPEP, there was higher resistance found within the doxycycline group compared to that of the standard of care group.[85,86] The clinical

Table 3
Summary of selected doxycycline postexposure prophylaxis trials

		Clinical Trials of Doxycycline Postexposure Prophylaxis				
		Any STI Rate[a,c]		Risk Reduction (%)[b]		
Study	Participants	Doxy-PEP	Standard of Care	Chlamydia	Syphilis	Gonorrhea
DoxyPEP	501 (PWH n = 174)	11.1/100 PQ	31.4/100 PQ	88	87	55
DOXYVAC	502	5.6/100 PY	35.4/100 PY	89	79	51
IPERGAY	232	37.7/100 PY	67.7/100 PY	70	73	17

Abbreviations: doxy, doxycycline; PEP, postexposure prophylaxis; PQ, per quarter; PY, per year.
[a] DoxyPEP rate includes combination of PrEP and PWH cohorts. DoxyPEP trial rate in PQ vs person-years (PY) in other 2 studies.
[b] Risk reduction calculated from relative risk in DoxyPEP and hazard ratio in DOXYVAC and IPERGAY.
[c] DOXYVAC STI rate only chlamydia and syphilis.

relevance of doxy-PEP use on *S aureus* and the broader microbiome continues to be an active area of ongoing investigation.

Vaccination

Beyond oral antibiotic prophylaxis, vaccination against *Neisseria* for meningitis has shown varying efficacy in preventing *N gonorrhea* infection. This was first supported within ecologic studies that revealed decreased rates of GC after administration of outer membrane vesicle serogroup B meningococcal vaccination.[88] This was redemonstrated in a retrospective case–control study in New Zealand where vaccination was also associated with decreased rates of GC.[89] More recently, the MenB-4C vaccine, which is available in the United States and contains the same outer membrane vesicle, was shown to be 40% effective in those receiving full (3 dose) vaccination series and 26% in those with a partial series.[90] Future studies look to exploit these data to develop a possible vaccine for GC prevention.

The FDA approved the use of the JYNNEOS vaccine for mpox (and smallpox) based on immunogenicity studies. A real-world analysis of the JYNNEOS vaccine effectiveness in the US mpox outbreak of 2022 estimated effectiveness of 41% after 1 dose and 73% after 2 doses of the vaccine among immunocompromised patients.[91] Two-dose mpox vaccine is, therefore, recommended for PWH.

Vaccine effectiveness for prevention of hepatitis A virus (HAV) and hepatitis B virus (HBV) as well as HPV is well established including in PWH. All sexually active patients with HIV found to be nonimmune and not chronically infected with HBV should be vaccinated with reinforced hepatitis B vaccine (40 mcg injections at 0, 1, and 6 months). Anti-HBV surface antibody titers should be checked 1 to 2 months after the last vaccine dose. Additionally, HAV vaccination is recommended for nonimmune persons who inject drugs, MSM, those with chronic liver disease, and patients who are experiencing homelessness. HPV vaccination is indicated for all patients aged between 9 and 26 years and can be considered (through shared decision-making) in patients aged up to 46 years. PWH should receive 3 doses of the 9 valent HPV vaccine.[7]

SUMMARY

Rates of STIs are increasing in the United States and are disproportionately higher in PWH. Many STIs are associated with increased rates of HIV acquisition and transmission. Thus, strategies to increase counseling, prevention, complete and regular screening, and evidence-based treatment including partner management are critical to the United States goal of getting to 0 new HIV infections. Molecular-based testing has expanded to include more pathogens and approval for use at nongenital sites and is becoming increasingly available at the point of clinical care. Increased adoption of self-testing will further decrease diagnostic barriers and expedite timely treatment. Large gains in decreasing the burden of STIs in PWH will come through routine testing and full implementation of prevention science, including established and emerging strategies such as vaccination and doxycycline PEP.

CLINICS CARE POINTS

- Routinize multisite STI screening including extragenital screening.
- Vaginal/endocervical swabs are preferred over urine chlamydia and GC NAATs in people with vaginas.
- Patients diagnosed with pharyngeal GC should have a test of cure 7 to 14 days after treatment.
- Syphilis diagnosis and accurate staging requires knowledge of a wide spectrum of manifestations including those that could affect treatment options (eg, ocular or otic symptoms and neurologic symptoms).
- STI prevention with doxycycline PEP holds promise in reducing incident chlamydia, GC, and syphilis in MSM and transgender women.

ACKNOWLEDGMENTS

M.M.G. is supported by Yale Infectious Diseases T32 training grant 5T32AI007517-23

DISCLOSURE

Dr J. Tuan: no conflicts; Dr W. Trebelcock: no conflicts; Dr D. Dunne's spouse holds stock in Pfizer, Inc.

REFERENCES

1. Sexually Transmitted Infections Surveillance, 2022. 2024. Available at: https://www.cdc.gov/std/statistics/2022/default.htm. [Accessed 2 February 2024].
2. Kreisel KM, Spicknall IH, Gargano JW, et al. Sexually transmitted infections among US women and men: prevalence and incidence estimates, 2018. Sex Transm Dis 2021;48(4):208–14.
3. Secco AA, Akselrod H, Czeresnia J, et al. Sexually transmitted infections in persons living with HIV infection and estimated HIV transmission risk: trends over time from the DC Cohort. Sex Transm Infect 2020;96(2):89–95.
4. Cohen MS, Hoffman IF, Royce RA, et al. Reduction of concentration of HIV-1 in semen after treatment of urethritis: implications for prevention of sexual transmission of HIV-1. AIDSCAP Malawi Research Group. Lancet Lond Engl 1997;349(9069):1868–73.
5. Jones J, Weiss K, Mermin J, et al. Proportion of incident human immunodeficiency virus cases among men who have sex with men attributable to gonorrhea and chlamydia: a modeling analysis. Sex Transm Dis 2019;46(6):357–63.

6. Rein MF. The Interaction Between HIV and the Classic Sexually Transmitted Diseases. Curr Infect Dis Rep 2000;2(1):87–95.

7. Thompson MA, Horberg MA, Agwu AL, et al. Primary Care Guidance for Persons With Human Immunodeficiency Virus: 2020 Update by the HIV Medicine Association of the Infectious Diseases Society of America. Clin Infect Dis 2021;73(11): e3572–605.

8. Workowski KA, Bachmann LH. Centers for Disease Control and Prevention's Sexually Transmitted Diseases Infection Guidelines. Clin Infect Dis 2022;74(74 Suppl 2):S89–94.

9. Marcus JL, Bernstein KT, Kohn RP, et al. Infections missed by urethral-only screening for chlamydia or gonorrhea detection among men who have sex with men. Sex Transm Dis 2011;38(10):922.

10. Farfour E, Dimi S, Chassany O, et al. Trends in asymptomatic STI among HIV-positive MSM and lessons for systematic screening. PLoS One 2021;16(6): e0250557.

11. Geba MC, Powers S, Williams B, et al. A Missed Opportunity: Extragenital Screening for Gonorrhea and Chlamydia Sexually Transmitted Infections in People With HIV in a Southeastern Ryan White HIV/AIDS Program Clinic Setting. Open Forum Infect Dis 2022;9(7):ofac322.

12. Kalichman SC, Pellowski J, Turner C. Prevalence of sexually transmitted co-infections in people living with HIV/AIDS: systematic review with implications for using HIV treatments for prevention. Sex Transm Infect 2011;87(3):183–90.

13. National Center for HIV/AIDS, Viral Hepatitis, STD, and TB Prevention (U.S.). Division of STD Prevention. *Sexually Transmitted Disease Surveillance 2018*. CDC 2019. https://doi.org/10.15620/cdc.79370.

14. de Vries HJC. Lymphoganuloma venereum in the Western world, 15 years after its re-emergence: new perspectives and research priorities. Curr Opin Infect Dis 2019;32(1):43–50.

15. Tuddenham S, Ghanem KG, Gebo KA, et al. Gonorrhoea and chlamydia in persons with HIV: number needed to screen. Sex Transm Infect 2019;95(5):322–7.

16. Collis TK, Celum CL. The clinical manifestations and treatment of sexually transmitted diseases in human immunodeficiency virus-positive men. Clin Infect Dis Off Publ Infect Dis Soc Am 2001;32(4):611–22.

17. Tuddenham S, Hamill MM, Ghanem KG. Diagnosis and Treatment of Sexually Transmitted Infections: A Review. JAMA 2022;327(2):161–72.

18. Geisler WM, Hocking JS, Darville T, et al. Diagnosis and Management of Uncomplicated Chlamydia trachomatis Infections in Adolescents and Adults: Summary of Evidence Reviewed for the 2021 Centers for Disease Control and Prevention Sexually Transmitted Infections Treatment Guidelines. Clin Infect Dis 2022; 74(Supplement_2):S112–26.

19. Rank RG, Yeruva L. Hidden in plain sight: chlamydial gastrointestinal infection and its relevance to persistence in human genital infection. Infect Immun 2014; 82(4):1362–71.

20. Soni S, White JA. Self-screening for Neisseria gonorrhoeae and Chlamydia trachomatis in the human immunodeficiency virus clinic–high yields and high acceptability. Sex Transm Dis 2011;38(12):1107–9.

21. Lunny C, Taylor D, Hoang L, et al. Self-collected versus clinician-collected sampling for chlamydia and gonorrhea screening: a systemic review and meta-analysis. PLoS One 2015;10(7):e0132776.

22. Pathela P, Jamison K, Kornblum J, et al. Lymphogranuloma venereum: an increasingly common anorectal infection among men who have sex with men attending New York City Sexual Health Clinics. Sex Transm Dis 2019;46(2):e14–7.

23. Bachmann LH, Johnson RE, Cheng H, et al. Nucleic acid amplification tests for diagnosis of Neisseria gonorrhoeae and Chlamydia trachomatis rectal infections. J Clin Microbiol 2010;48(5):1827–32.

24. Dombrowski JC, Wierzbicki MR, Newman LM, et al. Doxycycline versus azithromycin for the treatment of rectal chlamydia in men who have sex with men: a randomized controlled trial. Clin Infect Dis Off Publ Infect Dis Soc Am 2021;73(5):824–31.

25. Lau A, Kong FYS, Fairley CK, et al. Azithromycin or doxycycline for asymptomatic rectal chlamydia trachomatis. N Engl J Med 2021;384(25):2418–27.

26. Leeyaphan C, Ong JJ, Chow EPF, et al. Systematic review and meta-analysis of doxycycline efficacy for rectal lymphogranuloma venereum in men who have sex with men. Emerg Infect Dis 2016;22(10):1778–84.

27. Crew PE, Abara WE, McCulley L, et al. Disseminated gonococcal infections in patients receiving eculizumab: a case series. Clin Infect Dis 2019;69(4):596–600.

28. Centers for Disease Control and Prevention. Recommendations for the laboratory-based detection of Chlamydia trachomatis and Neisseria gonorrhoeae–2014. MMWR Recomm Rep Morb Mortal Wkly Rep Recomm Rep 2014; 63(RR-02):1–19.

29. St Cyr S, Barbee L, Workowski KA, et al. Update to CDC's Treatment Guidelines for Gonococcal Infection, 2020. MMWR Morb Mortal Wkly Rep 2020;69(50):1911–6.

30. Tully J, Cole R, Taylor-Robinson D, et al. A newly discovered mycoplasma in the human urogenital tract. Lancet 1981;317(8233):1288–91.

31. Chambers LC, Morgan JL, Lowens MS, et al. Cross-sectional study of urethral exposures at last sexual episode associated with non-gonococcal urethritis among STD clinic patients. Sex Transm Infect 2019;95(3):212–8.

32. Bachmann LH, Kirkcaldy RD, Geisler WM, et al. Prevalence of mycoplasma genitalium infection, antimicrobial resistance mutations, and symptom resolution following treatment of urethritis. Clin Infect Dis 2020;71(10):e624–32.

33. Lis R, Rowhani-Rahbar A, Manhart LE. Mycoplasma genitalium infection and female reproductive tract disease: a meta-analysis. Clin Infect Dis 2015;61(3): 418–26.

34. Bissessor M, Tabrizi SN, Bradshaw CS, et al. The contribution of Mycoplasma genitalium to the aetiology of sexually acquired infectious proctitis in men who have sex with men. Clin Microbiol Infect 2016;22(3):260–5.

35. Das K, De la Garza G, Siwak EB, et al. Mycoplasma genitalium promotes epithelial crossing and peripheral blood mononuclear cell infection by HIV-1. Int J Infect Dis 2014;23:31–8.

36. Napierala Mavedzenge S, Weiss HA. Association of Mycoplasma genitalium and HIV infection: a systematic review and meta-analysis. AIDS 2009;23(5):611.

37. Mahlangu MP, Müller EE, Venter JME, et al. The Prevalence of Mycoplasma genitalium and Association With Human Immunodeficiency Virus Infection in Symptomatic Patients, Johannesburg, South Africa, 2007–2014. Sex Transm Dis 2019;46(6):395–9.

38. Mavedzenge SN, Van Der Pol B, Weiss HA, et al. The association between Mycoplasma genitalium and HIV-1 acquisition in African women. AIDS Lond Engl 2012; 26(5):617–24.

39. Manhart LE, Mostad SB, Baeten JM, et al. High Mycoplasma genitalium Organism Burden Is Associated with Shedding of HIV-1 DNA from the Cervix. J Infect Dis 2008;197(5):733–6.

40. Roxby AC, Yuhas K, Farquhar C, et al. Mycoplasma genitalium infection among HIV-infected pregnant African women and implications for mother-to-child transmission of HIV. AIDS Lond Engl 2019;33(14):2211–7.

41. Gaydos CA, Manhart LE, Taylor SN, et al. Molecular Testing for Mycoplasma genitalium in the United States: Results from the AMES Prospective Multicenter Clinical Study. J Clin Microbiol 2019;57(11). 011255-e1219.

42. Unemo M, Salado-Rasmussen K, Hansen M, et al. Clinical and analytical evaluation of the new Aptima Mycoplasma genitalium assay, with data on M. genitalium prevalence and antimicrobial resistance in M. genitalium in Denmark, Norway and Sweden in 2016. Clin Microbiol Infect Off Publ Eur Soc Clin Microbiol Infect Dis 2018;24(5):533–9.

43. Bradshaw CS, Jensen JS, Tabrizi SN, et al. Azithromycin Failure in Mycoplasma genitalium Urethritis. Emerg Infect Dis 2006;12(7):1149–52.

44. Jensen JS, Bradshaw CS, Tabrizi SN, et al. Azithromycin Treatment Failure in *Mycoplasma genitalium* –Positive Patients with Nongonococcal Urethritis Is Associated with Induced Macrolide Resistance. Clin Infect Dis 2008;47(12):1546–53.

45. Machalek DA, Tao Y, Shilling H, et al. Prevalence of mutations associated with resistance to macrolides and fluoroquinolones in Mycoplasma genitalium: a systematic review and meta-analysis. Lancet Infect Dis 2020;20(11):1302–14.

46. Dionne-Odom J, Westfall AO, Van Der Pol B, et al. Sexually transmitted infection prevalence in women with hiv: is there a role for targeted screening? Sex Transm Dis 2018;45(11):762–9.

47. Waites KB, Crabb DM, Ratliff AE, et al. Latest advances in laboratory detection of mycoplasma genitalium. J Clin Microbiol 2023;61(3). 007900-e821.

48. Ghanem KG, Ram S, Rice PA. The Modern Epidemic of Syphilis. N Engl J Med 2020;382(9):845–54.

49. Ropper AH. Neurosyphilis. N Engl J Med 2019;381(14):1358–63.

50. Rompalo AM, Lawlor J, Seaman P, et al. Modification of syphilitic genital ulcer manifestations by coexistent HIV infection. Sex Transm Dis 2001;28(8):448–54.

51. Schöfer H, Imhof M, Thoma-Greber E, et al. Active syphilis in HIV infection: a multicentre retrospective survey. The German AIDS Study Group (GASG). Sex Transm Infect 1996;72(3):176–81.

52. Flood JM, Weinstock HS, Guroy ME, et al. Neurosyphilis during the AIDS epidemic, San Francisco, 1985-1992. J Infect Dis 1998;177(4):931–40.

53. Lukehart SA, Hook EW, Baker-Zander SA, et al. Invasion of the Central Nervous System by Treponema pallidum: Implications for Diagnosis and Treatment. Ann Intern Med 1988;109(11):855–62.

54. Marra CM, Maxwell CL, Smith SL, et al. Cerebrospinal fluid abnormalities in patients with syphilis: association with clinical and laboratory features. J Infect Dis 2004;189(3):369–76.

55. Papp JR, Park IU, Fakile Y, et al. CDC Laboratory Recommendations for Syphilis Testing, United States, 2024. MMWR Recomm Rep (Morb Mortal Wkly Rep) 2024; 73(1):1–32.

56. Tuddenham S, Ghanem KG. Management of Adult Syphilis: Key Questions to Inform the 2021 Centers for Disease Control and Prevention Sexually Transmitted Infections Treatment Guidelines. Clin Infect Dis 2022;74(Supplement_2): S127–33.

57. Syphilis | NIH. 2023. Available at: https://clinicalinfo.hiv.gov/en/guidelines/hiv-clinical-guidelines-adult-and-adolescent-opportunistic-infections/syphilis. [Accessed 27 October 2023].

58. Rolfs RT, Joesoef MR, Hendershot EF, et al. A randomized trial of enhanced therapy for early syphilis in patients with and without human immunodeficiency virus infection. The Syphilis and HIV Study Group. N Engl J Med 1997;337(5):307–14.

59. Ren M, Dashwood T, Walmsley S. The Intersection of HIV and Syphilis: Update on the Key Considerations in Testing and Management. Curr HIV AIDS Rep 2021; 18(4):280–8.

60. Tomkins A, Ahmad S, Cousins DE, et al. Screening for asymptomatic neurosyphilis in HIV patients after treatment of early syphilis: an observational study. Sex Transm Infect 2018;94(5):337–9.

61. Marchese V, Tiecco G, Storti S, et al. Syphilis infections, reinfections and serological response in a large italian sexually transmitted disease centre: a monocentric retrospective study. J Clin Med 2022;11(24):7499.

62. Nieuwenburg SA, Sprenger RJ, Schim van der Loeff MF, et al. Clinical outcomes of syphilis in HIV-negative and HIV-positive MSM: occurrence of repeat syphilis episodes and non-treponemal serology responses. Sex Transm Infect 2022; 98(2):95–100.

63. Kissinger P, Adamski A. Trichomoniasis and HIV interactions: a review. Sex Transm Infect 2013;89(6):426–33.

64. Masha SC, Cools P, Sanders EJ, et al. Trichomonas vaginalis and HIV infection acquisition: a systematic review and meta-analysis. Sex Transm Infect 2019; 95(1):36–42.

65. Kissinger P, Amedee A, Clark RA, et al. Trichomonas vaginalis treatment reduces vaginal HIV-1 shedding. Sex Transm Dis 2009;36(1):11–6.

66. Kissinger PJ, Gaydos CA, Seña AC, et al. Diagnosis and Management of Trichomonas vaginalis: Summary of Evidence Reviewed for the 2021 Centers for Disease Control and Prevention Sexually Transmitted Infections Treatment Guidelines. Clin Infect Dis 2022;74(Supplement_2):S152–61.

67. Sheele JM, Crandall CJ, Arko BL, et al. The OSOM® Trichomonas Test is unable to accurately diagnose Trichomonas vaginalis from urine in men. Am J Emerg Med 2019;37(5):1002–3.

68. Kissinger P, Mena L, Levison J, et al. A randomized treatment trial: single versus 7-day dose of metronidazole for the treatment of Trichomonas vaginalis among HIV-infected women. J Acquir Immune Defic Syndr 1999 2010;55(5):565–71.

69. Howe K, Kissinger PJ. Single-Dose Compared With Multidose Metronidazole for the Treatment of Trichomoniasis in Women: A Meta-Analysis. Sex Transm Dis 2017;44(1):29–34.

70. McQuillan G, Kruszon-Moran D, Flagg EW, et al. Prevalence of Herpes Simplex Virus Type 1 and Type 2 in Persons Aged 14-49: United States, 2015-2016. NCHS Data Brief 2018;304:1–8.

71. Wald A, Link K. Risk of human immunodeficiency virus infection in herpes simplex virus type 2-seropositive persons: a meta-analysis. J Infect Dis 2002;185(1):45–52.

72. Looker KJ, Elmes JAR, Gottlieb SL, et al. Effect of HSV-2 infection on subsequent HIV acquisition: an updated systematic review and meta-analysis. Lancet Infect Dis 2017;17(12):1303–16.

73. Keller MJ, Huber A, Espinoza L, et al. Impact of Herpes Simplex Virus Type 2 and Human Immunodeficiency Virus Dual Infection on Female Genital Tract Mucosal Immunity and the Vaginal Microbiome. J Infect Dis 2019;220(5):852–61.

74. Tobian AAR, Grabowski MK, Serwadda D, et al. Reactivation of Herpes Simplex Virus Type 2 After Initiation of Antiretroviral Therapy. J Infect Dis 2013;208(5):839–46.

75. Ashley-Morrow R, Krantz E, Wald A. Time course of seroconversion by HerpeSelect ELISA after acquisition of genital herpes simplex virus type 1 (HSV-1) or HSV-2. Sex Transm Dis 2003;30(4):310–4.

76. Agyemang E, Le QA, Warren T, et al. Performance of commercial enzyme-linked immunoassays for diagnosis of herpes simplex virus-1 and herpes simplex virus-2 infection in a clinical setting. Sex Transm Dis 2017;44(12):763–7.

77. Saldana CS, Kelley CF, Aldred BM, et al. Mpox and HIV: a Narrative Review. Curr HIV AIDS Rep 2023;20(4):261–9.

78. Clinical Considerations for Treatment and Prophylaxis of Mpox Infection in People Who are Immunocompromised| Mpox | Poxvirus | CDC. 2023. Available at: https://www.cdc.gov/poxvirus/mpox/clinicians/people-with-HIV.html. [Accessed 30 October 2023].

79. Mitjà O, Alemany A, Marks M, et al. Mpox in people with advanced HIV infection: a global case series. Lancet Lond Engl 2023;401(10380):939–49.

80. Rao AK. Interim Clinical Treatment Considerations for Severe Manifestations of Mpox — United States, February 2023. MMWR Morb Mortal Wkly Rep 2023;72.

81. Magaret AS, Mujugira A, Hughes JP, et al. Effect of Condom Use on Per-act HSV-2 Transmission Risk in HIV-1, HSV-2-discordant Couples. Clin Infect Dis Off Publ Infect Dis Soc Am 2016;62(4):456–61.

82. Loveless JA, Denton W. The Oral Use of Sulfathiazole as a Prophylaxis for Gonorrhea: Preliminary Report. J Am Med Assoc 1943;121(11):827–8.

83. Bolan RK, Beymer MR, Weiss RE, et al. Doxycycline Prophylaxis to Reduce Incident Syphilis among HIV-Infected Men Who Have Sex With Men Who Continue to Engage in High-Risk Sex: A Randomized, Controlled Pilot Study. Sex Transm Dis 2015;42(2):98.

84. Molina JM, Charreau I, Chidiac C, et al. Post-exposure prophylaxis with doxycycline to prevent sexually transmitted infections in men who have sex with men: an open-label randomised substudy of the ANRS IPERGAY trial. Lancet Infect Dis 2018;18(3):308–17.

85. Luetkemeyer AF, Donnell D, Dombrowski JC, et al. Postexposure Doxycycline to Prevent Bacterial Sexually Transmitted Infections. N Engl J Med 2023;388(14):1296–306.

86. Molina J, Bercot B, Assoumou A, et al. ANRS 174 DOXYVAC: an open-label randomized trial to prevent STIs in MSM on PrEP. Seattle, WA: Presented at: Conference on Retroviruses and Opportunistic Infections; 2023.

87. Stewart J, Oware K, Donnell D, et al. Doxycycline Postexposure Prophylaxis for Prevention of STIs Among Cisgender Women. Seattle, WA: Presented at: Conference on Retroviruses and Opportunistic Infections; 2023.

88. Whelan J, Kløvstad H, Haugen IL, Holle MRDR van B, Storsaeter J. Ecologic Study of Meningococcal B Vaccine and Neisseria gonorrhoeae Infection, Norway - Volume 22, Number 6—June 2016 - Emerging Infectious Diseases journal - CDC.

89. Petousis-Harris H, Paynter J, Morgan J, et al. Effectiveness of a group B outer membrane vesicle meningococcal vaccine against gonorrhoea in New Zealand: a retrospective case-control study. Lancet 2017;390(10102):1603–10.

90. Abara WE, Bernstein KT, Lewis FMT, et al. Effectiveness of a serogroup B outer membrane vesicle meningococcal vaccine against gonorrhoea: a retrospective observational study. Lancet Infect Dis 2022;22(7):1021–9.

91. Deputy NP, Deckert J, Chard AN, et al. Vaccine Effectiveness of JYNNEOS against Mpox Disease in the United States. N Engl J Med 2023;388(26):2434–43.

Human Immunodeficiency Virus in the South

An Epidemic Within an Epidemic

Carlos S. Saldana, MD[a,b,*], Wendy S. Armstrong, MD[a,b]

KEYWORDS

- HIV • Disparities • Southern United States • Health care access • Stigma
- Syndemics • Social determinants of health • Health care policy

KEY POINTS

- The Southern region of the United States bears a disproportionate burden of the human immunodeficiency virus (HIV) epidemic, with higher incidence rates and a significant impact on marginalized communities, particularly racial, ethnic, and sexual minorities.
- Socioeconomic disparities, limited health care access (including Medicaid non-expansion), and stigma play a crucial role in shaping HIV outcomes.
- HIV criminalization and anti-lesbian, gay, bisexual, transgender, and queer+ legislation exacerbate stigma and create barriers to health care by deterring testing, treatment, and open discussion about harm reduction and prevention.
- Syndemics, involving the interaction of HIV with co-occurring health issues like sexually transmitted infections, substance-use disorders, and serious mental illness, compounds these challenges and exacerbates the overall impact of the HIV epidemic.
- There is a need for further advocacy, community engagement, and multifaceted strategies, including policy reforms and health care system enhancements to effectively address the HIV epidemic in the South.

INTRODUCTION

The global impact of human immunodeficiency virus (HIV) is profound. Since the beginning of the epidemic in the 1980s, more than 85 million people have acquired HIV, and about 40 million people have died of HIV.[1] Globally as of the end of 2022, more than 39 million people were with HIV.[1] In the United States, as of 2021, over a million individuals live with HIV, and the Southern region (as defined by the U.S. Census Bureau) bears a significant burden of the disease (**Fig. 1**).[2,3] Men who have sex with men from racial and ethnic minorities are markedly overrepresented in these

[a] Division of Infectious Diseases, Department of Medicine, Emory University School of Medicine, Atlanta, GA, USA; [b] Ponce de Leon Center, Grady Health System, Atlanta, GA, USA
* Corresponding author. 341 Ponce de Leon Ave Northeast, Atlanta, GA, 30308.
E-mail address: Cssalda@emory.edu

Infect Dis Clin N Am 38 (2024) 581–598
https://doi.org/10.1016/j.idc.2024.06.002
0891-5520/24/© 2024 Elsevier Inc. All rights reserved, including those for text and data mining, AI training, and similar technologies.

id.theclinics.com

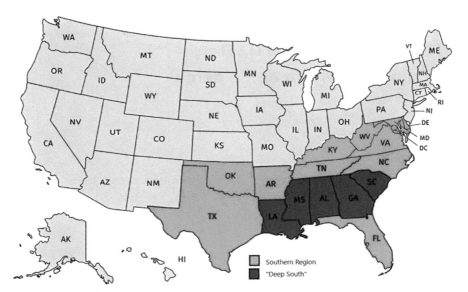

Fig. 1. Map of the United States highlighting the Southern region in orange color. States in dark red color are considered "Deep South" within the region. (*Sources*: Centers for Disease Control and Prevention. HIV Surveillance Report, 2021; vol. 34. http://www.cdc.gov/hiv/library/reports/hiv-surveillance.html. U.S. Census Bureau. Census Regions and Divisions of the United States, 2023. https://www2.census.gov/geo/pdfs/maps-data/maps/reference/us_regdiv.pdf.)

statistics, underscoring the intersecting influences of sexual orientation, race, ethnicity, and geography in the epidemiologic landscape of HIV.[4]

The HIV epidemic in the South is closely tied to systemic challenges, including socioeconomic disparities, limited access to affordable health care, restrictive legislation, and prevailing stigma associated with sexual and reproductive health.[5] This review aims to examine the HIV epidemic in the Southern United States, often characterized as an "epidemic within an epidemic." The authors discuss the complex and intertwined barriers that exacerbate the prevalence and impact of HIV in this region. The authors dissect the intersectional dynamics of affected populations, socioeconomic determinants, and other systemic barriers. Additionally, the authors highlight pathways for potential interventions aimed at improving health outcomes in populations that are disproportionately impacted.

EPIDEMIOLOGY OF THE SOUTHERN EPIDEMIC

A recent report from the Centers for Disease Control and Prevention (CDC) highlights significant disparities in HIV prevalence and incidence within the United States.[2] Despite a national 12% decrease in new HIV infections from 2017 to 2021, the Southern region bore a disproportionate disease burden. In 2021, of the 1.1 million people with HIV (people with HIV [PWH]) in the United States, 493,000 or 45% resided in Southern states, despite the region representing only 38% of the US population.[3,6] During the same year, there were an estimated 36,000 new infections reported in the United States and dependent areas, and more than half of those diagnoses (18,700) were in the South.[2] These have primarily impacted adolescents and young adults who report male-to-male sexual contact (67%) from Black (40%) and Hispanic/Latino/a/e (29%) groups.[2]

Similar trends are seen in HIV-related mortality, with over half of the deaths (55%) occurring in the South and 49% occurring in Black individuals.[7] A majority (73%) of deaths occurred among individuals aged 45 years and older; however, for PWH between the ages of 25 and 44 years, 36% of deaths occurred in Black individuals, compared to 24% in Whites. Additionally, HIV continues to be a major overall cause of death for individuals aged 25 to 44 years, ranking as the 13th most common cause of death in 2021 among all persons, but the 7th among Black/African American male individuals and the 12th among Black female individuals within this age group.[7]

An in-depth look at HIV-related health metrics and social determinants across states in the Southern region is presented in **Table 1**. We highlight HIV prevalence and incidence,[2] HIV mortality,[7] and care continuum data,[8] in addition to HIV

Table 1
Key health metrics for US states in the Southern region, focusing on HIV, social determinants, Medicaid expansion status, and syphilis rates

STATE	HIV Prevalence 2021	HIV Incidence 2021	% Linked To Care 2021	% Retained In Care 2021	% Virally Suppressed 2021	PrEP-to-Need Ratio 2022	HIV Deaths 2021	% Unemployment 2021	% Housing Instability 2021	% Poverty 2021	% Uninsured 2021	Median Income**	Medicaid Expansion	Cong. Syph[a]
AL	14,436	625	80.3	71.9	59.1	5.44	331	3.4	11.9	15.8	11.6	54,943	NoA	63.7
AR	6,225	338	77.2	67	52.5	5.05	124	4.1	10.8	16	10.3	52,123	AAI	139
DC	13,672	197	73.6	69.2	54.9	39.32	265	6.8	16.9	15.4	3.8	93,547	AAI	69
DE	3,515	81	84	82.1	73.4	10.35	75	5.5	13.2	11.4	7.1	72,724	AAI	9.5
FL	117,244	4,072	82.7	77.6	68.7	11.2	2,429	4.6	17	13.1	15.6	61,777	NoA	83.2
GA	59,422	2,371	81.6	72.7	62.1	5.79	967	3.9	13.7	13.9	15.1	65,030	NoA	75
KY	8,137	390	74.1	80.4	65.2	7.63	152	4.4	11.3	16.3	6.9	55,454	AAI	47.9
LA	21,552	899	80.6	78.6	68.9	5.42	501	5.6	14.3	18.8	9.7	53,571	AAI	191.5
MD	33,467	749	86.8	72	61.8	9.63	692	5.3	14	9.2	6.9	91,431	AAI	NR
MS	9,873	419	71.4	71	59.6	3.96	197	5.5	12.7	19.4	14.3	49,111	NoA	182
NC	34,327	1,390	80.2	77.4	68	7.06	654	4.9	12.5	13.7	12.7	60,516	ANI	34.9
OK	6,948	387	78.3	71.7	61.4	7.15	147	4	11.1	15.2	16.8	56,956	AAI	175.6
SC	18,109	652	85.4	81.9	72.6	5.83	411	3.9	12.7	14.5	12.6	58,234	NoA	33.2
TN	18,738	831	70.2	78.8	66.9	10.78	439	4.5	11.9	14.3	11.9	58,516	NoA	47.7
TX	100,700	4,363	78.6	75	62.8	9.49	1,748	5.6	13.7	14	19.8	67,321	NoA	182
VA	24,411	792	79.9	71.8	65.1	9.79	351	3.9	12.5	9.9	9.2	80,615	AAI	18.8
WV	2,196	149	71.8	68.9	54.4	6.25	56	5.1	10.3	16.9	7.9	50,884	AAI	87.2

NoA, not adopted, ANI, adopted not implemented, AAI, Adopted and implemented, Cong. Syph, congenital syphilis.

Color coding: For General Data (Yellow to Red): Shades transition from yellow to red, where yellow denotes better outcomes and red signifying worse outcomes, with intermediate shades denote a gradation of moderate outcomes. For HIV Care Continuum Data and Medicaid expansion status (Green to Red): Green indicating better outcomes and red indicating worse outcomes across various metrics. Intermediate shades represent varying outcomes levels.

Centers for Disease Control and Prevention. HIV Care Continuum, 2019. https://www.cdc.gov/hiv/pdf/library/factsheets/cdc-hiv-care-continuum.pdf. AIDSVu. New Data on Inequities in PrEP use, June 21, 2023. https://aidsvu.org/aidsvu-releases-new-data-highlighting-ongoing-inequities-in-prep-use-among-black-and-hispanic-people-and-across-regions-of-the-county/. Healthy People 2030, U.S. department of health, and Human Services. https://health.gov/healthypeople/objectives-and-data/social-determinants-health. Centers for Disease Control and Prevention. Congenital Syphilis—United States, 2021. https://www.cdc.gov/std/statistics/2021/tables/20.htm.
[a]Rates per 100,000, NR= Not reported.
Sources: Centers for Disease Control and Prevention. HIV Surveillance Report, 2021; vol. 34. http://www.cdc.gov/hiv/library/reports/hiv-surveillance.html. 7. Centers for Disease Control and Prevention. HIV Mortality 2021. https://www.cdc.gov/hiv/pdf/library/slidesets/cdc-hiv-surveillance-slideset-mortality-2021.pdf.

preexposure prophylaxis (PrEP)-to-need ratios (PNRs) per state,[9] as well as relevant social determinants of health,[10] and syphilis burden,[11] providing insights into broader public health challenges.

DETERMINANTS INFLUENCING THE HIV EPIDEMIC IN THE SOUTHERN REGION

Several factors directly and negatively influence HIV disparities and outcomes in the South (**Fig. 2**). These include access to health care, HIV scale and associated workforce challenges, stigma, and discrimination, use of and access to HIV prevention options, social determinants of health, including poverty, food, and housing insecurity, income inequality and educational attainment, co-occurring syndemics, HIV criminalization legislation, and lagging political will. Influencing all these factors is systemic racism, an important foundational effect that cannot be underestimated.

Limited Access to Comprehensive Health Care

Enhancing HIV care continuum outcomes in the Southern United States hinges on improved health care access, particularly for treatment and prevention tools. Despite this need, access barriers persist. In 2021, the *uninsured rate for individuals under 65 years in the Southern region was 14.1%, higher than the national average* of 10.3%.[6] Medicaid, as the primary funding source for PWH in the United States, provides coverage for 40% of nonelderly adults with HIV, compared to 15% of the nonelderly population overall.[12]

Medicaid expansion, under the Affordable Care Act, aims to extend coverage to adults under 65 years with incomes up to 138% of the federal poverty level, regardless of family status or health conditions. This expansion has been adopted by 41 states, including Washington DC. However, *among the 10 states that have not, 7 are in the South*. In states that expanded Medicaid, PWH generally have better health outcomes including improved viral suppression, and fewer are uninsured (6% compared to 20% in non-expansion states).[12] Furthermore, those living in Medicaid expansion states also experience higher HIV/sexually transmitted infection (STI) awareness and PrEP usage, fewer health disparities, and increased HIV testing rates, particularly in marginalized areas.[13,14]

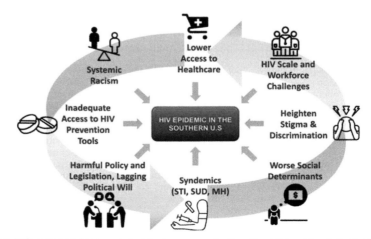

Fig. 2. Multifaceted and interrelated factors exacerbating the HIV epidemic in the Southern United States.

Despite the positive perceptions among PWH regarding Medicaid,[15] patients still face *challenges with enrollment and navigating bureaucratic hurdles, especially those with behavioral health needs.*[16] Section 1115 waivers have allowed states to experiment with Medicaid programs beyond federal rules, fostering innovation in health care delivery, eligibility, and payment systems. These waivers are tools for states to tailor Medicaid to local needs, subject to federal approval and oversight. While 1115 waivers represent an alternative to support PWH in lieu of Medicaid expansion, attempts to enact such measures in some states have been defeated and 1115 waivers with work requirements in states heavily impacted by HIV do not exclude medically frail patients.[17]

Non-expansion states rely heavily on key federally funded HIV programs, like the Health Resources and Services Administration's Ryan White HIV/AIDS Program (RWHAP) and the AIDS Drug Assistance Program (ADAP), which play a crucial role in offering health care support to individuals with low income without an alternative payer source[18]; however, these are *not a comprehensive substitute for health care insurance.* These programs face limitations like dependency on annual congressional funding and restrictions on the types of care they cover.[19] Furthermore, the effectiveness of these initiatives *varies significantly across states due to differing local policies and practices.* For example, states may have different requirements for laboratory testing and reporting under RWHAP. Similarly, the criteria for income eligibility, as well as medication formularies and authorization processes for ADAP, differ from state to state.[19]

These differences in policies and eligibility criteria across various regions lead to *uneven resource allocation* for federally funded programs.[19] For example, RWHAP funding per PWH per year varies considerably among cities: In Atlanta, GA, funding is $1919/PWH; in Miami, FL, funding is $2053/PWH; and in New York City, NY, funding is $2350/PWH. The disparities are even more striking in Medicare/Medicaid funding per PWH, with Atlanta receiving $4,408, Miami $3,403, and New York City a staggering $22,329 per person.[19] This inequitable distribution of funds is especially concerning in those *cities with the highest needs and inequities,* yet the available funding is most limited. Such imbalance leads to significant disparities in health care resources including medication access and safety net support systems creating considerable challenges for caregivers and patients.[20]

HIV Scale in the South and Associated Workforce Challenges

Providing care for the growing and aging population of PWH necessitates a comprehensive, well-trained, and multidisciplinary workforce (Nolan and Colleagues, "Training the Next Generation of the HIV Workforce: Needs, Challenges, and Opportunities"). However, the United States is currently grappling with a *significant shortage of physicians*, including those specializing in infectious diseases and HIV care. Alarmingly, over 80% of US counties lack an infectious disease physician (Nolan and Colleagues, "Training the Next Generation of the HIV Workforce: Needs, Challenges, and Opportunities").[21,22] These projections indicate that the demand for HIV providers will continue to exceed the supply. This situation is compounded by the recent "End the HIV Epidemic" initiative with an important focus on diagnosing and retaining PWH in care that will further amplify the demand for skilled HIV clinicians.[23]

In Southern states, an analysis of Medicaid claims and clinician characteristics from 2009 to 2011 revealed a concerning shortage of experienced HIV care providers.[24] Out of 5012 identified primary care and infectious disease clinicians, only 28% had considerable experience in HIV management, defined as caring for 10 or more

Medicaid enrollees with HIV over 3 years. These experienced clinicians were located in urban areas, leading to a notable absence in rural regions. In fact, 81% of rural counties lacked any experienced HIV clinicians.[24] These findings are consistent with other studies, highlighting that in every Southern state, *the average number of experienced providers in rural counties is 0*. Similarly, across all counties in the Southern states, the mean number of HIV care providers is also 0 except for Delaware, Florida, and Washington DC.[25,26] This shortage is particularly alarming considering that 9 of the 10 US counties with the highest HIV incidence rates are in the South. Unlike other regions, *the South faces a significant disparity in the availability of providers, particularly in the areas where they are most urgently needed.*

This crisis in rural HIV care takes on an additional dimension when considering accessibility challenges faced by the majority (54%) of PWH in these areas.[27] For these individuals, reaching health care facilities often means *traveling distances up to 6 times greater than their urban counterparts*.[27] While telemedicine has been proposed as a potential solution,[28] its effectiveness is hampered by the "digital divide." This term refers to unequal access to digital technologies, influenced by factors such as cost, comfort with technology, and the availability of broadband services. Rural and underserved communities are particularly impacted by this gap in digital infrastructure, complicating the deployment of telemedicine services for PWH in these areas. Thus, *while digital solutions offer promise, their successful implementation in these communities remains a significant challenge.*

Complicating these challenges are reports that *health care workers in the South are leaving* Southern states and others are reluctant to move to Southern states. This is particularly notable among those whose practice environment is impacted by restrictive legislation influencing sexual and reproductive health rights, and anti-lesbian, gay, bisexual, transgender, and queer (LGBTQ) laws, particularly targeting transgender youth.[29] These laws not only undermine the principles of medical ethics and patient autonomy but also impose moral and professional dilemmas on providers. As a result, many are compelled to migrate to more progressive environments where comprehensive and inclusive care is endorsed. This can only exacerbate the existing shortfall in the HIV workforce in the South.[29]

The *understaffing of the public health workforce* poses a significant challenge, especially in areas of high demand. This issue is particularly evident in roles such as disease intervention specialists, linkage coordinators, and patient navigators, who are crucial in conducting case investigations for HIV/STI. These positions often experience high turnover rates, a situation that was exacerbated during the COVID-19 pandemic.[30] In the South, where the incidence of HIV is notably higher than in other regions, the demand for case investigations and referrals to medical and social services significantly strain the public health workforce.[31]

Disparities in public health funding make the recruitment and retention of public health workers difficult. The per capita public health spending in Southern states is lower than the national average. In fact, states in the South allocate approximately 18% less in health spending per capita compared to those in the Northeast.[32] These disparities limit the South's ability to recruit and retain skilled public health professionals, directly impacting the effectiveness of disease management programs. Additionally, federal funding through the CDC for public health, which often supplements state budgets, has been distributed unevenly. *The Southern region has the highest population, but not the highest funding* (the Northeast region does), suggesting that other factors beyond population size influence the allocation of funding across these regions.[33] This inequity in funding and spending highlights a critical need for increased investment in the South's public health infrastructure, specifically prioritizing workforce development and disease intervention programs, to mitigate the impact of HIV and ensure equitable health outcomes across regions.

Stigma and Discrimination Predominate in the South

Stigma emerges as the true "silent killer" for PWH. This is particularly pronounced in the Southern United States, where *LGBTQ+ individuals face heightened levels of discrimination and stigma,*[34,35] which manifests as social ostracism, verbal abuse, and unequal treatment in employment, housing, and lower access to HIV prevention and care.[36] LGBTQ+ individuals grapple with increased stigma, especially in the South, due to entrenched conservative cultural norms and religious beliefs that view non-heteronormative orientations and identities unfavorably.[34–36] Studies have shown a *significant presence of internalized stigma among these sexual minorities,* leading to mental health challenges and reduced self-esteem.[34–36]

Legislation in many Southern states exacerbates this situation by imposing constraints on LGBTQ+ interests.[37] Laws that restrict transgender rights, allow the denial of treatment (such as gender-affirming care) or services based on conservative and religious beliefs, and curtail LGBTQ+ education in schools, negatively impact the mental health and welfare of LGBTQ+ individuals.[38] Professional organizations have highlighted that these laws not only reinforce stigma but significantly harm the mental and emotional well-being of LGBTQ+ people.[39]

Stigma and discrimination create formidable barriers to health care, especially in HIV and STI testing and treatment. The fear of judgment and discrimination often dissuades individuals from seeking essential health care services. This is evidenced by the Southern LGBTQ Health Survey, including 5617 participants, and represents the largest survey on LGBTQ+ health in the South.[40] More than half of the respondents reported challenges in accessing quality medical care, attributing this difficulty to their residence in the South. Many *felt uneasy about seeking medical care locally,* with transgender individuals endorsing more discomfort and obstacles in accessing health care compared to their cisgender counterparts.

The South Has Worse Social Health Determinants Compared Nationally

Social determinants of health (SDoH) are particularly challenging in the South, creating barriers for PWH in accessing and maintaining health care. Factors like food and housing insecurity, difficulties in medication storage, transportation issues, demanding employment schedules, and caregiver responsibilities for multigenerational families significantly hinder PWH from obtaining consistent, long-term health care.[20]

In comparison to national averages, *the Southern region shows notable disparities in key health determinants.* The *poverty* rate in the South, at 13.9%, is higher than the national level of 12.6%.[41] This disparity is even more pronounced in nonmetropolitan areas of the South, where 19.7% live in poverty, compared to just 12.9% in the Northeast.[41] *Food insecurity* is also more prevalent in the South, with a rate of 11.4% versus the national average of 10.2%.[42] The *median household income* in the South is lower at $63,524 (compared to $74,580 nationally in 2022), and the rate of *high school educational attainment* is also below the national average (87.9% compared to 88.9%).[43] Although minor, differences in high school attainment and food insecurity contribute to the HIV epidemic in the South but are not primary drivers of disparities.

Housing insecurity is a significant issue in southern metropolitan areas where PWH reside. Thirty-one percent of Southern residents who are behind on rent or mortgage payments fear losing their homes. This statistic rises to over 41% in Kentucky,

Georgia, Alabama, and Tennessee.[44] Furthermore, *income inequality* in the South is significant, as measured by the Gini coefficient.[45] Southern cities feature prominently among those with the highest rates of income inequality in the country. In 2022, Miami Beach, FL, and Atlanta, GA, were the cities with the highest Gini coefficients in the United States, with 8 of the top 10 cities with high-income inequality located in the Deep South, areas that also have significant HIV incidence rates.[46]

These challenges underscore the need for more comprehensive supportive services for PWH, including tangible resources like transportation, food, and housing, as well as additional personnel such as social workers, case managers, and peer navigators. However, this need arises in the context of state governments offering fewer safety net services and resources to PWH. Consequently, *health care providers and systems are stretched thin, struggling to deliver adequate care with limited resources.*

Syndemics Exacerbate Health Challenges in Southern Region

A syndemic refers to the interaction of 2 or more concurrent diseases, worsening each other's progression. This effect is amplified by social, economic, political, and environmental factors impacting the population.[47] For example, the combination of HIV, non-HIV/STIs, respiratory illnesses, viral hepatitis, substance-use disorders (SUD), and mental health disorders, particularly in socioeconomically challenged areas, leads to worse health outcomes. The coexistence of multiple diseases accelerates each one's progression, complicates treatment, and exacerbates social and economic difficulties. This phenomenon is notably evident in the Southern United States.

The prevalence of *STIs* is higher in the Southern United States compared to national averages.[48] In 2021, chlamydia and gonorrhea rates were 545.3 and 242.9 per 100,000 individuals in the South, respectively, compared to the national rates of 495.5 for chlamydia and 214.0 for gonorrhea.[48] Mississippi, Louisiana, Georgia, and South Carolina have the highest rates for both. Interestingly, the rates of syphilis in the South are similar to national averages, at 16.7 per 100,000 in the South versus 16.2 per 100,000 nationally[11]; however, a recent report highlights a substantial increase in congenital syphilis cases nationally. Most cases (1,981) were in the South with inadequate treatment accounting for most missed opportunities in the region (54.5%), followed by non-timely testing (23.7%).[49]

The 2021 and 2022 National Surveys on Drug Use and Health reveal that LGBTQ+ adults face *higher risks of SUD, serious mental health issues, and suicidal thoughts* compared to their heterosexual peers.[50] A study in the US Deep South found that only 20% of treatment facilities offer specialized programs for older adults,[51] despite rising opioid use and overdoses nationwide.[52] This shortage of SUD treatment is worsened by poverty, rural settings, stigma, *and lack of treatment options and harm reduction resources* (such as syringe exchange services, clean supplies, and safe consumption facilities) in the region. These factors are critical in HIV care and prevention, as the presence of mental health disorders and SUD, compounded with limited treatment and harm reduction resources can increase HIV risk, complicate treatment adherence, and lead to HIV clusters and outbreaks.[53]

During the COVID-19 pandemic, HIV services in the United States faced challenges, as a 2021 survey conducted in the South revealed issues like *financial strain, staff mental health problems, and technological gaps within HIV care organizations, along with patients reporting worsening issues related to mental health, substance use, and housing instability.*[54] A study conducted in a Texas clinic noted reduced HIV care visits and virologic suppression but more mental health service utilization.[55] The period during the pandemic also saw telemedicine's beneficial role in HIV care in the South, emphasizing the need for enhanced organizational support and adaptation to new care delivery models.[28,55]

Harmful Legislation and Policy, Lagging Political Will

A commitment from political leadership can facilitate progress even in States with significant barriers to care. Political will could lead to advocacy for expansion in health care access, support for public health infrastructure, and policies to prioritize a syndemic approach to health such as syringe services legislation.[56] In addition, political will can lead to policies and priorities that reduce stigma and abolish HIV criminalization. As of 2022, 35 states across the United States have implemented laws criminalizing HIV exposure. Notably, *over half of the Southern states have established specific criminal statutes or sentencing enhancements targeting PWH.*[57] These laws and practices can deter testing or engagement in health care among already marginalized, over-policed, and/or immigrant communities, exacerbating the existing mistrust in the health care system.[57]

Laws fueled by stigma, particularly those *criminalizing SUD*, critically hinder access to essential SUD treatment and associated harm reduction resources.[58,59] These restrictions have led to limited availability of safe drug supplies, clean needles, and syringes, thereby increasing the risk of HIV transmission among people who use drugs. In addition, many Southern states are enacting new *anti-LGBTQ+ legislation*, which poses a significant threat to the well-being of already vulnerable communities overrepresented in the HIV epidemic.[37] Finally, *anti-LGBTQ+ legislation severely impacts comprehensive sexual health education* in the South.[60] This scarcity of sexual health education and promotion is linked to higher incidences of HIV/STIs and teenage pregnancies in the Southern region.[48,49]

Inadequate Access to HIV Prevention and Newer Treatment Modalities

One of the most effective tools to end the HIV epidemic is increasing access and education related to PrEP. The PNR[9] measures the alignment between PrEP usage relative to new HIV diagnoses in a determined area. A lower PNR indicates a larger unmet need. Data reveal substantial disparities in PrEP use across different racial/ethnic groups, genders, and regions.[9] Despite the overall growth in PrEP use nationally since its introduction in 2012, *the rate of PrEP uptake is lower in the South compared to other regions and has not kept pace with the rate of improved uptake in other regions.*[61] Black and Hispanic populations, as well as women, have lower usage rates relative to the proportion they represent of new HIV diagnoses, often compounded by systemic barriers. Black individuals are the least represented group among PrEP users. Mississippi, South Carolina, Alabama, and West Virginia, all Southern states, have the highest unmet needs for PrEP.[9]

Long-acting injectable (LAI) PrEP (currently LA-cabotegravir) offers an alternative prevention modality. LAI for treatment also offers an exciting opportunity to improve health outcomes, particularly for those who have trouble with daily adherence to oral medications.[62] Many are concerned that clinicians will see disparities widen instead of narrow with these new modalities because of high cost, logistical challenges in clinics that are often overstretched and inadequately equipped or staffed to handle the distribution and administration of these medications, and the reality that the patients with the greatest self-advocacy often have access to new therapies earliest.[63]

Systemic Racism, the Critical Determinant in HIV Health Disparities, and Outcomes

The impact of systemic racism on HIV outcomes cannot be overestimated, particularly among sexual minority men within Black and Hispanic communities. The Southern

United States has a higher proportion of Black/African American residents, especially in major cities like Atlanta, Houston, and New Orleans, which have significant rates of new HIV infections nationally.[64] Historical and ongoing social inequities, such as the effects of slavery, Jim Crow laws, redlining, and a lack of intergenerational wealth, exacerbate these disparities. Moreover, the southern states' proximity to Latin America and the Caribbean draws a growing Hispanic immigrant population, introducing unique social vulnerabilities. These factors collectively heighten the challenges these groups face in the HIV epidemic.

Qualitative research highlighting the voices of African American/Black and Latino groups reveals persistent racial and ethnic disparities in HIV care and prevention.[65,66] These perspectives highlight the complex interplay of societal structures, rooted in those systemic barriers, within health care, economic systems, language justice, and legal frameworks. Finally, poverty is a critical factor, affecting various aspects of life such as housing stability, insurance coverage, and access to HIV care and prevention methods.[41–45]

PATHS FORWARD

To effectively end the HIV epidemic for all, the ongoing challenges in the South must be addressed by all. The HIV Medicine Association has compiled a set of strategies and recommendations to achieve this goal. Additionally, lessons from the COVID-19 pandemic such as rapid adaptation and technological integration should be leveraged to better address the challenges the South faces.[67,68] **Table 2** provides an overview of the various barriers and opportunities identified for addressing the HIV epidemic in the Southern United States, highlighting key challenges and potential strategies for mitigating disparities.

Affordable universal health care in the United States that includes comprehensive access to HIV prevention, mental health resources, and SUD treatments. Continued advocacy to include expanding Medicaid and ensuring sustained federal support for programs like RWHAP and ADAP. Furthermore, reducing administrative barriers to accessing such programs, and expanding innovative care models, such as telemedicine and mobile health.[67–69]

Strengthening the Southern HIV workforce. Addressing the shortage of health care providers in the South requires boosting training, recruitment, and retention. Prioritizing the hiring of community representative and bilingual professionals and ensuring fair wages for all health care roles. Additionally, expanding visa options and eligibility for training grants for international medical trainees can help fill gaps and foster health care innovation.[67,68,70]

Addressing social determinants impacting HIV. Efforts to end the HIV epidemic must prioritize SDoH. This involves funding for standardized data collection and recognizing the importance of housing and supplemental services like transportation and legal aid as part of health care. Supporting peer navigators and basing services on SDoH and epidemiologic data are critical to improving access and outcomes.[20,68]

Empowerment and support, not stigma. Community education and outreach are essential to reduce HIV-related stigma, especially in conservative and religious communities. Tailored educational efforts, collaborations with faith-based leaders, and training health care providers in cultural sensitivity are key strategies. Advocating for supportive policies and leveraging social media to promote positive HIV messaging are also important.[71–73]

Promoting HIV prevention through reasonable drug pricing. Advocacy for lower drug prices and the use of Department of Health and Human Services guidelines for generic

Table 2

Summary of key factors influencing the HIV epidemic in the Southern region of the United States, contrasted with potential opportunities aimed at mitigating the impact of HIV in this region

	Barriers	Opportunities
Access to Health Care	Higher uninsured rates than national averages	Advocating for universal access to health care
	Seven out of 10 States that have not expanded Medicaid in the United States are in the South	Advocate for Medicaid expansion
	High reliance on federally funded HIV programs in non-expansion states coupled with limitations and variability in requirement for eligibility and enrollment across states	Standardize subsidy program policies and eligibility for HIV care and prevention. Implement interventions to waive, remove or streamline service eligibility, enrollment, and recertification
	Uneven resource allocation in the South compared to other regions	Fund innovative health delivery models that leverage mobile health, telehealth, etc.
		Boost funding for community health centers to enhance care for underserved groups
Scale and Workforce	Severe shortage of physicians and HIV specialists affecting the South	Invest in training and recruiting more health care professionals, particularly in identification, incentivizing compensation, and loan repayment strategies
	Lack of experienced HIV care providers, including nurses, social workers, care managers, mental health providers, particularly in rural areas of the South	Develop incentives to attract and retain health care professionals in underserved and rural areas.
		Offer consistent funding for care providers at all levels, including those with lived experiences at a living wage
	PWH in rural areas endure greater travel distances to health care facilities	Expand eligibility for training grants with more flexible visa policies that include international medical trainees.
	Understaffing of the public health workforce	Increase and equate public health funding to bolster the workforce in the South
	Disparity in public health funding and spending	
Stigma and Discrimination	Heightened levels of discrimination and stigma	Foster community-based initiatives to reduce stigma and promote inclusivity
	Legislative constraints regarding LGBTQ+ matters in many Southern states	Implement comprehensive anti-discrimination policies and laws to protect marginalized groups
	Impact of stigma and discrimination on health care access	Educate health care providers on cultural competency and sensitivity toward marginalized communities
		Increase investment in affordable housing, food security programs, and transportation services for PWH

(continued on next page)

Table 2
(*continued*)

	Barriers	Opportunities
Social Determinants of Health	Higher rates of poverty, food and housing insecurity, and transportation issues lead to barriers to health care access	Develop employment, educational, and vocational programs prioritizing impoverished communities
	Income inequality and disparities in social determinants of health between metropolitan and nonmetropolitan areas	Enhance social support systems, including case management and peer navigation services
Syndemics	Compounded impact of multiple coexisting diseases, including STIs, addiction and mental health illnesses with HIV	Integrate HIV care with other free or low-cost medical services to address co-occurring conditions such as SUD and mental illness
	Higher prevalence of STIs in the South	Increase funding and resources for STI testing, treatment and education in high-prevalence areas
	Limited SUD treatment facilities, particularly for LBGTQ+ individuals	Expand culturally sensitive SUD treatment facilities and programs, including syringe exchange programs, particularly in areas with limited resources
Political Will, Legislation, and Policy	Widespread HIV criminalization legislation in over half of the Southern states	Advocate for the repeal of HIV criminalization laws and policies that negatively impact PWH
		Engage policymakers to ensure HIV-related legislation is based on scientific evidence and public health principles
	Insufficient testing and treatment within jails and prisons, coupled with inadequately funded programs to facilitate connections upon release	Promote policies that safeguard the health of PWH in the justice system, during incarceration and transition periods
	Insufficient state-level prioritization regarding the end of the HIV epidemic initiative	Advocating for policies that support Ending the HIV Epidemic, by presenting data demonstrating cost savings for states and improved outcomes for PWH
	Limitations on access to sexual and reproductive health and education	Promote policies that allow sexual health education in schools and communities and fund programs
Inadequate Access to HIV Prevention	Disparities in awareness and access to HIV prevention methods, especially among racial and ethnic minorities	Enhance education and awareness campaigns about HIV prevention methods
	Challenges in accessing cutting-edge prevention tools like long-acting injectables due to cost and health care system limitations	Fund programs to ensure access to long-acting injectables and oral HIV prevention therapies in low-insurance areas. Crucial since Ryan White programs do not cover these costs at present
		Collaborate with stakeholders from pharmaceutical companies, lawmakers, and health care providers to reduce medication costs and improve distribution
Systemic Racism	Racial and ethnic disparities in HIV care and prevention, exacerbated by systemic barriers in health care, economic systems, and legal frameworks	Address systemic racism through policy changes, educational initiatives, and community engagement.
		Focus on culturally sensitive health care services and research to address the unique needs of marginalized communities

drugs are crucial to making these drugs more affordable and accessible. Savings from reduced drug costs should be reinvested into expanding HIV prevention and care, enhancing access to resources like PrEP, and supporting home HIV and STI screening initiatives.[66–68,73]

Inclusive policies and driving political change. Repealing laws that criminalize HIV exposure and advocating for evidence-based public health policies are fundamental. Expanding access to substance use treatment, harm reduction programs, and reforming sexual and reproductive health education to include comprehensive topics holds promise in improving health outcomes. Legal protections for marginalized groups, particularly those engaged in the correctional system settings, should also be strengthened.[29,68]

SUMMARY

In summary, the authors highlight the higher burden of HIV in the Southern United States, with particular emphasis on the disparities affecting Black and Hispanic/Latino/a/e populations, adolescents, and young adults. These disparities are rooted in interrelated issues such as restricted health care access, systemic racism, and various social determinants of health including higher rates of poverty, housing instability, and educational barriers. The South's unique struggles are further complicated by an HIV workforce shortage, especially in rural locales, along with pervasive stigma and discrimination against LGBTQ+ communities. Compounding these challenges are coexisting syndemics like STIs, SUDs, and other mental health illnesses that further challenge HIV care and retention. This review underscores the necessity for comprehensive approaches that encompass expanding health care including Medicaid expansion, strengthening the HIV workforce, confronting stigma, addressing SDoH, syndemic approaches, broadening the availability of HIV prevention tools, and revising policies to bolster HIV prevention and treatment efforts. Implementing these strategies is crucial for closing the care gaps and enhancing health outcomes for PWH in the Southern United States.

CLINICS CARE POINTS

- Identify and address social determinants like food and/or housing insecurity and transportation that often impact health outcomes.

- Provide community education to reduce HIV-related stigma and train in cultural sensitivity to support inclusive care environments.

- Advocate for recruitment and retention strategies to expand the pool of skilled HIV care providers, especially in underserved areas.

- Support Medicaid expansion and policies that reduce barriers to continuous and comprehensive health care coverage.

- Manage HIV in context with coexisting conditions such as STIs and substance use, utilizing integrated screening and treatment strategies.

- Promote and prescribe HIV prevention resources in its many available forms.

DISCLOSURE

The authors declare that they have no conflicts of interest and nothing to disclose regarding the content presented in this review article.

FUNDING

Dr Saldana receives grant funding for CDC, NIH and is consultant for ViiV Healthcare. No conflicts to report for Dr Armstrong.

REFERENCES

1. World Health Organization. WHO HIV Epidemiology Fact Sheet, Available at: https://cdn.who.int/media/docs/default-source/hq-hiv-hepatitis-and-stis-library/j0294-who-hiv-epi-factsheet-v7.pdf. Accessed December 1 2023.
2. Centers for Disease Control and Prevention. HIV Surveillance Report, 34. Available at: http://www.cdc.gov/hiv/library/reports/hiv-surveillance.html, 2021.Accessed December 1 2023.
3. U.S. Census Bureau. Census Regions and Divisions of the United States, Available at: https://www2.census.gov/geo/pdfs/maps-data/maps/reference/us_regdiv.pdf, 2023. Accessed December 1 2023.
4. Centers for Disease Control and Prevention. Estimated HIV Incidence and Prevalence in the United States, 2017–2021, *HIV Surveillance Supplemental Report*, 28 (3), 2023, Available at: http://www.cdc.gov/hiv/library/reports/hiv-surveillance.html. Accessed December 1 2023.
5. Gant Z, Dailey A, Wang S, et al. Trends in HIV care outcomes among adults and adolescents in the U.S. South, 2015-2019. Ann Epidemiol 2022;71:15–22.
6. AIDSVu. Emory University, Rollins School of Public Health, Available at: https://aidsvu.org/. Accessed December 1 2023.
7. Centers for Disease Control and Prevention. HIV Mortality, Available at: https://www.cdc.gov/hiv/pdf/library/slidesets/cdc-hiv-surveillance-slideset-mortality-2021.pdf, 2021. Accessed December 1 2023.
8. Centers for Disease Control and Prevention. HIV Care Continuum, Available at: https://www.cdc.gov/hiv/pdf/library/factsheets/cdc-hiv-care-continuum.pdf, 2019. Accessed December 1 2023.
9. AIDSVu. New Data on Inequities in PrEP Use, Available at: https://aidsvu.org/aidsvu-releases-new-data-highlighting-ongoing-inequities-in-prep-use-among-black-and-hispanic-people-and-across-regions-of-the-county/, 2023. Accessed December 1 2023.
10. Healthy people 2030, U.S. Department of health, and Human services, Available at: https://health.gov/healthypeople/objectives-and-data/social-determinants-health. Accessed December 1 2023.
11. Centers for Disease Control and Prevention. Congenital Syphilis — United States, Available at: https://www.cdc.gov/std/statistics/2021/tables/20.htm, 2021. Accessed December 1 2023.
12. Dawson L., Kates J., Roberts T., et al., Medicaid, and people with HIV. KFF, Available at: https://www.kff.org/hivaids/issue-brief/medicaid-and-people-with-hiv/, 2023. Accessed December 1 2023.
13. Gai Y, Marthinsen J. Medicaid expansion, HIV Testing, and HIV-Related Risk Behaviors in the United States, 2010-2017. Am J Public Health 2019;109(10):1404–12.
14. Fayaz Farkhad B, Holtgrave DR, Albarracín D. Effect of medicaid expansions on HIV diagnoses and pre-exposure prophylaxis use. Am J Prev Med 2021;60(3):335–42.
15. McManus KA, Schurman E, An Z, et al. Patient perspective of people with HIV who gained medicaid through medicaid expansion: a cross-sectional qualitative study. AIDS Res Hum Retroviruses 2022;38(7):580–91.

16. Arnold EA, Fuller S, Kirby V, et al. The impact of medicaid expansion on people living with HIV and seeking behavioral health services. Health Aff 2018;37(9): 1450–6.

17. "Medicaid Waiver Tracker: Approved and Pending Section 1115 Waivers by State." KFF, Available at: https://www.kff.org/medicaid/issue-brief/medicaid-waiver-tracker-approved-and-pending-section-1115-waivers-by-state/, 2023. Accessed December 1 2023.

18. Doshi RK, Milberg J, Jumento T, et al. For many served by the Ryan White HIV/AIDS program, disparities in viral suppression decreased, 2010-14. Health Aff 2017;36(1):116–23.

19. Panagiotoglou D, Olding M, Enns B, et al. Building the case for localized approaches to HIV: Structural Conditions and Health System Capacity to Address the HIV/AIDS Epidemic in Six US Cities. AIDS Behav 2018;22(9):3071–82.

20. Sullivan PS, Satcher Johnson A, Pembleton ES, et al. Epidemiology of HIV in the USA: Epidemic burden, inequities, contexts, and responses. Lancet 2021; 397(10279):1095–106.

21. Walensky RP, McQuillen DP, Shahbazi S, et al. Where is the ID in COVID-19? Ann Intern Med 2020;173(7):587–9.

22. Armstrong WS. The human immunodeficiency virus workforce in crisis: an urgent need to build the foundation required to end the epidemic. Clin Infect Dis 2021; 72(9):1627–30.

23. Fauci AS, Redfield RR, Sigounas G, et al. Ending the HIV epidemic: a plan for the United States. JAMA 2019;321(9):844–5.

24. Bono RS, Dahman B, Sabik LM, et al. Human immunodeficiency virus-experienced clinician workforce capacity: urban-rural disparities in the Southern United States. Clin Infect Dis 2021;72(9):1615–22.

25. Gilman B., Bouchery E., Barrett K., et al., HIV clinician workforce study, *Mathematica Policy Res*, 2013, Available at: https://www.mathematica.org/our-publications-and-findings/publications/hiv-clinician-workforce-study. Accessed December 1 2023.

26. Weiser J, Beer L, West BT, et al. Qualifications, demographics, satisfaction, and future capacity of the HIV care provider workforce in the United States, 2013-2014. Clin Infect Dis 2016;63:966–75.

27. Kimmel AD, Masiano SP, Bono RS, et al. Structural barriers to comprehensive, co-ordinated HIV care: geographic accessibility in the US South. AIDS Care 2018; 30(11):1459–68.

28. Salgado S, Felzien G, Brumbeloe J. Georgia leverages telehealth to expand HIV care management in underserved areas. Am J Prev Med 2021;61(5 Suppl 1): S55–9.

29. Person AK, Terndrup CP, Jain MK, et al. "Do we stay or do we go?" the impact of anti-LGBTQ+ legislation on the HIV Workforce in the South. Clin Infect Dis 2023.

30. Kintziger KW, Stone KW, Jagger MA, et al. The impact of the COVID-19 response on the provision of other public health services in the U.S.: A cross-sectional study. PLoS One 2021;16(10):e0255844.

31. Stone KW, Kintziger KW, Jagger MA, et al. Public health workforce burnout in the COVID-19 response in the U.S. Int J Environ Res Public Health 2021;18(8):4369.

32. Centers for Medicare & Medicaid Services. State Residence. CMS.gov, Available at: https://www.cms.gov/data-research/statistics-trends-and-reports/national-health-expenditure-data/state-residence. Accessed December 1 2023.

33. CDC. Fiscal Year 2022 Grant Funding By State. FundingProfiles.CDC.gov, Available at: https://fundingprofiles.cdc.gov/. Accessed December 1 2023.

34. Berg RC, Ross MW. The second closet: a qualitative study of HIV Stigma Among Seropositive Gay Men in a Southern U.S. City. Int J Sex Health 2014;26(3): 186–99.

35. Stringer KL, Turan B, McCormick L, et al. HIV-related stigma among healthcare providers in the deep South. AIDS Behav 2016;20(1):115–25.

36. Babel RA, Wang P, Alessi EJ, et al. Stigma, HIV Risk, and Access to HIV Prevention and Treatment Services Among Men Who have Sex with Men (MSM) in the United States: A Scoping Review. AIDS Behav 2021;25(11):3574–604.

37. ACLU. Legislative Attacks on LGBTQ Rights. ACLU.org, Available at: https://www.aclu.org/legislative-attacks-on-lgbtq-rights. Accessed December 1 2023.

38. American Bar Association. Impact of Anti-LGBTQ Legislative and Executive Branch Action on Children's Well-Being. ABA.org, Available at: https://www.americanbar.org/groups/litigation/resources/newsletters/childrens-rights/impact-anti-lgbtq-legislative-executive-branch-action-childrens-well-being/. Accessed December 1 2023.

39. Association of American Medical Colleges (AAMC). The Current Wave of Anti-LGBT Legislation: Historical Context and Implications for LGBT Health. AAMC.org, Available at: https://www.aamc.org/what-we-do/equity-diversity-inclusion/lgbt-health-resources/reports/anti-lgbt-legislation. Accessed December 1 2023.

40. Harless C, Nanney M, Johnson AH, et al. Southern LGBTQ health survey. Asheville, NC: Campaign for Southern Equality; 2019.

41. U.S. Department of Agriculture, Economic Research Service. Poverty, Available at: https://data.ers.usda.gov/reports.aspx?ID=17826. Accessed December 1 2023.

42. U.S. Department of Agriculture, Economic Research Service. Key Statistics & Graphics, Available at: https://www.ers.usda.gov/topics/food-nutrition-assistance/food-security-in-the-us/key-statistics-graphics/. Accessed December 1 2023.

43. U.S. Trustee Program, Department of Justice. Census Bureau Median Family Income By Family Size, Available at: https://www.justice.gov/ust/eo/bapcpa/20220401/bci_data/median_income_table.htm. Accessed December 1 2023.

44. Pandemic to Prosperity. Likelihood of eviction or foreclosure, by state, Available at: https://www.pandemictoprosperity.org/onepagers/housing-insecurity-apr2023, 2023. Accessed December 1 2023.

45. U.S. Census Bureau. Gini Index, Available at: https://www.census.gov/topics/income-poverty/income-inequality/about/metrics/gini-index.html. Accessed December 1 2023.

46. DePietro A., 20 Cities With The Worst Income Inequality In America In 2022. Forbes, Available at: https://www.forbes.com/sites/andrewdepietro/2022/03/31/20-cities-with-the-worst-income-inequality-in-america-in-2022/. Accessed December 1 2023.

47. Bromberg DJ, Mayer KH, Altice FL. Identifying and managing infectious disease syndemics in patients with HIV. Curr Opin HIV AIDS 2020;15(4):232–42.

48. Centers for Disease Control and Prevention. Sexually Transmitted Disease Surveillance 2021: STDs in Adolescents and Young Adults, Available at: https://www.cdc.gov/std/statistics/2021/tables/2.html. Accessed December 1 2023.

49. McDonald R, O'Callaghan K, Torrone E, et al. Vital signs: missed opportunities for preventing congenital syphilis — United States, 2022. MMWR Morb Mortal Wkly Rep 2023;72:1269–74.

50. U.S. Department of Health and Human Services, Substance Abuse and Mental Health Services Administration, Center for Behavioral Health Statistics and

Quality, *National Survey on Drug Use and Health*, 2022, Available at: https://datafiles.samhsa.gov/. Accessed December 1 2023.

51. Mumba MN, Jaiswal J, Bui C, et al. Substance use treatment services for older adults in five states in the Southern United States: a state-by-state comparison of available treatment services. Aging Ment Health 2023;27(5):1028–36.

52. Tanz LJ, Dinwiddie AT, Mattson CL, et al. Drug overdose deaths among persons aged 10–19 years — United States, July 2019–December 2021. MMWR Morb Mortal Wkly Rep 2022;71:1576–82.

53. McClung RP, Atkins AD, Kilkenny M, et al. Response to a Large HIV Outbreak, Cabell County, West Virginia, 2018-2019. Am J Prev Med 2021;61(5 Suppl 1): S143–50.

54. Cooper H, Reif S, Wilson E, et al. The COVID-19 Pandemic: Impact on Southern HIV Service Organizations, Staff, and Clients. AIDS Educ Prev 2022;34(4): 333–47.

55. Norwood J, Kheshti A, Shepherd BE, et al. The Impact of COVID-19 on the HIV Care Continuum in a Large Urban Southern Clinic. AIDS Behav 2022;26(8): 2825–9.

56. Adimora AA, Ramirez C, Schoenbach VJ, et al. Policies and politics that promote HIV infection in the Southern United States. AIDS 2014;28(10):1393–7.

57. U.S. Department of Justice. Justice Department Releases Best Practices Guide to Reform HIV-Specific Criminal Laws, Available at: https://www.justice.gov/opa/pr/justice-department-releases-best-practices-guide-reform-hiv-specific-criminal-laws-align. Accessed December 1 2023.

58. Bratberg JP, Simmons A, Arya V, et al. Support, don't punish: Drug decriminalization is harm reduction. J Am Pharm Assoc (2003) 2023;63(1):224–9.

59. NIDA. Punishing drug use heightens the stigma of addiction, Available at: https://nida.nih.gov/about-nida/noras-blog/2021/08/punishing-drug-use-heightens-stigma-addiction, 2021. Accessed December 1 2023.

60. Kline NS, Griner SB, Neelamegam M, et al. Responding to "Don't Say Gay" Laws in the US: research priorities and considerations for health equity. Sex Res Social Policy 2022;19(4):1397–402.

61. Musoke LS, Shumaker A, Wilson B, et al. PrEP inequity across geographic, racial and sex groups in a Nationwide US veteran cohort. Open Forum Infect Dis 2023; 10(Suppl 2). ofad500.169.

62. Landovitz RJ, Donnell D, Clement ME, et al. Cabotegravir for HIV prevention in cisgender men and transgender women. N Engl J Med 2021;385(7):595–608.

63. Collins LF, Corbin-Johnson D, Asrat M, et al. Early experience implementing long-acting injectable cabotegravir/rilpivirine for human immunodeficiency virus-1 treatment at a ryan white-funded clinic in the US South. Open Forum Infect Dis 2022;9(9):ofac455.

64. U.S. Census Bureau. U.S. Census Bureau QuickFacts: United States, Available at: https://www.census.gov/quickfacts/fact/table/US/PST045222. Accessed December 1 2023.

65. Filippone P, Serrano S, Campos S, et al. Understanding why racial/ethnic inequities along the HIV care continuum persist in the United States: a qualitative exploration. Int J Equity Health 2023;22(1):168.

66. Saldana C, Philpott DC, Mauck DE, et al. Public Health Response to Clusters of Rapid HIV Transmission Among Hispanic or Latino Gay, Bisexual, and Other Men Who Have Sex with Men — Metropolitan Atlanta, Georgia, 2021–2022. MMWR Morb Mortal Wkly Rep 2023;72(10):261–4.

67. Person AK, Armstrong WS, Evans T, et al. Principles for Ending Human Immuno-deficiency Virus as an Epidemic in the United States: A Policy Paper. Clin Infect Dis 2023;76(1):1–9.
68. Armstrong WS, Agwu AL, Barrette EP, et al. Innovations in human immunodeficiency virus (HIV) care delivery during the coronavirus disease 2019 (COVID-19) Pandemic. Clin Infect Dis 2021;72(1):9–14.
69. Dawson L. and Kates J., Domestic HIV funding in the white house FY 2024 budget request. kaiser family foundation, Available at: https://www.kff.org/hivaids/issue-brief/domestic-hiv-funding-in-the-white-house-fy-2024-budget-request/, 2023. Accessed December 1 2023.
70. Saldana CS, Burkhardt E, Pennisi A, et al. Development of a machine learning modelling tool for predicting incident HIV using public health data from a County in the Southern United States. Open Forum Infect Dis 2023;10(Suppl 2). ofad500.168.
71. Pichon LC, Jewell EN, Williams Stubbs A, et al. An engaged community of faith to decrease HIV stigma in the U.S. South. Int J Environ Res Public Health 2023; 20(3):2100.
72. Chen D, Watson RJ, Caputi TL, et al. Proportion of U.S. Clinics Offering LGBT-Tailored Mental Health Services Decreased Over Time: A Panel Study. Ann LGBTQ Public Popul Health 2021;2(3):174–84.
73. Shah HS, Dolwick Grieb SM, Flores-Miller A, et al. Sólo Se Vive Una Vez: The Implementation and Reach of an HIV Screening Campaign for Latinx Immigrants. AIDS Educ Prev 2020;32(3):229–42.

HIV and Substance Use Disorders

Audun J. Lier, MD, MPH[a], Adati Tarfa, PharmD, MS, PhD[b],
Sheela V. Shenoi, MD, MPH[c,d], Irene Kuo, PhD, MPH[e],
Sandra A. Springer, MD[c,d],*

KEYWORDS

- HIV • Substance use disorder • Integrated care

KEY POINTS

- Untreated substance use disorder (SUD) increases the risk for human immunodeficiency virus (HIV) acquisition and leads to poor HIV outcomes in people with HIV.
- Treatment of concomitant SUD reduces the risk of HIV transmission in persons at risk for HIV and improves HIV outcomes in people with HIV.
- Persons with substance misuse and SUDs should be screened for HIV and be offered pre-exposure prophylaxis.
- People with HIV should be screened for substance misuse and SUDs.
- Screening for substance misuse and SUDs should be integrated into HIV prevention and treatment, SUD treatment, and harm reduction care settings.

BACKGROUND
The Current State of the Problem

Substance use disorder and human immunodeficiency virus

An estimated 11.1% of people with human immunodeficiency virus (HIV) (PWH) have a diagnosis of substance use disorder (SUD).[1] HIV may be transmitted by sharing injection drug equipments and high-risk sexual behaviors associated with substance use (eg, condomless or pre-exposure prophylaxis [PrEP]-less sexual intercourse, multiple partners, transactional sex, or commercial sex work).[2] Adults and adolescent persons who inject drugs (PWID) accounted for 8% of new HIV diagnoses in the United States

[a] Renaissance School of Medicine at Stony Brook University; Northport Veterans Administration Medical Center, 79 Middleville Road, Northport, NY 11768, USA; [b] Yale University School of Medicine, 135 College Street, Suite 280, New Haven, CT 06510, USA; [c] Veterans Administration Connecticut Healthcare System, 950 Campbell Avenue, West Haven, CT 06516, USA; [d] Yale University School of Medicine, 135 College Street, Suite 323, New Haven, CT 06510, USA; [e] Department of Epidemiology, The George Washington University, Milken Institute School of Public Health, 950 New Hampshire Avenue Northwest, Suite 500, Washington, DC 20052, USA
* Corresponding author.
E-mail address: Sandra.Springer@yale.edu

Infect Dis Clin N Am 38 (2024) 599–611
https://doi.org/10.1016/j.idc.2024.06.003
0891-5520/24/Published by Elsevier Inc.

id.theclinics.com

(US) in 2021, increasing since 2017.[3] Importantly, clusters of HIV outbreaks have occurred among PWID, for example, between 2014 and 2015, an HIV outbreak related to injection drug use in Scott County, Indiana, where 181 individuals were newly diagnosed.[4] Similarly, from 2015 through 2018, the communities of Lawrence and Lowell, Massachusetts experienced an outbreak of HIV among 129 PWID,[5] and in 2018 to 2019, Cabell County in West Virginia witnessed an outbreak among 14 PWID.[6] These outbreaks occurred even in communities with comprehensive harm reduction services, signifying important public health implications related to identifying drug-related outbreaks and the rapid implementation of screening, linkage to care, and harm reduction services to break the chains of transmission.[7] Further, persons with untreated SUD may have difficulty adhering to antiretroviral therapy (ART)[1] and often receive inadequate medical care, partly due to the traditional separation of HIV care and substance use services.

Substance use disorders among people with HIV and populations at risk for HIV

Opioid use disorder: background, epidemiology, and treatment. Opioid misuse and opioid use disorder (OUD) are associated with poor ART adherence[8] and HIV transmission via shared injection equipment associated with parenteral opioid (heroin, fentanyl, or its derivatives) use or through unprotected sexual intercourse while using opioids.[2] There are 3 medications for opioid use disorder (MOUD): buprenorphine, extended-release naltrexone (XR-NTX), and methadone.[9] Buprenorphine is a partial μ-receptor opioid-agonist approved for moderate to severe Diagnostic and Statistical Manual of Mental Disorders, Fifth Edition (DSM-5) OUD. Formulations of buprenorphine include daily sublingual tablets (Subutex), buccal film (Belbuca), extended-release subcutaneous monthly injection (Sublocade), and weekly and monthly injections (Brixadi). Buprenorphine and naloxone coformulations are available, including buccal film (Suboxone) and sublingual tablets (Zubsolv).[10] XR-NTX (Vivitrol), the only μ-receptor antagonist, is prescribed as an intramuscular injection every 28 days following a required 7-day period of opioid abstinence to avoid precipitated withdrawal.[9] Lastly, methadone is a long-acting full μ-receptor agonist that can only be prescribed for treatment of OUD within an authorized opioid treatment program (OTP), thus, limiting the accessibility of this medication.[9]

Alcohol use disorder: background, epidemiology, and treatment. An estimated 30% to 50% of PWH have an alcohol use disorder (AUD),[11] which increases the risk of poor linkage to HIV care and ART initiation in PWH, decreases adherence to ART and contributes to poor HIV treatment outcomes, including lack of viral suppression.[12]

Three medications are Food and Drug Administration (FDA)-approved for the treatment of DSM-5 moderate to severe AUD: acamprosate, disulfiram, and naltrexone (oral daily pills and monthly injections of XR-NTX). The American Psychiatric Association recommends that either naltrexone or acamprosate be offered as first-line treatment. Acamprosate is more efficacious in promoting abstinence,[13] while XR-NTX is more efficacious in reducing heavy drinking and total alcohol consumption.[14] Despite this efficacy, less than 9% of patients who undergo any form of AUD treatment receive pharmacotherapy.[14] Additionally, motivational enhancement therapy, cognitive behavioral therapy (CBT), and 12-step programs, such as Alcoholics Anonymous, are helpful alone or in combination with medication to reduce alcohol use for persons with AUD.[14]

Stimulant Use Disorder: Background, Epidemiology, and Treatment

Stimulant use (eg, methamphetamtine and cocaine) can negatively impact HIV prevention and treatment.[15] There are no current FDA-approved medications for stimulant use disorder (StUD), yet there are some medications, such as bupropion, modafinil, and topiramate, that may be helpful for cocaine and amphetamine-type StUD per current American Society of Addiction Medicine and American Academy of Addiction Psychiatry StUD Guidelines.[16] The most effective form of treatment that should be incorporated in any plan for StUD, thus, far is contingency management (CM),[17] where participants receive rewards or incentives for achieving reduced stimulant use or abstinence. CM has been shown to improve adherence to ART[18] and viral suppression in PWH who use stimulants.[19] CM plus a community reinforcement approach led to an increased number of abstinent patients and was more efficacious than CBT, non-contingent rewards, and 12-step program plus non-contingent rewards.[20] CM, however, may present multiple barriers for clinicians (eg, logistics of maintaining an adequate supply of behavior reinforcers) and barriers for clients (eg, transportation, housing instability, frequent appointments, or drug screens), leading to referral to specialty care.[21] The FDA has approved *Dynamicare*, a CM mobile application with live assistance[22] that is individualized to support people with StUD (See below under mobile device health).

Benzodiazepine Use Disorder: Background, Epidemiology, and Treatment

PWUD who use benzodiazepines may engage in risky behaviors including paying for sex, sharing injection equipment, increasing injection frequency, and injecting more heroin and amphetamines.[23] Further, benzodiazepines' impact on ART adherence and the potential cognitive implications for PWH is understudied.[24] Lastly, some benzodiazepines (eg, alprazolam, diazepam) are cytochrome P 3A4 substrates and when combined with ritonavir and cobicistat-boosted ART, may result in prolonged half-lives and increased concentrations that may cause enhanced and prolonged sedating effects.[25]

There is no specific pharmacotherapy to treat benzodiazepine use disorder. Behavioral interventions (eg, CBT) with stepwise withdrawal may be beneficial in reducing benzodiazepine use over short periods. Group or individual psychotherapy techniques may be more useful in outpatient withdrawal treatment.[26]

Club Drugs: Background and Treatment

The use of club drugs, including methylenedioxymethamphetamine (MDMA), gamma hydroxybutyrate (GHB), ketamine, mephedrone, inhaled nitrate ('poppers'), and phosphodiesterase inhibitors (PDE5), reduces ART adherence in PWH.[27] Further, in persons without HIV, club drug use increases risk-taking behavior and risk of HIV transmission.[27] Lastly, due to interactions with the cytochrome P oxidase 450 system[27] or PDE5,[28] overdoses from club drugs (eg, MDMA, GHB, ketamine) have been reported.

There are no recommended pharmacotherapies to treat club drug use disorders. Current treatment is limited to behavioral interventions developed for other SUD.[27]

Discussion: What can be Done?

Treatment of substance use disorder in people with human immunodeficiency virus can improve human immunodeficiency virus outcomes

Treatment of underlying SUDs can improve outcomes in PWH (**Table 1** for Diagnostic Measures and **Table 2** for SUD treatments). For OUD, all 3 MOUDs are effective in treating opioid craving, relapse, and overdose,[9] and maintenance of MOUD is associated with reduced HIV risk behaviors,[29,30] improved retention in HIV treatment, improved ART adherence, achieving and maintaining viral suppression, [31–33] and reduction in HIV transmission.[34] XR-NTX has been demonstrated to reduce alcohol consumption and improve viral load suppression in PWH with AUD who were being

Table 1
Substance use disorder screening and diagnostic assessments (adults)

Pre-screening Test

NIDA Single Question Screening test for Drug Use	"How many times in the past year have you used an illegal drug or used a prescription medication for non-medical reasons (for example, because of the experience or feeling it caused)?" Responses to one or both should be followed-up with a full screen
Drug Abuse Screening Test (DAST-1)	"In the last 12 mo, have you used drugs other than those required for medical reasons?". Positive response should be followed-up with a DAST-10 (also available in Spanish)
Alcohol Use Disorders Identification Test-Concise (AUDIT-C)	"How often do you have a drink containing alcohol?"; "How many standard drinks containing alcohol do you have on a typical day?"' "How often do you have 4 or more drinks on one occasion?" Positive responses should be followed-up with a 10-question AUDIT assessment
Substance Use Brief Screen (SUBS)	"How many times in the past year have you used a recreational drug or used a prescription medication for non-medical reasons?" Positive responses should be followed by a full screen.
Older Adult Brief Screen (Age 60 and older)	"How often do you have a drink containing alcohol?"; "How many standard drinks containing alcohol do you have on a typical day of drinking?"; 'How often do you have 4 or more drinks on one occasion?"; "How many times in the past year have you used an illegal drug or used a prescription medication for non-medical reasons (for example, because of the experience or feeling it caused)?"'; "Have you used any cannabis over the past 6 months?". Positive responses should be followed by ASSIST-LITE full screen.
Rapid Opioid Use Disorder Assessment (ROUDA)	8-question diagnostic tool to assess DSM-5 moderate to severe OUD provides diagnosis in 2–4 min with a score of 3 or greater and can be given by non-clinicians. Captures long-term and short-term remission
Rapid Stimulant Use Disorder Assessment (RSUDA)	8-item diagnostic tool to assess DSM-5 moderate to severe stimulant use disorder diagnosis in 2–4 min with a score of 3 or greater and can be given by non-clinicians. Captures long-term and short-term remission

(continued on next page)

Table 1 (continued)	
Full screening test	
Alcohol Use Disorder Identification Test (AUDIT)	10-question screening tool to assess risky alcohol use across age, cultures, and gender
Alcohol, Smoking, and Substance Abuse Involvement Screen Test (ASSIST)	8-question assessment of risky substance use covering alcohol, amphetamine-type stimulants, cannabis, cocaine, hallucinogens, inhalants, opioids, sedatives, tobacco
ASSIST-LITE	6-question assessment of commonly used substances, including alcohol, cannabis, opioids, sedatives, stimulants, and tobacco (simplified version of ASSIST)
Tobacco, Alcohol, Prescription Medication, and Other Substance Use Tool (TAPS)	An adaptation of ASSIST-LITE, this tool is a two-stage screen for commonly used substances (screening and brief intervention)
Drug Abuse Screening Test (DAST-10)	10-item self-reported instrument that assesses drug use over the preceding 12 m (excludes alcoholic drinks)
The Cannabis Use Disorders Identification Test (CUDIT-R)	8-item tool used to assess for cannabis use disorder

Pre-screening and full screening instruments for substance use disorder.
Adapted from [SBIRT: Screening, Brief Intervention and Referral to Treatment. New York State Office of Addiction Services and Supports. Accessed November 30, 2023. https://oasas.ny.gov/sbirt and Di Paola and colleagues Validation of Two Diagnostic Assessment for Opioid and Stimulant Use Disorder for Use by Non-Clinicians. Psych Res Clin Pract. 2023;5:78–83; https://doi.org/10.1176/appi.prcp.20230022].

released from prisons or jails into the community.[35,36] Medication treatment for other SUD is limited, especially concerning HIV outcomes, and remains a major gap in HIV care.[37]

Pre-exposure propylaxis for people who use drugs who are at risk for human immunodeficiency virus

Despite International Acquired Immunodeficiency Syndrome (AIDS) Society (IAS)-USA recommendations for PrEP among PWID and who use drugs (PWUD) with sexual risk, global PrEP implementation has been slow.[37] Increasing access via integrating PrEP into MOUD programs is an additional opportunity to engage PWID and PWUD in HIV prevention.[38] Low-risk perception[39] and poor access to PrEP[40] may partly explain low utilization rates in addition to physicians' explicit or implicit bias against prescribing PrEP for PWID, mainly due to suspicion of medication non-adherence.[40] New PrEP delivery advances may help address these adherence concerns. Long-acting injectable (LAI) cabotegravir PrEP, injected every 2 months, has demonstrated superiority in preventing HIV compared to daily, oral PrEP and is now recommended for men who have sex with men, transgender, and cis-women.[41] Reducing provider bias and overcoming structural barriers to expand LAI PrEP access to all at risk for HIV are critical in engaging PWID and PWUD in highly effective biomedical interventions. Lastly, nearly one-third of PWID is also at risk for HIV via sexual behaviors[42] and should be screened for bacterial sexually transmitted infections (STIs).

Table 2
Substance use disorder treatments

Substance Use Disorder	Treatment	ART Interactions
Alcohol use disorder		
Acamprosate	666 mg PO three times a day or 333 mg PO three times a day for patients with CrCl 30–50 mL/min	None
Disulfiram	250 mg PO once daily	Use caution when prescribing ART that contain ethanol or propylene glycol (eg, FPV, LPV/r, RTV)
Naltrexone	50–100 mg PO once daily or 380 mg intramuscular suspension every 28–30 d	None
Opioid use disorder		
Buprenorphine	Individualize buprenorphine doses based on patients' prior opioid use. Suggested dose range is 4–32 mg sublingually tablet or film, once or twice daily; subcutaneously (Sublocade 300 mg once monthly for 2 months, then 100 mg monthly maintenance dose); Weekly or monthly injections, Brixadi (multiple dose formulations)	Potential interactions with ART regimens that are CYP inhibitors or inducers
Extended-release naltrexone	380 mg intramuscular suspension every 28–30 d	None
Methadone (oral daily)	Individualized dosed regimens; patients who received higher doses (eg, >100 mg) are more likely to remain in treatment	Potential interactions with ART regimens that are CYP inhibitors or inducers
Sedative use disorder (Benzodiazepines)		
	Cognitive behavioral therapy, Group or individual psychotherapy, Slow supervised taper	N/A
Stimulant use disorder		
	Medications not FDA approved but available. (Refer to the ASAM/AAAP guideline) Cognitive behavioral therapy, Contingency management, Motivational interviewing	N/A

Abbreviations: ART, antiretroviral therapy; CrCl, creatinine clearance; CYP, cytochrome P45; FPV, fosamprenavir; LPV/r, lopinavir-ritonavi; mg, milligra; min, minut; mL, milliliter; PO, by mouth; RTV, ritonavi.

Substance use disorder treatments and HIV antiretroviral interactions.

Adapted from [Guidelines for the Use of Antiretroviral Agents in Adults and Adolescents with HIV. HIV.gov. Updated June 3, 2021. Accessed November 30, 2023. https://clinicalinfo.hiv.gov/en/guidelines/hiv-clinical-guidelines-adult-and-adolescent-arv/substance-use-disorders-and-hiv].

Ending the human immunodeficiency virus epidemic via substance use disorder treatment

Ending the HIV Epidemic (EHE) is the US national plan for HIV aiming to reduce new HIV infections by 75% by 2025 and 90% by 2030 through 4 key strategies: (1) universal HIV testing; (2) rapid treatment of new HIV diagnoses and ensuring viral suppression, (3) prevention of HIV via provisions of rapid PrEP for those who test HIV negative and syringe services for PWID, and (4) responding rapidly to new HIV outbreaks by providing needed preventive and treatment services.[43] However, the EHE plan did not include specific guidance or goals targeted for PWUD who are at high risk for HIV acquisition or transmission. Further, the EHE plan relies on persons to attend traditional brick-and-mortar clinics, overlooking barriers to care that can be exacerbated in settings, where care is not integrated, as patients often have to go to multiple providers for different care needs.[44] PWUD are, therefore, a high-risk group that would benefit greatly from interventions that reduce barriers to accessing care. In order to address this important limitation in the EHE initiative, the National Institute on Drug Abuse issued a Note of Special Interest in December 2022 to support research that expands the EHE scope to include PWUD who are with, or at risk for, HIV.[45]

Human immunodeficiency virus and substance use disorder integrated care models

Given the overlapping barriers that hinder access to health care for PWUD and PWH, there is a substantial need for integrating care for SUD and HIV.[46] Indeed, the National Academies of Science, Engineering, and Medicine (NASEM) identified opportunities to integrate care for PWH and OUD (which could also be applied to AUD and StUD), including removing limits on harm reduction services such as syringe services programs (SSPs), removal of state-level prior authorization policies to prescribe buprenorphine, elimination of the DATA Drug Enforcement Administration (DEA) X-Waiver, removal of same-day billing restriction for behavioral and physical health care, expansion of Medicaid health insurance in states that have not already done so, reduction of stigma, and inclusion of integrated care into medical education.[47,48] As of this NASEM report, the requirement of an X-waiver has been removed in order to prescribe buprenorphine, which is an improvement, although that has only led to a modest increase in the number of patients receiving buprenorphine.[49] Additionally, the Medication Access and Training Expansion Act, which requires applicants for a new or renewed DEA license to complete at least 8 hours of training on treating and managing patients with OUD or other SUD, can contribute to the expansion of providers who can prescribe buprenorphine but may also not necessarily lead to patients receiving the medication. Unfortunately, integrated care models have largely focused on brick-and-mortar clinical settings, which may not be a realistic option for many PWH with concomitant SUD.[37,47]

Brick-and-mortar facilities. In these traditional settings, best practices recommend that patients be offered routine screening for both SUD and HIV testing, with the provision of PrEP or ART as appropriate.[37] In addition, due to the increased risk of acquiring bacterial STIs among PWUD,[50] the provision of STI screening should also be offered in these settings. Further, all PWH with OUD or AUD should be offered medication treatment.[37] Next, all health care professionals who provide care for PWH should be trained to identify, screen, and treat SUDs, regardless of their training background.[37,51] It is insufficient to refer patients to addiction medicine specialists or psychiatrists simply. Instead, PWH who are diagnosed with SUDs should be assessed for treatment readiness in-clinic by providers and be offered medications to reduce symptoms of withdrawal.[47]

Access to SUD treatment, particularly MOUD, has often been challenging for PWUD in brick-and-mortar settings due to factors such as stigma,[51] incarceration, and lack of transportation.[37] As such, brick-and-mortar facilities should prioritize expanding staff, SUD training, utilizing peer/patient navigators, and integrating HIV and SUD care.[37]

Mobile health clinics. In response to the structural barriers that prevent optimal SUD service delivery in brick-and-mortar facilities, mobile health clinics (MHC) may bridge this gap by meeting patients "where they are".[52] MHC brings clinical services to the community level, providing health services in locations and times that may not be available in traditional health care facilities. MHC models can overcome transportation issues, health insurance, stigma, and discomfort around traditional health care settings.[52] MHC may most benefit justice-involved persons, rural communities, transgender persons, women, unhoused, and uninsured persons.[52] Despite increased interest,[53] MHCs face limited pharmacy access since mobile retail pharmacies are either illegal or heavily regulated within the US, requiring an established OTP. Thus, to allow MHC to be truly successful in meeting PWUD where they are, state or federal-level legislation allowing for the provision of PrEP and ART within mobile retail pharmacies and DEA approval of buprenorphine in non-traditional settings must be permitted.[52]

Prisons or jails. Justice-involved persons have higher rates of HIV and SUD than the general population yet is often not provided with sufficient care for these 2 conditions in US carceral settings.[54] For instance, justice-involved persons often are unable to access testing treatment or PrEP care.[54] Expanding integrated SUD and HIV treatment and prevention services within these settings is paramount. Further, implementation of evidence-based preventive care, including PrEP and MOUD, prior to prison release for people with OUD is critical for improving individual and public health outcomes. Further, post-release linkage to SUD and HIV care is vital in order to ensure that patients continue to have access to ART, PrEP, and SUD treatment and remain retained in care.[47]

Harm reduction programs. Harm reduction program services provide syringe exchange and sterile injection equipment (eg, water, syringes, and cotton), naloxone, fentanyl test strips, barrier protection, and basic wound care[55] are well-positioned to provide integrated care for PWUD with HIV or at risk for HIV. In addition to SUD care and screening, they can be utilized to provide rapid HIV, Hepatitis C virus (HCV), bacterial STI testing, and PrEP. The Veterans Health Administration (VHA) SSP, an excellent example, engaged over 400 Veterans and dispelled confusion around legal considerations regarding the federal purchase of syringes. There are now 10 successfully implemented SSPs within the VHA, with 12 more "in progress". These programs have distributed 10,000 syringes, 2,500 fentanyl test strips, 50 wound care kits, and 45 safer sex kits while providing HIV and HCV testing.[56] Unfortunately, outside of the VHA, community harm reduction programs have not been legalized in every state.

Mobile device health. Mobile device health (mHealth) has the potential to provide holistic, patient-centered, integrated care for PWUD with HIV and at-risk for HIV. For example, a pilot HIV and Hepatitis education initiative was associated with increased and sustained improvements in knowledge regarding HCV and HIV transmission and risk behaviors in participants with OUD.[57] Further, mHealth applications are integrating HIV and SUD, such as ART-CHESS (Antiretroviral Therapy-Comprehensive Health Enhancement Support System)[58] for people with HIV and OUD and

PositiveLinks for people with HIV and PWUD application, which has shown significant improvement in HIV virologic suppression.[59] *DynamiCare Health* mobile application is feasible and acceptable for CM related to AUD, OUD, cannabis, nicotine, and StUD and is now FDA-approved to provide incentivized mobile application provided CM treatment for SUDs.[22] Lastly, the CARE + Corrections for PWH, recently released to the community from carceral settings, improved the proportion of participants virologically suppressed.[60] For PWUD at risk for HIV, a mHealth approach to remind individuals to use PrEP and educate them on HIV risk reduction is feasible and acceptable.[61]

SUMMARY

The intricate nature of SUD underscores the necessity for specialized expertise in managing each unique SUD. However, amid the current deficit in such expertise and the absence of tailored treatment guidelines, there are actionable steps at a fundamental level. This involves acknowledging the nuanced intersection of HIV and substance use and subsequently integrating HIV assessment within SUD disciplines and addressing SUD within HIV disciplines to reduce care silos. This integrated approach ensures a holistic response to each epidemic—HIV and SUD—by recognizing and addressing their interconnected challenges from the outset of assessment, through treatment, and into management.

CLINICS CARE POINTS

- People with SUD should be tested for HIV and offered PrEP (oral or LAI) if negative.
- HIV sex risk behaviors should be assessed in all PWUDs, and PrEP (oral or LAI) should be offered.
- PWH should be screened for SUD, and ART integrated with their treatment for SUDs.
- MHC and mHealth are opportunities to engage people in care without traditional structures of care and improve HIV clinical outcomes.
- Buprenorphine and other forms of MOUD and other SUD treatments should be expanded beyond traditional brick-and-mortar facilities.
- Harm reduction services should be integrated into clinical settings.
- LAI-ART may be offered to PWH who are already taking LAI forms of medication for SUD.

DISCLOSURE

Author S.A. Springer has provided paid scientific consultation to Alkermes Inc. S.A. Springer has received in-kind study drug donations from Alkermes Inc and Indivior Pharmaceutical Company for NIH-funded research. Work related to this manuscript was funded by National Institute on Drug Abuse, United States (NIDA; DP1DA056106, Springer). The funder was not involved in the research design, analysis or interpretation of the data or the decision to publish the manuscript.

REFERENCES

1. Substance Abuse and Mental Health Services Administration. Prevention and Treatment of HIV Among People Living with Substance Use and/or Mental Disorders. Publication No. PEP20-06-03-001. National Mental Health and Substance Use Policy

Laboratory, Substance Abuse and Mental Health Services Administration. 2020. Available at: https://store.samhsa.gov/product/Prevention-and-Treatment-of-HIV-Among-People-Living-with-Substance-Use-and-or-Mental-Disorders/PEP20-06-03-001. [Accessed 30 November 2023].

2. Levitt A, Mermin J, Jones CM, et al. Infectious Diseases and Injection Drug Use: Public Health Burden and Response. J Infect Dis 2020;222(Suppl 5):S213–7.

3. HIV.gov. Data and trends: U.S. Statistics. 2023. Available at: https://hiv.gov/hiv-basics/overview/data-and-trends/statistics. [Accessed 31 October 2023].

4. Peters PJ, Pontones P, Hoover KW, et al. HIV Infection Linked to Injection Use of Oxymorphone in Indiana, 2014–2015. N Engl J Med 2016;375(3):229–39.

5. Cranston K. Notes from the field: HIV diagnoses among persons who inject drugs—Northeastern Massachusetts, 2015–2018. MMWR Morbidity and mortality weekly report 2019;68.

6. Atkins A, McClung RP, Kilkenny M, et al. Notes from the field: outbreak of human immunodeficiency virus infection among persons who inject drugs - Cabell County, West Virginia, 2018-2019. MMWR Morb Mortal Wkly Rep 2020;69(16): 499–500.

7. Lyss SB, Buchacz K, McClung RP, et al. Responding to outbreaks of human immunodeficiency virus among persons who inject drugs-United States, 2016-2019: perspectives on recent experience and lessons learned. J Infect Dis 2020;222(Suppl 5):S239–49.

8. Azar P, Wood E, Nguyen P, et al. Drug use patterns associated with risk of non-adherence to antiretroviral therapy among HIV-positive illicit drug users in a Canadian setting: a longitudinal analysis. BMC Infect Dis 2015;15:193.

9. Substance Abuse and Mental Health Services Administration. Medications for opioid use disorder: treatment improvement protocol (TIP) series 63, full document. HHS Publication No.18-5063 FULLDOC. 2021. Available at: https://store.samhsa.gov/sites/default/files/pep21-02-01-002.pdf. Accessed November 28, 2023.

10. Poliwoda S, Noor N, Jenkins JS, et al. Buprenorphine and its formulations: a comprehensive review. Health Psychol Res 2022;10(3):37517.

11. Duko B, Ayalew M, Ayano G. The prevalence of alcohol use disorders among people living with HIV/AIDS: a systematic review and meta-analysis. Subst Abuse Treat Prev Policy 2019;14(1):52.

12. Azar MM, Springer SA, Meyer JP, et al. A systematic review of the impact of alcohol use disorders on HIV treatment outcomes, adherence to antiretroviral therapy and health care utilization. Drug Alcohol Depend 2010;112(3):178–93.

13. Maisel NC, Blodgett JC, Wilbourne PL, et al. Meta-analysis of naltrexone and acamprosate for treating alcohol use disorders: when are these medications most helpful? Addiction 2013;108(2):275–93.

14. Fairbanks J, Umbreit A, Kolla BP, et al. Evidence-based pharmacotherapies for alcohol use disorder: clinical pearls. Mayo Clin Proc 2020;95(9):1964–77.

15. Carrico AW, Woolf-King SE, Neilands TB, et al. Stimulant use and HIV disease management among men in same-sex relationships. Drug Alcohol Depend 2014;139:174–7.

16. American Society of Addiction Medicine and American Academy of Addiction Psychiatry (ASAM/AAAP). Clinical practice guideline on the management of stimulant use disorder. Available at: https://downloads.asam.org/sitefinity-production-blobs/docs/default-source/quality-science/stud_guideline_document_final.pdf?sfvrsn=71094b38_1. [Accessed 30 April 2024].

17. Ronsley C, Nolan S, Knight R, et al. Treatment of stimulant use disorder: a systematic review of reviews. PLoS One 2020;15(6):e0234809.

18. Ribeiro A, Pinto DGA, Trevisol AP, et al. Can contingency management solve the problem of adherence to antiretroviral therapy in drug-dependent individuals? Health Educ Behav 2023;50(6):738–47.

19. Cunningham CO, Arnsten JH, Zhang C, et al. Abstinence-reinforcing contingency management improves HIV viral load suppression among HIV-infected people who use drugs: A randomized controlled trial. Drug Alcohol Depend 2020;216: 108230.

20. De Crescenzo F, Ciabattini M, D'Alo GL, et al. Comparative efficacy and acceptability of psychosocial interventions for individuals with cocaine and amphetamine addiction: A systematic review and network meta-analysis. PLoS Med 2018;15(12):e1002715.

21. National Mental Health and Substance Use Policy Laboratory. Treatment of stimulant use disorders. SAMHSA Publication No. PEP20-06-01-001. substance abuse and mental health services administration, 2020. June 2020. Available at: https://store.samhsa.gov/sites/default/files/pep20-06-01-001.pdf. [Accessed 3 November 2023].

22. DeFulio A, Brown HD, Davidson RM, et al. Feasibility, acceptability, and preliminary efficacy of a smartphone-based contingency management intervention for buprenorphine adherence. Behav Anal Pract 2023;16(2):450–8.

23. Darke S, Hall W, Ross M, et al. Benzodiazepine use and HIV risk-taking behaviour among injecting drug users. Drug Alcohol Depend 1992;31(1):31–6.

24. Newville H, Roley J, Sorensen JL. Prescription medication misuse among HIV-infected individuals taking antiretroviral therapy. J Subst Abuse Treat 2015; 48(1):56–61.

25. Bruce RD, Altice FL, Friedland GH. Pharmacokinetic drug interactions between drugs of abuse and antiretroviral medications: implications and management for clinical practice. Expert Rev Clin Pharmacol 2008;1(1):115–27.

26. Soyka M. Treatment of benzodiazepine dependence. N Engl J Med 2017; 376(12):1147–57.

27. Colfax G, Guzman R. Club drugs and HIV infection: a review. Clin Infect Dis 2006; 42(10):1463–9.

28. Bracchi M, Stuart D, Castles R, et al. Increasing use of 'party drugs' in people living with HIV on antiretrovirals: a concern for patient safety. AIDS 2015;29(13): 1585–92.

29. McNamara KF, Biondi BE, Hernandez-Ramirez RU, et al. A Systematic review and meta-analysis of studies evaluating the effect of medication treatment for opioid use disorder on infectious disease outcomes. Open Forum Infect Dis 2021; 8(8):ofab289.

30. Lier AJ, Seval N, Vander Wyk B, et al. Maintenance on extended-release naltrexone is associated with reduced injection opioid use among justice-involved persons with opioid use disorder. J Subst Abuse Treat 2022;142:108852.

31. Fanucchi L, Springer SA, Korthuis PT. Medications for treatment of opioid use disorder among persons living with HIV. Curr HIV AIDS Rep 2019;16(1):1–6.

32. Springer SA, Qiu J, Saber-Tehrani AS, et al. Retention on buprenorphine is associated with high levels of maximal viral suppression among HIV-infected opioid dependent released prisoners. PLoS One 2012;7(5):e38335.

33. Springer SA, Di Paola A, Azar MM, et al. Extended-release naltrexone improves viral suppression among incarcerated persons living with HIV with opioid use

disorders transitioning to the community: results of a double-blind, placebo-controlled randomized trial. J Acquir Immune Defic Syndr 2018;78(1):43–53.

34. MacArthur GJ, Minozzi S, Martin N, et al. Opiate substitution treatment and HIV transmission in people who inject drugs: systematic review and meta-analysis. BMJ 2012;345.

35. Springer SA, Di Paola A, Barbour R, et al. Extended-release naltrexone improves viral suppression among incarcerated persons living with HIV and alcohol use disorders transitioning to the community: results from a double-blind, placebo-controlled trial. J Acquir Immune Defic Syndr 2018;79(1):92–100.

36. Springer SA, Di Paola A, Azar MM, et al. Extended-release naltrexone reduces alcohol consumption among released prisoners with HIV disease as they transition to the community. Drug Alcohol Depend 2017;174:158–70.

37. Gandhi RT, Bedimo R, Hoy JF, et al. Antiretroviral Drugs for Treatment and Prevention of HIV Infection in Adults: 2022 Recommendations of the International Antiviral Society-USA Panel. JAMA 2023;329(1):63–84.

38. Streed CG Jr, Morgan JR, Gai MJ, et al. Prevalence of HIV preexposure prophylaxis prescribing among persons with commercial insurance and likely injection drug use. JAMA Netw Open 2022;5(7):e2221346.

39. Champion JD, Recto P. An assessment of HIV risk, perceptions of risk, and potential adherence to preexposure prophylaxis among HIV-negative people with injection drug use who access mobile outreach services. J Addict Nurs Apr-Jun 01 2023;34(2):101–10.

40. Dubov A, Krakower DS, Rockwood N, et al. provider implicit bias in prescribing HIV pre-exposure prophylaxis (PrEP) to people who inject drugs. J Gen Intern Med 2023;38(13):2928–35.

41. Landovitz RJ, Donnell D, Clement ME, et al. Cabotegravir for HIV prevention in cisgender men and transgender women. N Engl J Med 2021;385(7):595–608.

42. Picard J, Jacka B, Hoj S, et al. Real-world eligibility for HIV pre-exposure prophylaxis among people who inject drugs. AIDS Behav 2020;24(8):2400–8.

43. Fauci AS, Redfield RR, Sigounas G, et al. Ending the HIV epidemic: a plan for the United States. JAMA 2019;321(9):844–5.

44. Lancaster KE, Endres-Dighe S, Sucaldito AD, et al. Measuring and addressing stigma within HIV interventions for people who use drugs: a scoping review of recent research. Curr HIV AIDS Rep 2022;19(5):301–11.

45. National Insitute of Drug Abuse. Notice of special interest (NOSI): research to address 'ending the HIV epidemic' initiative goals relevant to substance using populations at-risk for or living with HIV. https://grants.nih.gov/grants/guide/notice-files/NOT-DA-23-013.html.

46. Hill K, Kuo I, Shenoi SV, et al. Integrated care models: HIV and substance use. Curr HIV AIDS Rep 2023;20(5):286–95.

47. Springer SA, Merluzzi AP, Del Rio C. Integrating responses to the opioid use disorder and infectious disease epidemics: a report from the national academies of sciences, engineering, and medicine. JAMA 2020;324(1):37–8.

48. Springer SA, Barocas JA, Wurcel A, et al. Federal and state action needed to end the infectious complications of illicit drug use in the United States: IDSA and HIV-MA's Advocacy Agenda. J Infect Dis 2020;222(Suppl 5):S230–8.

49. Chua KP, Bicket MC, Bohnert ASB, et al. Buprenorphine dispensing after elimination of the waiver requirement. N Engl J Med 2024;390(16):1530–2.

50. Brookmeyer KA, Haderxhanaj LT, Hogben M, et al. Sexual risk behaviors and STDs among persons who inject drugs: A national study. Prev Med 2019;126:105779.

51. Springer SA, Korthuis PT, Del Rio C. Integrating treatment at the intersection of opioid use disorder and infectious disease epidemics in medical settings: a call for action after a national academies of sciences, engineering, and medicine workshop. Ann Intern Med 2018;169(5):335–6.
52. Malone NC, Williams MM, Smith Fawzi MC, et al. Mobile health clinics in the United States. Int J Equity Health 2020;19(1):40.
53. Springer SA, Nijhawan AE, Knight K, et al. Study protocol of a randomized controlled trial comparing two linkage models for HIV prevention and treatment in justice-involved persons. BMC Infect Dis 2022;22(1):380.
54. Springer SA, Pesanti E, Hodges J, et al. Effectiveness of antiretroviral therapy among HIV-infected prisoners: reincarceration and the lack of sustained benefit after release to the community. Clin Infect Dis 2004;38(12):1754–60.
55. National Institute of Drug Abuse. Harm reduction. 2022. Available at: https://nida. nih.gov/research-topics/harm-reduction. [Accessed 31 October 2023].
56. VA Diffusion Marketplace. Expanding harm reduction services and implementation of syringe services programs (SSP) within veterans health administration (VHA). Veterans Health Administration 2023. Available at: https://marketplace. va.gov/innovations/implementation-of-syringe-services-programs-within-the-va. [Accessed 30 November 2023].
57. Ochalek TA, Heil SH, Higgins ST, et al. A novel mHealth application for improving HIV and Hepatitis C knowledge in individuals with opioid use disorder: a pilot study. Drug Alcohol Depend 2018;190:224–8.
58. Yang F, Shah DV, Tahk A, et al. mHealth and social mediation: mobile support among stigmatized people living with HIV and substance use disorder. New Media Soc 2023/04/01 2023;25(4):702–31.
59. Dillingham R, Ingersoll K, Flickinger TE, et al. PositiveLinks: A mobile health intervention for retention in HIV care and clinical outcomes with 12-month follow-up. AIDS Patient Care STDS 2018;32(6):241–50.
60. Kuo I, Liu T, Patrick R, et al. Use of an mHealth intervention to improve engagement in HIV community-based care among persons recently released from a correctional facility in Washington, DC: a pilot study. AIDS Behav 2019;23(4): 1016–31.
61. Shrestha R, Altice FL, DiDomizio E, et al. Feasibility and acceptability of an mHealth-based approach as an HIV prevention strategy among people who use drugs on pre-exposure prophylaxis. Patient Prefer Adherence 2020;14: 107–18.

Operationalization of Status Neutral Human Immunodeficiency Virus Care for Criminal-Legal Involved Populations

Ruchi Vyomesh Shah, DO[a], Alysse G. Wurcel, MD, MS[b],*

KEYWORDS

- HIV • Jails • Prisons • Carceral settings • Correctional settings • PrEP
- Status neutral HIV care • Harm reduction

KEY POINTS

- People who are incarcerated are at increased risk of human immunodeficiency virus (HIV) but face barriers in receiving HIV testing and tools to prevent HIV.
- HIV testing, treatment, and prevention should be offered in carceral settings.
- The Status Neutral HIV Care Framework should be operationalized in carceral settings to increase access to HIV prevention tools.

BACKGROUND

Criminal-legal involved populations are at an increased risk for human immunodeficiency virus (HIV). The United States has the highest per capita incarceration rate in the world, with an estimated 2 million people confined in jails or prisons.[1] Prisons typically detain people following conviction of a crime, and the periods of detention are upwards of 2 years.[2] Jails—run at the city or county level—usually have shorter maximum periods of detention (<2 years) and also house people who have "pre-trial" status, meaning they have not been convicted of a crime.[3] An estimated 3.9 million people in the U.S. are on probation or parole—not detained in a correctional facilities but still under systems of carceral control.[4]

While the prevalence of HIV in the U.S. has decreased by 12% overall from 2017 to 2021, this degree of change is not reflected in people with HIV in the custody of federal

[a] Boston Medical Center, Grayken Center for Addiction, Boston, MA, USA; [b] Division of Infectious Diseases and Geographic Medicine, Tufts Medicine, 800 Washington Street, Boston, MA 02111, USA
* Corresponding author.
E-mail address: Alysse.wurcel@tuftsmedicine.org

Infect Dis Clin N Am 38 (2024) 613–625
https://doi.org/10.1016/j.idc.2024.04.008
0891-5520/24/© 2024 Elsevier Inc. All rights reserved.

and state correctional facilities.[5,6] There are multiple underlying reasons that continue to drive increased risk and prevalence of HIV in criminal-legal involved populations including racism, stigma and discrimination, homophobia, misogyny, anti-immigrant sentiment, poverty, and other barriers to quality health care access.[7–9] Criminalization of people who use drugs (PWUD) has significantly contributed to HIV incidence in this group and racial/ethnic minority groups. These populations have disparate rates of incarceration.

The Ending the HIV Epidemic (EHE), launched in 2019 by the U.S. Department of Health and Human Services, presents a multi-agency approach toward the goal of reducing new HIV infections in the U.S. by 90% by 2030. This initiative focuses on 4 pillars—diagnosis, prevention, treatment, and outbreak.[10] These pillars need to be fully incorporated into carceral settings in order to mitigate infections and work toward ending the HIV epidemic. There have been incredible strides in the HIV testing, treatment, and prevention in carceral settings; however, the available data about HIV-related care in U.S. jails and prisons reveal that incarceration remains a "missed opportunity."[11–13]

The gap can be addressed through the implementation of a Status Neutral HIV Care Framework across the broad spectrum of criminal-legal settings, including jails, prisons, and community supervision sites. The Status Neutral Care Framework for HIV care was first introduced by the New York City Department of Health and Mental Hygiene to address gaps in the traditional HIV care continuum model.[14] The Status Neutral HIV framework uses the HIV test as a starting point and engages people who have positive *and* negative tests. The Status Neutral Framework has been endorsed by the Centers for Disease Control and Prevention (CDC),[15] and has increasingly been used to operationalize greater HIV-prevention efforts for people who are at risk for HIV but test negative. The goal of this chapter is to review the history of HIV testing and treatment in carceral settings, the current guidelines for HIV-related care in carceral settings, and outline ideas for how the Status Neutral Framework can be used to improve HIV care in carceral settings (**Fig. 1**).

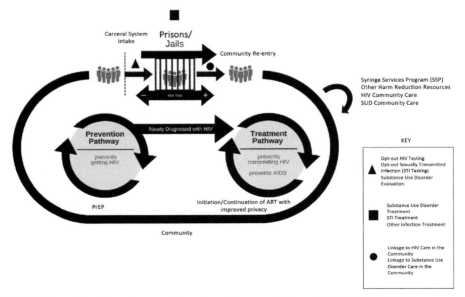

Fig. 1. Examples of how to operationalize status neutral care in jails and prisons.

HISTORY OF HUMAN IMMUNODEFICIENCY VIRUS TESTING IN CARCERAL SETTINGS

Although there are several reasons why carceral settings are important places to offer HIV care, it is worth pausing to reflect on the early days of the HIV epidemic, when people incarcerated in prison and jail who tested positive for HIV faced segregation, intense stigma and involuntary disclosure of HIV status.[16–18] Mandatory testing was common practice, especially in prisons, although several experts cited ethical objections.[16,19,20] Other methods of testing included voluntary testing (eg, the person asked for a test) and "opt-out" testing, where people were told that testing was offered to everyone and given the opportunity to opt out.[16,21,22] In 2006, the CDC published guidelines for one-time HIV testing for all people engaged in health care, including correctional facilities as a place where health care is delivered and HIV testing should be offered.[23]

GUIDELINES AND BEST PRACTICES FOR HUMAN IMMUNODEFICIENCY VIRUS TESTING IN CARCERAL SETTINGS

The current CDC guidelines released in April 2022 recommend HIV testing during the intake process in jails and prisons using the opt-out method.[24] Intake is one of the only interactions where individuals who are newly detained in a jail or prison are required to discuss health issues. The intake process was originally instituted to screen for severe psychiatric illness and to understand the current acute and chronic health care conditions of the newly-detained person.[25] In 2011, all jails and prisons were advised to implement HIV testing programs at intake.[26] Although most prisons have systems of offering HIV testing, usually at intake,[27] operationalization of HIV testing in line with CDC guidelines has been suboptimal in jails.[28,29]

There are several barriers to HIV testing that manifest in jail settings, where the average length of detention is less than in prisons. Jail clinicians and administrators are often burdened by competing priorities including management of addiction and mental health.[30] As of 2018, HIV medications in jails and prisons should be covered by Ryan White funding but several jails are unaware of this change, leading to hesitancy to offer HIV testing for fear of needing to pay for costly medications.[31] A strategy developed to circumvent this barrier is exit testing, when people are tested close to the date of re-entry (the time when someone leaves jail or prison) with focus on linkage to care in the community.[32] Another barrier in jail is the time needed to draw blood, send for analysis, and then coordinate delivery of test results.[33] Rapid HIV testing has been used in jails for nearly 20 years.[34] However, some health departments do not allow rapid HIV testing in jails or prisons because of concerns for false results (both negatives and positives[35]). Additionally, given the overlap of HIV with other infections, health departments have developed preferred testing algorithms with several tests (HIV, HCV, and syphilis) run on one venipuncture sample.[36] Another barrier to HIV testing at intake may be the individual's relationship to the person offering the HIV test. Intake processes ideally are performed by clinicians, although a recent study found that 46% of jails use non-clinical staff such as corrections officers to offer infectious diseases testing.[37] There are several reasons why incarcerated people would be unlikely to request HIV testing from correctional officers. Finally, despite evolution in consent requirements for HIV,[38] several jails (including jails in Massachusetts) still require written consent even though the state laws only require verbal consent. Written consent is a barrier both as an additional administrative task and also because it elevates stigma by creating an "exceptionalism" to HIV testing when it should be considered a routine test.[39]

HUMAN IMMUNODEFICIENCY VIRUS TREATMENT IN CARCERAL SETTINGS

A 1990 report found through a survey of jails and prisons, most reported AZT was available to people with symptomatic AIDS,[40] although there are several law suits and policy reports that document inconsistent AZT availability.[41] Notably, people who were incarcerated were not allowed to participate in clinical trials on HIV medications. Although this protection was intended to protect individuals who were vulnerable to coercion, the impact was that about incarcerated individuals did not have equal access to potentially life-saving medications.[40] To most in the HIV community, this advent of "highly-active anti-retroviral treatment" marked a transition in HIV from being a death sentence to a chronic disease.[42] Protease inhibitors were not readily available in many prisons and jails because of the cost.[43] Incarceration was a risk for missing doses.[44] Several prisons required those incarcerated to purchase their own HIV medications—a financial burden that often proved to be impossible.[45]

The initial introduction of protease inhibitors posed a challenge in prisons and jails due to the demanding dosing schedule, which required multiple administrations throughout the day.[46,47] A majority of carceral facilities had 1 of 2 methods of HIV medication distribution: Directly observed therapy (DOT) or Keep-On-Person (KOP), also known as self-administration.[48] For the DOT method, people with HIV line up at either a medication window or a medication cart to get their medications. Both methods present privacy concerns.[49] There should be strict protocols in place to prevent nurses from announcing the name of the medication or what it is for, to prevent breaches in privacy for people who are getting HIV medications.[50] Similarly, pill containers could be viewed by other people in jail through the KOP method. Randomized controlled trials of KOP and DOT found no difference in viral suppression.[51,52]

With increasing support for HIV care delivery in jails and prisons, as well as political and legal pressure, systems of HIV care improved. Cohort studies showed that "optimization" of care occurred with incarceration, as most people with HIV/AIDS entered jail/prison with detectable HIV virus and left jail/prison with undetectable virus.[53,54] Challenges persist in ensuring consistent access to HIV medications for people who are incarcerated,[55] but advancements including once daily regimens, lower prices, and support from state and public health with costs of medications and national correctional credentialing requirements have led to more consistent availability of HIV medications in most U.S. carceral systems. As HIV advances continue, a delay between the availability of treatment in the community and the carceral setting lingers. For example, the availability of long-acting injectable HIV medications in jails and prisons has not yet been studied.

The major issue people with HIV detained in carceral settings face is linkage to HIV care in the community.[56,57] People with untreated HIV[58] and substance use disorder (SUD),[59] in particular, are populations at risk for fragmented care when transitioning to the community. One of the largest retrospective cohort studies followed people with HIV incarcerated in Connecticut and found that about 2/3 of people were engaged in HIV care 1 year after re-entry to community.[60] Factors associated with linkage to care within 14 days of re-entry to the community included longer incarceration, transitional case management, HIV medications during incarceration, and 2 or more comorbidities. Factors that emerged in the analysis as associated with post-release HIV care engagement included receiving greater than 30 case management visits,[60] receiving antiretroviral therapy and being treated for a medical comorbidity during incarceration.[60] Community workers, mobile health technologies and co-location of HIV care with SUD treatment are strategies that have been studied as ways to support engagement in HIV care following re-entry to the community.[61–64] Barriers to linkage include lack of insurance, housing instability, limited transportation options, paucity of HIV clinicians, and sub-optimally treated mental illness and SUD.[65-68] Research on the use of long-acting HIV medications in jails and prisons as a strategy to support individuals transitioning back into the community is an area that warrants further investigation.

One of the most effective strategies to date in supporting criminal-legal involved populations with taking HIV medications and linkage to HIV care has been offering SUD medications. The HIV epidemic, hepatitis epidemics, and SUD have been described as linked epidemics, or a "syndemic".[69] Medications for opioid use disorder (M-OUD), especially methadone and buprenorphine, are evidence-based pharmacologic interventions that prevent drug use, overdose, and death.[70,71] People with HIV, in particular, benefit from M-OUD not only as a method of supporting recovery, but also because it helps support HIV medication adherence.[72] Advances in M-OUD availability in the community and in carceral settings have occurred over the past decade, but a recent survey reported that M-OUD were only available in 32% of jails.[73] We will discuss strategies to address gaps in M-OUD treatment later in this chapter.

Another strategy to support HIV treatment in carceral settings is a waiver to the Medicaid Inmate Exemption Policy (MIEP). When Congress passed the Social Security Act to create Medicare and Medicaid in 1965, it simultaneously created the Medicaid Inmate Exclusion Policy (also known as the "inmate exception"), prohibiting Medicaid reimbursement for health care services in jails and prisons except for hospital stays that are more than 24 hours.[74] When people leave jail or prison, they often enter into the community without medical insurance and can face barriers getting medications for chronic diseases and scheduling health care appointments.[75] The Medicaid Reentry Section 1115 Demonstration allows state Medicaid programs to expand coverage to incarcerated individuals 90 days prior to their release for chronic health conditions including SUD and HIV.[75] Several states have submitted applications to the federal government to waive the MIEP. To date, California and Washington have been granted these 90 day waivers and Massachusetts had a 30 day waiver which can be resubmitted to request 90 day coverage. The 1115 MIEP waiver will enable effective strategies to link criminal-legal involved individuals to HIV and SUD care in the community post-release.[75] Medications across the spectrum of HIV care, from treatment to prevention could be initiated during the pre-release period and supported by robust linkage to care programs after release.

STATUS NEUTRAL HUMAN IMMUNODEFICIENCY VIRUS CARE IN CARCERAL SETTINGS

The intervention goals of status neutral HIV care outlined by the CDC are as follows: eliminating stigma, making services more accessible, helping people achieve optimal health and well-being, efficiencies in service delivery, and greater health equity.[15] The Status Neutral Framework uses the HIV test as an opportunity to engage in not only HIV treatment if positive, but also is a path toward Pre-Exposure Prophylaxis (PrEP), treatment for SUDs, testing for other sexually transmitted diseases, and linkage to harm reduction tools.

Pre-exposure Prophylaxis Prescribing in Carceral Settings

Key HIV risk factors for incarcerated individuals include sex and injection drug use.[76,77] If people test negative for HIV while in jail or prison, it provides the opportunity to discuss initiation of PrEP for HIV prevention.[78] PrEP access, both prescriptions in carceral settings and programs linking people on release to PrEP, is rare.[79] There are several vulnerable communities who are at increased risk of incarceration as well, including people who use drugs, people who do sex work, transgender people, and individuals who are racially and ethnically minoritized.[80,81] Key decision makers in jail and prison administration and clinical care have expressed concerns about PrEP prescriptions including cost and concern it will increase sexual activity inside carceral settings, reminiscent of the misguided argument against providing sexual education, and birth control in schools.[82,83] Ongoing trials are assessing interventions that could increase PrEP prescription to people who are in jails and prisons.[84,85] Rhode Island Department of Corrections implemented a statewide PrEP initiation program with linkage to PrEP care in the community post-release from November 2019 to April 2022.[86] Based on their experience, the department has published guidance about how to implement PrEP programs through a phased approach including increasing PrEP awareness, uptake, and adherence.[87]

Treatment for Substance Use Disorders

Treatment for SUD should be incorporated into both arms of the status neutral HIV pathway for those who test positive and negative. Medications for OUD (M-OUD) should be available in all jails and prisons as it align with evidence based practices for the prevention of overdose, reduces rates of re-incarceration, and improves the overall environment in the facility.[88–90] In 2019, 63% of jails screened for opioid use disorder (OUD) and 20% of jails offered M- OUD.[91] Concerns about diversion of medications for OUD may deter carceral settings from providing M-OUD, however there is evidence that diversion is rare.[92] The data supporting clinical outcomes after initiation of M-OUD are overwhelming, and there is substantial evidence that medications work even when not paired with psychotherapy.[93] Carceral settings should not require engagement in personalized or group therapy as a requirement for M-OUD. Extended-release buprenorphine is an effective, but underused, medication for people with OUD.[94,95] Methamphetamine use disorder highly prevalent in carceral settings, but treatment options are more limited than for OUD.[96] Contingency management strategies are evidence-based methods of treating methamphetamine use, but to our knowledge, they have not been used in jails or prisons.[97] As there new treatments for methamphetamine use disorder emerge, these treatments should be offered in carceral settings.[98]

Sexually Transmitted Infections

The Status Neutral framework provides opportunities for testing for sexually transmitted infections (STIs)—an important pillar of ending the HIV epidemic. There are high rates of chlamydia, gonorrhea, and syphilis in people who are incarcerated, and the diagnosis and treatment of STIs decreases risk of HIV transmission.[99,100] The CDC correctional guidelines recommend STI testing for everyone in carceral settings.[24] STIs facilitate HIV infection.[101] Several jails and prisons have standardized chlamydia and gonorrhea testing for women with urine samples.[102–104] However, testing of men is not routine and despite high rates of extra genital STIs,[105] extragenital swabbing is not widely available in carceral settings.[106] Nationally, syphilis rates are rising,[107] there have been several reports of syphilis increases in people who use drugs[108] and people incarcerated in jails and prisons.[109] Increasing access to HIV care for criminal-legal involved populations should be coupled with opportunities for STI testing.

Harm Reduction

Ideally, everyone who is at risk for infections will have access to systems, tools, and education to reduce that risk. This can be challenging in jails and prisons, when the activities of sex and drug use are banned but still occur, and harm reduction is practiced. An early 1996 study found that people who are incarcerated were using rubber gloves and plastic wrap during sex and used syringes, pieces of pens, and lightbulbs to inject drugs due to lack of access to harm reduction supplies.[110] Programs to reduce HIV risk in carceral settings through condom distribution have been reported,[111,112] although broad implementation of condom availability in prisons and jails will likely be met with resistance. A more feasible approach is the referral of people from jail or prisons to harm reduction services following release, including syringe exchange programs or mobile vans that provide harm reduction equipment. There are several communities across the U.S. that have established linkage to care programs for people at risk for HIV who are leaving jails and prison.[113–115]

SUMMARY

Ensuring access to comprehensive HIV care–including HIV testing, treatment, and prevention–within carceral facilities is crucial in addressing the health care needs of criminal-legal involved populations. Providing adequate HIV care in these settings plays a vital role in promoting public health and reducing the transmission of the virus both within correctional facilities and the broader community. Status Neutral HIV Care should be operationalized in carceral settings, with prioritization of offering PrEP, treatment of SUDs, testing and treatment of STIs, and harm reduction practices.

CLINICS CARE POINTS

- Despite CDC recommendations, HIV testing is sup-optimally implemented in jails.
- Opt-out HIV testing should be offered to people who are entering jails and prisons at intake.
- People who are incarcerated lose their health insurance. Repealing the Medicaid Inmate Exclusion policy is one way to support linkage to HIV care on re-entry.
- Treatment of SUD improves outcomes for people with HIV. SUD evaluation and treatment should be offered at all jails and prisons.

DISCLOSURE

The authors have nothing to disclose.

REFERENCES

1. Joe S. Analyzing mass incarceration. Science 2021;374(6565):237.
2. Carson EA. Prisoners in 2022 – Statistical tables. In: Statistics BoJ. 2023. NCJ Number 307086.
3. Zeng Z. Jail Inmates in 2022. In: Statistics BoJ. 2023.
4. Kaeble D. Probation and parole in the United States, 2020. US department of Justice, office of justice programs. USA: Bureau of Justice Stastics; 2021.
5. CDC. Estimated HIV Incidence and Prevalence in the United States 2017-2021. Available at: https://www.cdc.gov/hiv/library/reports/hiv-surveillance/vol-28-no-3/index.html.
6. Spaulding AC, Seals RM, Page MJ, et al. HIV/AIDS among inmates of and releasees from US correctional facilities, 2006: declining share of epidemic but persistent public health opportunity. PLoS One 2009;4(11):e7558.

7. Brewer R, Ramani SL, Khanna A, et al. A systematic review up to 2018 of HIV and associated factors among criminal justice-involved (CJI) black sexual and gender minority populations in the United States (US). J Racial Ethn Health Disparities 2022;9(4):1357–402.

8. Bromberg DJ, Mayer KH, Altice FL. Identifying and managing infectious disease syndemics in patients with HIV. Curr Opin HIV AIDS 2020;15(4):232–42.

9. Rice WS, Logie CH, Napoles TM, et al. Perceptions of intersectional stigma among diverse women living with HIV in the United States. Soc Sci Med 2018;208:9–17.

10. Fauci AS, Redfield RR, Sigounas G, et al. Ending the HIV epidemic: a plan for the United States. JAMA 2019;321(9):844–5.

11. Flanigan TP, Zaller N, Beckwith CG, et al. Testing for HIV, sexually transmitted infections, and viral hepatitis in jails: still a missed opportunity for public health and HIV prevention. J Acquir Immune Defic Syndr (1999) 2010;55(Suppl 2): S78–83.

12. Levano SR, Epting ME, Pluznik JA, et al. HIV testing in jails: Comparing strategies to maximize engagement in HIV treatment and prevention. PLoS One 2023; 18(6):e0286805.

13. NCCHC. Administrative Management for People Living With HIV in Correctional Institutions (2020). 2022.

14. Myers JE, Braunstein SL, Xia Q, et al. Redefining prevention and care: a status-neutral approach to HIV. Open Forum Infect Dis 2018;5(6):ofy097.

15. CDC. Status Neutral HIV Prevention and Care. 2023. Available at: https://www. cdc.gov/hiv/effective-interventions/prevent/status-neutral-hiv-prevention-and-care/index.html.

16. Basu S, Smith-Rohrberg D, Hanck S, et al. HIV testing in correctional institutions: evaluating existing strategies, setting new standards. AIDS Public Policy J 2005; 20(1–2):3–24.

17. Harris v. Thigpen. Fed Suppl 1990;727:1564–83.

18. Mtr La Rocca v. Dalsheim, 120 697(NY: Supreme Court, Dutchess 1983).

19. Andrus JK, Fleming DW, Knox C, et al. HIV testing in prisoners: is mandatory testing mandatory? Am J Publ Health 1989;79(7):840–2.

20. Starchild A. Mandatory testing for HIV in federal prisons. N Engl J Med 1989; 320(5):315–6.

21. Kavasery R, Maru DS, Cornman-Homonoff J, et al. Routine opt-out HIV testing strategies in a female jail setting: a prospective controlled trial. PLoS One 2009;4(11):e7648.

22. Lucas KD, Eckert V, Behrends CN, et al. Evaluation of routine HIV opt-out screening and continuum of care services following entry into eight prison reception centers–California, 2012. MMWR Morbidity and mortality weekly report 2016; 65(7):178–81.

23. Branson BM, Handsfield HH, Lampe MA, et al. Revised recommendations for HIV testing of adults, adolescents, and pregnant women in health-care settings. MMWR Recomm Rep (Morb Mortal Wkly Rep) 2006;55(Rr-14):1–17, quiz CE11-14.

24. CDC. At-a-glance: CDC recommendations for correctional and detention settings. 2022. Available at: https://www.cdc.gov/correctionalhealth/rec-guide.html# recommended-actions.

25. Martin MS, Potter BK, Crocker AG, et al. Mental health treatment patterns following screening at intake to prison. J Consult Clin Psychol 2018;86(1):15.

26. HIV screening of male inmates during prison intake medical evaluation–Washington, 2006-2010. MMWR Morb Mortal Wkly Rep 2011;60(24):811–3.

27. Maruschak LM. HIV in prisons, 2020-statistical tables. USA: Bureau of Justice Statistics; 2022.
28. Wurcel AG, Chen G, Zubiago JA, et al. Heterogeneity in jail nursing medical intake forms: a content analysis. J Correct Health Care 2021;27(4):265–71.
29. Levano SR, Epting ME, Pluznik JA, et al. HIV testing in jails: comparing strategies to maximize engagement in HIV treatment and prevention. PLoS One 2023;18(6):e0286805.
30. Sabharwal CJ, Muse KH, Alper H, et al. Jail-based providers' perceptions of challenges to routine HIV testing in New York City jails. J Correct Health Care 2010;16(4):310–21.
31. The Use of Ryan White HIV/AIDS Program Funds for Core Medical Services and Support Services for People Living with HIV Who Are Incarcerated and Justice Involved In: HRSA, ed2018.
32. Simonsen KA, Shaikh RA, Earley M, et al. Rapid HIV screening in an urban jail: how testing at exit with linkage to community care can address perceived barriers. J Prim Prev 2015;36(6):427–32.
33. Routine jail-based HIV testing - Rhode Island, 2000-2007. MMWR Morbidity and mortality weekly report 2010;59(24):742–5.
34. Beckwith CG, Atunah-Jay S, Cohen J, et al. Feasibility and acceptability of rapid HIV testing in jail. AIDS Patient Care STDS 2007;21(1):41–7.
35. Johnson CC, Fonner V, Sands A, et al. To err is human, to correct is public health: a systematic review examining poor quality testing and misdiagnosis of HIV status. J Int AIDS Soc 2017;20(Suppl 6):21755.
36. Fukuda HD, Randall LM, Meehan T, et al. Leveraging Health Department Capacities, Partnerships, and Health Insurance for Infectious Disease Response in Massachusetts, 2014-2018. Publ Health Rep 2020;135(1_suppl):75s–81s.
37. Maner M, Omori M, Brinkley-Rubinstein L, et al. Infectious disease surveillance in U.S. jails: findings from a national survey. PLoS One 2022;17(8):e0272374.
38. Tarver BA, Sewell J, Oussayef N. State laws governing HIV testing in correctional settings. J Correct Health Care 2016;22(1):28–40.
39. Blain M, Wallace SE, Tuegel C. Shadow of HIV exceptionalism 40 years later. J Med Ethics 2021;47(11):727–8.
40. Hammett TM, Dubler NN. Clinical and epidemiologic research on HIV infection and AIDS among correctional inmates: Regulations, ethics, and procedures. Eval Rev 1990;14(5):482–501.
41. Warren N, Bellin E, Zoloth S, et al. Human immunodeficiency virus infection care is unavailable to inmates on release from jail. Arch Fam Med 1994;3(10):894–8.
42. Hirschel B, Francioli P. Progress and problems in the fight against AIDS. N Engl J Med 1998;338(13):906–8.
43. Zaller N, Thurmond P, Rich JD. Limited spending: an analysis of correctional expenditures on antiretrovirals for HIV-infected prisoners. Publ Health Rep 2007; 122(1):49–54.
44. Kerr T, Marshall A, Walsh J, et al. Determinants of HAART discontinuation among injection drug users. AIDS Care 2005;17(5):539–49.
45. Wright P, Herivel T, editors. Prison Nation: The Warehousing of America's Poor. 1st edition. New York: Routledge; 2003. https://doi.org/10.4324/9780203952627.
46. Cohen CJ, Piliero PJ, Pile OH. Increasing treatment adherence in the correctional setting: current efforts to simplify protease inhibitor dosing regimens. J Correct Health Care 2000;7(1):61–90.
47. Culbert G J. Violence and the perceived risks of taking antiretroviral therapy in US jails and prisons. Int J Prison Health 2014;10(2):94–110.

48. Springer SA, Altice FL. Managing HIV/AIDS in correctional settings. Curr HIV AIDS Rep 2005;2(4):165–70.

49. Roberson DW. Medical privacy and antiretroviral therapy among HIV-infected female inmates. J Nurs Law 2012;15(1):3.

50. Emanuele P. Antiretroviral treatment in correctional facilities. HIV Clin Trials 2005; 6(1):25–37.

51. White BL, Golin CE, Grodensky CA, et al. Effect of directly observed antiretroviral therapy compared to self-administered antiretroviral therapy on adherence and virological outcomes among hiv-infected prisoners: a randomized controlled pilot study. AIDS Behav 2015;19(1):128–36.

52. Wohl DA, Stephenson BL, Golin CE, et al. Adherence to directly observed antiretroviral therapy among human immunodeficiency virus—infected prison inmates. Clin Infect Dis 2003;36(12):1572–6.

53. Meyer JP, Cepeda J, Wu J, et al. Optimization of human immunodeficiency virus treatment during incarceration: viral suppression at the prison gate. JAMA Intern Med 2014;174(5):721–9.

54. Springer SA, Pesanti E, Hodges J, et al. Effectiveness of antiretroviral therapy among HIV-infected prisoners: reincarceration and the lack of sustained benefit after release to the community. Clin Infect Dis 2004;38(12):1754–60.

55. Blue C, Buchbinder M, Brown ME, et al. Access to HIV care in jails: Perspectives from people living with HIV in North Carolina. PLoS One 2022;17(1):e0262882.

56. Iroh PA, Mayo H, Nijhawan AE. The HIV care cascade before, during, and after incarceration: a systematic review and data synthesis. Am J Publ Health 2015; 105(7):e5–16.

57. MacGowan RJ. HIV testing implementation guidance for correctional settings 2009.

58. Loeliger KB, Altice FL, Ciarleglio MM, et al. All-cause mortality among people with HIV released from an integrated system of jails and prisons in Connecticut, USA, 2007-14: a retrospective observational cohort study. Lancet HIV 2018; 5(11):e617–28.

59. Merrall EL, Kariminia A, Binswanger IA, et al. Meta-analysis of drug-related deaths soon after release from prison. Addiction 2010;105(9):1545–54.

60. Loeliger KB, Meyer JP, Desai MM, et al. Retention in HIV care during the 3 years following release from incarceration: A cohort study. PLoS Med 2018;15(10): e1002667.

61. Avery A, Ciomica R, Gierlach M, et al. Jail-based case management improves retention in HIV care 12 months post release. AIDS Behav 2019;23(4):966–72.

62. Brantley AD, Page KM, Zack B, et al. Making the connection: using videoconferencing to increase linkage to care for incarcerated persons living with HIV postrelease. AIDS Behav 2019;23(Suppl 1):32–40.

63. Uhrig Castonguay BJ, Cressman AE, Kuo I, et al. The implementation of a text messaging intervention to improve HIV continuum of care outcomes among persons recently released from correctional facilities: randomized controlled trial. JMIR Mhealth Uhealth 2020;8(2):e16220.

64. Dauria EF, Kulkarni P, Clemenzi-Allen A, et al. Interventions designed to improve HIV continuum of care outcomes for persons with HIV in contact with the carceral system in the USA. Curr HIV AIDS Rep 2022;19(4):281–91.

65. Mohammad S, Bahrani A, Kim M, et al. Barriers and facilitators to health during prison reentry to Miami, FL. PLoS One 2023;18(10):e0285411.

66. Loeliger KB, Altice FL, Desai MM, et al. Predictors of linkage to HIV care and viral suppression after release from jails and prisons: a retrospective cohort study. Lancet HIV 2018;5(2):e96–106.
67. Tiruneh YM, Li X, Bovell-Ammon B, et al. Falling through the cracks: risk factors for becoming lost to HIV care after incarceration in a southern jail. AIDS Behav 2020;24(8):2430–41.
68. Wiersema JJ, Teixeira PA, Pugh T, et al. HIV Care Engagement Among Justice-Involved and Substance Using People of Puerto Rican Origin Who are Living with HIV. J Immigr Minor Health 2021. https://doi.org/10.1007/s10903-021-01191-x.
69. Sanchez MA, Scheer S, Shallow S, et al. Epidemiology of the viral hepatitis-HIV syndemic in San Francisco: a collaborative surveillance approach. Publ Health Rep 2014;129(Suppl 1):95–101.
70. Olsen Y, Fitzgerald RM, Wakeman SE. Overcoming barriers to treatment of opioid use disorder. JAMA 2021;325(12):1149–50.
71. Linas BP, Savinkina A, Madushani R, et al. Projected estimates of opioid mortality after community-level interventions. JAMA Netw Open 2021;4(2):e2037259.
72. Thakarar K, Walley AY, Heeren TC, et al. Medication for addiction treatment and acute care utilization in HIV-positive adults with substance use disorders. AIDS Care 2020;32(9):1177–81.
73. Sufrin C, Kramer C, Terplan M, et al. Availability of medications for opioid use disorder in U.S. Jails. J Gen Intern Med 2023;38(6):1573–5.
74. Khatri UG, Winkelman TNA. Strengthening the medicaid reentry act - supporting the health of people who are incarcerated. N Engl J Med 2022;386(16):1488–90.
75. Wurcel AG, London K, Crable EL, et al. Medicaid inmate exclusion policy and infectious diseases care for justice-involved populations. Emerg Infect Dis 2024;30(13):S94–9.
76. Khan MR, Doherty IA, Schoenbach VJ, et al. Incarceration and high-risk sex partnerships among men in the United States. J Urban Health 2009;86:584–601.
77. Favril L. Drug use before and during imprisonment: Drivers of continuation. Int J Drug Pol 2023;115:104027.
78. da Silva DT, Bachireddy C. To End The HIV Epidemic, Implement Proven HIV Prevention Strategies In The Criminal Justice System. Health Affairs Forefront 2021.
79. Siegler AJ, Mouhanna F, Giler RM, et al. The prevalence of pre-exposure prophylaxis use and the pre-exposure prophylaxis–to-need ratio in the fourth quarter of 2017, United States. Ann Epidemiol 2018;28(12):841–9.
80. Brinkley-Rubinstein L, Peterson M, Arnold T, et al. Knowledge, interest, and anticipated barriers of pre-exposure prophylaxis uptake and adherence among gay, bisexual, and men who have sex with men who are incarcerated. PLoS One 2018;13(12):e0205593.
81. Knittel A, Ferguson E, Jackson J, et al. The role of relationships in decision-making about pre-exposure prophylaxis (PrEP) for HIV among women who have experienced incarceration. Am J Obstet Gynecol 2020;223(6):979.
82. Parsons J, Cox C. PrEP in Prisons: HIV prevention in incarcerated populations. Int J Prison Health 2020;16(2):199–206.
83. Chimoyi L, Charalambous S. The case for pre-exposure prophylaxis in prison settings. The Lancet HIV 2023;10(1):e3–4.
84. Edwards GG, Reback CJ, Cunningham WE, et al. Mobile-enhanced prevention support study for men who have sex with men and transgender women leaving

jail: protocol for a randomized controlled trial. JMIR research protocols 2020; 9(9):e18106.

85. LeMasters K, Oser C, Cowell M, et al. Longitudinal pre-exposure prophylaxis (PrEP) acceptability, initiation and adherence among criminal justice-involved adults in the USA: the Southern PrEP Cohort Study (SPECS) protocol. BMJ Open 2021;11(7):e047340.

86. Murphy M, Rogers BG, Ames E, et al. Implementing Preexposure Prophylaxis for HIV Prevention in a Statewide Correctional System in the United States. Public Health Rep 2024;139(2):174–9.

87. Murphy M, Sosnowy C, Rogers B, et al. Defining the Pre-exposure Prophylaxis Care Continuum Among Recently Incarcerated Men at High Risk for HIV Infection: Protocol for a Prospective Cohort Study. JMIR Res Protoc 2022;11(2): e31928.

88. Brinkley-Rubinstein L, Peterson M, Clarke J, et al. The benefits and implementation challenges of the first state-wide comprehensive medication for addictions program in a unified jail and prison setting. Drug Alcohol Depend 2019; 205:107514.

89. Evans EA, Stopka TJ, Pivovarova E, et al. Massachusetts justice community opioid innovation network (MassJCOIN). J Subst Abuse Treat 2021;128:108275.

90. Friedmann PD, Dunn D, Michener P, et al. COVID-19 impact on opioid overdose after jail release in Massachusetts. Drug Alcohol Depend Rep 2023;6:100141.

91. Maruschak LM, Minton TD, Zeng Z. Opioid use disorder screening and treatment in local jails, 2019. Department of justice, office of justice programs. USA: Bureau of Justice Statistics; 2023. p. 3.

92. Evans EA, Pivovarova E, Stopka TJ, et al. Uncommon and preventable: Perceptions of diversion of medication for opioid use disorder in jail. J Subst Abuse Treat 2022;138:108746.

93. Friedmann PD, Schwartz RP. Just call it "treatment". Addiction Sci Clin Pract 2012;7:1–3.

94. Lee JD, Malone M, McDonald R, et al. Comparison of treatment retention of adults with opioid addiction managed with extended-release buprenorphine vs daily sublingual buprenorphine-naloxone at time of release from jail. JAMA Netw Open 2021;4(9):e2123032.

95. Whaley S, Bandara S, Taylor K, et al. Expanding buprenorphine in US jails: One county's response to addressing the fears of diversion. Journal of Substance Use and Addiction Treatment 2023;146:208944.

96. Cumming C, Kinner SA, McKetin R, et al. The health needs of people leaving prison with a history of methamphetamine and/or opioid use. Drug Alcohol Rev 2023;42(4):778–84.

97. Roll JM. Contingency management: an evidence-based component of methamphetamine use disorder treatments. Addiction 2007;102(Suppl 1):114–20.

98. Acheson LS, Williams BH, Farrell M, et al. Pharmacological treatment for methamphetamine withdrawal: A systematic review and meta-analysis of randomised controlled trials. Drug Alcohol Rev 2023;42(1):7–19.

99. Desai J, Krakower D, Harris B-L, et al. HIV/sexually transmitted infection screening and eligibility for HIV preexposure prophylaxis among women incarcerated in an urban county jail. Sex Transm Dis 2023;50(10):675–9.

100. Spaulding AC, Rabeeah Z, Del Mar González-Montalvo M, et al. Prevalence and Management of Sexually Transmitted Infections in Correctional Settings: A Systematic Review. Clin Infect Dis 2022;74(Suppl_2):S193–217.

101. Celum CL. Sexually transmitted infections and HIV: epidemiology and interventions. Top HIV Med 2010;18(4):138–42.
102. Javanbakht M, Boudov M, Anderson LJ, et al. Sexually transmitted infections among incarcerated women: findings from a decade of screening in a Los Angeles County Jail, 2002-2012. Am J Publ Health 2014;104(11):e103–9.
103. Owusu-Edusei Jr K, Gift TL, Chesson HW, et al. Investigating the potential public health benefit of jail-based screening and treatment programs for chlamydia. Am J Epidemiol 2013;177(5):463–73.
104. Krieger D, Abe C, Pottorff A, et al. Sexually transmitted infections detected during and after incarceration among people with human immunodeficiency virus: prevalence and implications for screening and prevention. Sex Transm Dis 2019;46(9):602–7.
105. Abara WE, Llata EL, Schumacher C, et al. Extragenital gonorrhea and chlamydia positivity and the potential for missed extragenital gonorrhea with concurrent urethral chlamydia among men who have sex with men attending sexually transmitted disease clinics-sexually transmitted disease surveillance network, 2015-2019. Sex Transm Dis 2020;47(6):361–8.
106. Ybarra AC, Benjamins LJ. Extragenital sexually transmitted infections testing during COVID-19 pandemic among youth involved in the juvenile justice system. J Correct Health Care 2023;29(5):324–8.
107. Ramchandani MS, Cannon CA, Marra CM. Syphilis: a modern resurgence. Infectious Disease Clinics 2023;37(2):195–222.
108. Carlson JM, Tannis A, Woodworth KR, et al. Substance use among persons with syphilis during pregnancy—Arizona and Georgia, 2018–2021. MMWR (Morb Mortal Wkly Rep) 2023;72(3):63.
109. Lin CH, Henderson SO. Not a rare disease anymore? a case of ocular syphilis at the correctional facility. J Correct Health Care 2023;29(5):311–3.
110. Mahon N. New York inmates' HIV risk behaviors: the implications for prevention policy and programs. Am J Publ Health 1996;86(9):1211–5.
111. McCuller WJ, Harawa NT. A condom distribution program in the Los Angeles Men's Central Jail: Sheriff deputies' attitudes and opinions. J Correct Health Care 2014;20(3):195–202.
112. Lucas KD, Bick J, Mohle-Boetani JC. California's prisoner protections for family and community health act: implementing a mandated condom access program in state prisons, 2015-2016. Publ Health Rep 2020;135(1_suppl):50S–6S.
113. Voss MWW, Ciciurkaite G, Huntington M, et al. Impact of an opioid harm reduction consortium: emergency and justice engagement. Outcomes and Impact Quarterly 2023;3(3):4.
114. Clark AE. Building a bigger tent: a grant proposal to integrate harm reduction into orange county care systems. Long Beach: California State University; 2023.
115. Singer AJ, Kopak AM. Jail reentry and gaps in substance use disorder treatment in rural communities. Corrections 2023;8(5):505–27.

Training the Next Generation of the Human Immunodeficiency Virus Workforce

Needs, Challenges, and Opportunities

Nathanial S. Nolan, MD, MPH, MHPE[a,b,]*, Katherine Promer, MD[c],
Michael Tang, MD[c], Darcy Wooten, MD, MS[c]

KEYWORDS

- HIV • Workforce • EHE

KEY POINTS

- Major challenges in patient care for the future human immunodeficiency virus (HIV) workforce include a growing population of older patients with associated medical complexities and a marginalized patient population with substantial barriers to care.
- The supply of HIV specialists and other clinicians who will provide care to PWH is not keeping pace with demand, and disparities in access to care continue to widen.
- Efforts to recruit additional clinicians to the field include expanding HIV training models, providing trainees with earlier exposure to the field, and aligning generational values with the values of our specialty.
- Retention efforts should focus on improving remuneration, providing loan forgiveness, optimizing team-based care, and supporting low-volume providers with clinical management decisions via access to experts.

INTRODUCTION

Over the past 40 years, the field of HIV medicine has changed dramatically due to notable advances in disease diagnosis, management, and prevention. We now have the tools to effectively end the HIV epidemic through both treatment of patients with HIV (PWH) and prevention of future infections.[1] Among these tools are multiple well-tolerated antiretrovirals (ARVs) with high barriers to resistance, long-acting injectable agents for individuals with barriers to daily oral medications, and effective options for

[a] Division of Infectious Disease, Washington University School of Medicine, St. Louis, MO, USA; [b] Division of Infectious Disease, VA St. Louis Health Care, St. Louis, MO, USA; [c] Division of Infectious Disease, US San Diego School of Medicine, 9500 Gilman Drive, La Jolla, CA 92093, USA
* Corresponding author. JC/111 915 North Grand Boulevard, St. Louis MO 63106.
E-mail address: nolann@wustl.edu

Infect Dis Clin N Am 38 (2024) 627–639
https://doi.org/10.1016/j.idc.2024.06.004
0891-5520/24/Published by Elsevier Inc.

id.theclinics.com

both pre-exposure prophylaxis (PrEP) and post-exposure prophylaxis.[2] With these tools, US public health agencies have redoubled their efforts to eliminate HIV transmission through the Ending the HIV Epidemic (EHE) initiative, which hinges on disease identification, engagement in treatment, provision of prophylactic therapies, and public health responses to new outbreaks.[3] Not explicit in this public health campaign is the acknowledgment of the workforce that will be required to implement these initiatives and provide ongoing care for people already infected with HIV.[4]

STATE OF THE HUMAN IMMUNODEFICIENCY VIRUS EPIDEMIC IN THE UNITED STATES

Despite a steady decline in new infections, more people are with HIV than ever before. This is in part due to the dramatic improvements in life expectancy that have come with modern ARVs.[5,6] It is estimated that individuals aged 50 years and older will represent more than 70% of the population of PWH by 2030.[7] This represents an increasingly medically and psychosocially complex population, with a higher proportion of comorbidities traditionally related to aging, including cardiovascular disease, malignancy, and cognitive decline, compared to age-matched controls.[8,9]

Additionally, certain populations remain disproportionately impacted by HIV.[10] In the United States, of the estimated 32,100 new HIV infections that occurred in 2021, approximately 40% occurred in Black individuals and 29% in Hispanic/Latino individuals, as compared to 26% occurring in White individuals.[11] Despite the increased risk of HIV acquisition among Black and Hispanic/Latino populations, there is significantly less PrEP usage among these groups.[12] There is also dramatic regional variation, with the highest rate of new HIV cases in the United States occurring in the South, where there is a mismatch among available providers, preventative services, and population need.[13-15]

The HIV care cascade relies on not only diagnosis, but access to treatment, and retention in care. While close to 90% of PWH in the United States know their status, only about 66% are virally suppressed.[16] Comorbid mental health conditions, ongoing substance use, and social/financial concerns remain significant barriers to retention in care and virologic suppression.[17] Recognition of these challenges has led many thought leaders to suggest newer and novel mechanisms for delivering care, frequently in low-barrier and nontraditional settings.[18,19] Thus, the current HIV care workforce in the United States now contends with two simultaneous challenges—navigating chronic disease care for an aging population and engaging with marginalized communities that struggle to access traditional models of care.

STATE OF THE US HUMAN IMMUNODEFICIENCY VIRUS WORKFORCE

The HIV workforce is composed of an array of health professionals, from primary care physicians (such as internal medicine and family practice physicians) and advanced practice providers (APPs) to infectious disease (ID) and HIV specialists. This workforce is supported by nurses, clinical pharmacists, social workers, case managers, and peer navigators. According to 2010 estimates, approximately 4,937 clinicians were identified as providing HIV care in the United States, including internal medicine physicians (55%), family practice providers (37%), and ID-trained specialists (8%).[20] Based on these data, and subsequent clinician surveys, it was predicted that by 2019, there would be a widening mismatch between supply and demand for HIV medical services.[20,21] Though more recent figures have yet to be published, the COVID-19 public health crisis may have exacerbated this shortage, with multiple studies citing increasing rates of burnout and intention to leave the practice of medicine.[22,23] A

2023 AIDS Education and Training Centers (AETC) survey, presented to the Health Resources and Services Administration (HRSA) last year, reported that approximately 10.5% of ARV prescribers planned to stop treating patients with HIV and 7.3% planned to decrease their panel of PWH over the next 5 years.[24]

There is also concern about the pipeline of providers into HIV care. Infectious disease physicians continue to provide a significant amount of primary care to PWH[25]; however in recent years, the number of applicants entering the field of infectious diseases has stagnated (**Table 1**).[26] Increasingly, HIV care is provided by internal medicine and family medicine providers, yet there are limited opportunities for trainees in these specialties to gain expertise in caring for PWH.[27,28] Because it has become increasingly clear that primary care providers need to have skills related to the care of PWH, specific HIV training pathways in internal medicine and family medicine residency programs have been developed, though these remain limited in scope.[29–31]

Recent data have also highlighted the significant mismatch between provider practice location and incidence of new HIV infections. Although 52% of new HIV infections occur in the South,[13] 81% of Southern counties have no HIV-experienced clinicians, leading to significant limitations in access to care in rural settings.[32] Further, the HIV workforce lacks the diversity that represents its patient population. While 40% of new infections occur in Black individuals,[11] only 8% of HIV providers identify as Black compared to 67% identifying as White.[20]

DISCUSSION
Recruiting the Next Generation

Perhaps the most urgent step in addressing the HIV workforce shortage is inspiring a wider breadth of clinicians (ID specialists, internists, family medicine physicians, nurse practitioners, physician assistants, clinical pharmacists) to integrate care for PWH into their clinical career. The recent signal for decreased interest in infectious diseases by graduating trainees, in combination with the number of HIV clinicians planning to leave the field or retire soon, creates concern for an enlarging void of HIV specialists. Recruiting new clinicians into this workforce will rely on a multipronged approach that includes increased exposure to HIV care in medical training, demonstration of the values and priorities of the field, and increased practice incentives.[33]

Historically, infectious disease-trained physicians have significantly contributed to the HIV workforce.[25] In recent years, there has been a widening mismatch between training slots and applicants to the ID workforce, with the most recent fellowship match signaling a decline in the overall number of applicants.[34,35] While this decline in interest is multifactorial, there is an urgent need to address this shortage, not only for HIV primary care but also for hospital-based ID physicians who manage the acute care needs of PWH. Early specialty exposure may be related to eventual interest in the

Table 1
Six year trends in US ID fellowship training program match results

Year	2019	2020	2021	2022	2023	2024
Number of ID Fellowship Applicants	356	352	404	387	353	305
Number of ID Fellowship Positions Available	401	406	416	436	441	450
Percent of Fellowship Positions NOT Filled	18.7	20.7	12.2	17.9	25.6	32.2

Source: Joseph A. Limits of 'Fauci effect': infectious disease applicants plummet, and hospitals are scrambling. STAT News. Published online December 7, 2022. Accessed October 5, 2023. https://www.statnews.com/2022/12/07/infectious-disease-fellowship-drop-in-applicants/

field of ID and HIV medicine. Retrospective studies have suggested that when medicine interns rotate on infectious disease clinical services in the first 6 months of their training, they are subsequently more likely to apply to infectious disease fellowships.[36] Similarly, a survey of internal medicine residents suggested that pre-residency factors, such as medical school and undergraduate experiences, influenced their ultimate specialty choice.[37] This suggests that upstream interventions, such as improved pedagogy or visible role models, may be beneficial in increasing interest in HIV care. Indeed, creating clinical rotations in HIV primary care has been shown to increase trainee interest in an HIV career path,[38] though this effect has not been universally demonstrated.[39] Based on available data, it is likely that increased exposure to foundational HIV content, which is relevant to all clinicians no matter their chosen specialty or area of focus, would increase interest in HIV care and increase the pool of HIV competent clinicians in practice across specialties and clinical access points.

Given the current barriers in infectious disease fellowship recruitment, and the increasing breadth of subspecialties within the field of infectious diseases (eg, antimicrobial stewardship, infectious disease/critical care, and transplant ID), alternative pathways for HIV training will need to be expanded. Currently, several organizations, including the HIV Medical Association (HIVMA), offer HIV Clinical fellowships that support noninfectious disease physicians in gaining the experience necessary to become expert HIV clinicians.[40,41] Limited evidence suggests these fellowship programs can be successful in contributing meaningfully to the HIV workforce.[42] Some residency programs have alternatively developed HIV clinical training tracts, which are integrated into primary care residencies and do not require additional years of training.[43] Unfortunately, many of these programs exist outside of regions with the greatest disparities of care, that is, the US South. There are also limited data regarding subsequent entry into the HIV workforce, with less than half of surveyed graduates going on to care for 20 or more PWH.[43] Focused training programs should be created in areas that lack a robust HIV workforce, with incentives for subsequent care of that population. Further investment in these programs is likely to improve the overall capacity of the health care system to care for patients with HIV.

Similar expanded training opportunities are needed for APPs and clinical pharmacists interested in pursuing a career in HIV Medicine. This includes establishing advanced HIV specialization within traditional training programs for nurse practitioners (NPs), physician assistants (PAs), and clinical pharmacists, extended training options (ie, a 1 year clinical HIV fellowship after standard training is completed) as well as opportunities for externships and other clinical rotation experiences for NPs/PAs and clinical pharmacists already in practice. These expanded training opportunities must come with financial support, scholarships, and other incentives so that additional training is not disincentivized from a financial perspective. A recent position paper by the Infectious Diseases Society of America and HIVMA supports the use of team-based models that expand care through the use of specialized pharmacists and APPs.[44]

There has also been increasing recognition that a diverse workforce is necessary to serve a diverse population. Substantial investment has been placed into efforts to recruit underrepresented minoritized groups into HIV clinical training pathways. For example, the Centers for AIDS Research Diversity, Equity and Inclusion Pathway Initiative has partnered with historically Black colleges and universities as well as other institutions to foster a continuum of training opportunities, from high school to postdoctoral levels, to support trainees from underrepresented backgrounds.[45] Early evaluation suggests success in engaging interested learners, though longitudinal data will be needed.[46] Future work will need to focus not only on ethnic and racial diversity, but also on promoting diversity in training locale and practice location. The Southern United States, including many rural areas, faces a mismatch between the burden of HIV and access to HIV providers.[32,47] Future diversity efforts should seek to include trainees from rural Southern communities as a means of supporting a future workforce.

Workforce Retention

Despite interventions to increase trainees entering the pipeline, without changes in practice incentives, the field will likely lose high-quality trainees and clinicians. Relatively lower financial income coupled with high student loan debt can dissuade interested trainees from pursuing cognitive subspecialties, such as HIV care.[48,49] The HIV Epidemic Loan-Repayment Program Act was introduced initially in 2020 to provide loan repayment to those providing care to PWH in health professional-shortage areas or at Ryan White-funded clinics. Despite being introduced again in 2021, it ultimately never passed Congress.[50] The recently passed Bio-Preparedness Workforce Act has the potential to offer loan repayment to those ID and HIV professionals working in health professional-shortage areas or federally funded programs; however, it is not specific to the HIV workforce and has as of this writing not been funded by Congress.[51]

Remuneration is another significant consideration in bolstering the HIV workforce. HIV specialists remain poorly compensated compared to many of their medicine subspecialty colleagues.[48] This is in part due to a lack of revenue-generating procedures. HIV care is also socially complex, with many patients receiving their medical coverage via Medicaid or the Ryan White HIV/AIDS Program. While funding for the Ryan White HIV/AIDS program increases yearly, compared to inflation, the funding stream has remained flat or even declined.[52] Without ongoing support, HIV-focused clinics will struggle to offer compensation to the wide range of staff required to deliver essential primary care and wrap-around services.

In the recent AETC workforce survey, two factors associated with clinicians planning to leave the HIV workforce included administrative burden and burnout.[24] The HIV workforce is persistently confronted with the manifestations of social and structural health inequities, which contribute to many of the disparities facing PWH. Recent laws challenging reproductive rights for women and health care access for transgender individuals have highlighted the difficulties in providing evidence-based care to PWH. It is notable that many of these legislative actions have occurred in the US South, prompting concerns that disparities in this region could be worsened. HIV practitioners in this region have identified these laws as reasons that some may leave the area.[53] Visible advocacy efforts from regional and national organizations create the opportunity validate and support HIV clinicians as well as provide the opportunity for HIV providers to elevate their voice. Efforts should be made to provide HIV clinicians the tools to organize and advocate for their patients, and themselves.

New Models of Care

It is unlikely that the expansion of the HIV provider pipeline will satisfy the current and future workforce needs. New and innovative models of care will also be necessary to expand the reach of expert clinicians and ensure basic competencies for clinicians who care for a lower volume of PWH. Significant disparities in access to HIV care exist in rural communities and in the US South, where support is urgently needed.

As a means to expand the HIV workforce, Armstrong has described parallel strategies for providers caring for a low volume versus high volume of patients with HIV (**Fig. 1**).[4] For primary care providers practicing in a low patient volume setting, where maintenance of HIV specialty care knowledge may be challenging, it will be critical to

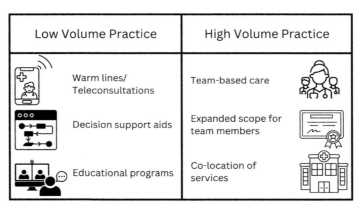

Low Volume Practice	High Volume Practice
Warm lines/ Teleconsultations	Team-based care
Decision support aids	Expanded scope for team members
Educational programs	Co-location of services

Fig. 1. Caring for a low volume versus high volume of patients with HIV.

have access to experts who can provide guidance, mentorship, and support. This can be accomplished through a combination of strategies, including access to HIV experts through Warmlines,[54] teleconsultation,[55,56] and education from HIV experts, as has been demonstrated in Project Echo.[57,58] Crucial to the addition of these nontraditional models of care is a plan to expand support, funding, and reimbursement for these consultative services in order to grow and sustain these programs.

Newer technological tools will also aid clinicians practicing in low-volume settings to effectively care for PWH. Decision-support software and artificial intelligence can help guide less experienced prescribers to appropriate first-line regimens. In a study where trainees without HIV clinical experience were provided patient scenarios, they were more frequently able to accurately prescribe ARV regimens using the online HIV-ASSIST tool as compared to using the US Department of Health and Human Services guidelines.[59] Though these tools are unlikely to replace expert HIV clinicians, they may serve as point-of-care support to facilitate more immediate treatment decisions as providers seek expert advice.

For providers with HIV expertise working in high patient volume settings, expansion and optimization of team-based care should be a priority (**Fig. 2**). The inclusion and expansion of roles for nurses, pharmacists, social workers, case managers, financial counselors, behavioral health counselors, mental health providers, and patient navigators will allow all parties to practice at the top of their license and maximize the time provided to HIV primary care clinicians to care for more complex patients. HIV primary care providers are frequently tasked with the role of serving in many capacities, including that of social worker, mental health provider, financial counselor and so forth. By expanding the number and scope of clinical support staff, lower complexity and administrative responsibilities can be offloaded from HIV providers. Continuing education programs aimed at chronic disease management will likely be needed to aid HIV-focused clinicians in managing PWH who have a higher burden of chronic illness. This work might also be supported by population health monitoring programs, which can support cancer screenings, management of cardiometabolic risk factors, and more rapid uptake of guideline-directed care. Finally, optimizing tools in the electronic health record that can automatize routine health care maintenance (ie, vaccinations, cancer screenings), support linkage and retention in care efforts, and decrease the amount of time providers spend on clinical documentation, will help improve patient outcomes and quality of care while reducing provider burnout.

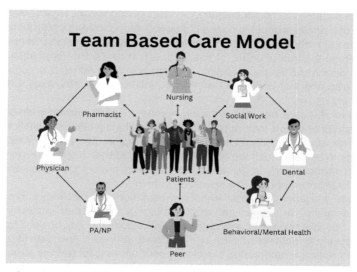

Fig. 2. Team-based care model.

Implicit in these recommendations is the need for increased and flexible funding. Adequate reimbursement for services, including nonclinical services such as peer-navigation, will be necessary to ensure sustainability and to promote innovation. Flexibility in resource utilization will also be required to create new and low-barrier opportunities for care. For example, a recently published novel telehealth harm-reduction program has shown promise in being able to deliver HIV care to patients who inject drugs, a population that has been historically difficult to engage in care.[60] These types of innovations, which will be necessary to support the HIV workforce in EHE, will require sustained funding (**Fig. 3**).

The Future

Despite many hurdles, there is room for optimism when considering the HIV workforce. More than ever before the health care system is realigning to recognize systemic

Building the HIV Workforce

Provider Level

- Increase trainee exposure to HIV earlier in education
- Create longitudinal pathways that promote diversity in the field
- Expand training opportunities for primary care physicians, APPs, PharmDs
- Facilitate the development of practice incentives (e.g., loan repayment, compensation initiatives)

System Level

- Optimize team based practices
- Participate in supportive services (i.e., TeleEcho)
- Remove barriers to alternative models of care (i.e., street medicine)
- Advance technologic solutions to facilitate/automate routine care
- Implement decision support aids for non-specialists caring for PLWH

Regional Level

- Facilitate practice incentives in regions with greatest disparities
- Invest in training programs in underserved regions
- Create support networks, such as teleconsultation or teleEcho to support rural providers
- Focus advocacy on state laws that may impact health equity

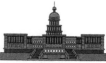

National Level

- Improve funding mechanisms for innovative models of care
- Create further reimbursement mechanisms for teleconsultation services
- Dedicate funding to compensation and loan repayment programs
- Advocate for pay parity with HIV and Infectious Disease specialists
- Ensure Ryan White funding keeps pace with inflation

Fig. 3. Building the HIV workforce.

and structural causes of health inequity.[61,62] Though significant work remains, a new generation of trainees is developing in a time when advocacy and social justice are being normalized in medical education. Perhaps one way to appeal to this new generation is to signal the true priorities of this field, which centers on equitable care for a historically disenfranchised population. Though HIV care remains a cognitive specialty, it is also one that is deeply centered on relationships, advocacy, and fighting for healthy equity.

The field of HIV care has an increasing number of tools and an ever-broadening scope of practice, which may appeal to intellectually stimulated health professions students. The workforce should highlight and champion the opportunities that exist for clinicians to serve a multitude of roles in the care of their patients. From addiction medicine to endocrinology to geriatrics, HIV providers are uniquely positioned to provide a wide spectrum of care in a specialist setting.

There is also evidence of realignment of payment models, which may improve access to care for many socially complex patients. For example, in 2023 the Centers for Medicare & Medicaid Services released a new point-of-service code that can be used for outreach work, particularly for patients who live in unsheltered settings.[63] And state Medicaid programs are increasingly recognizing the role of peers, allowing for reimbursement in some instances.[64] Though much work remains, there is recognition from payers that new alternative funding streams will be needed to provide effective care.

Though much has been written about the struggle of caring for PWH, the authors believe that a career in HIV Medicine provides a substantial amount of purpose, meaning, and joy which we must make visible to the next generations of clinicians. Many challenges lie ahead, but there are just as many opportunities for success. The vision of ending the epidemic has never been clearer and, with the right workforce, it is within reach.

SUMMARY

The United States has the tools to end the transmission of HIV. Despite a plethora of well-tolerated antiviral therapies, a significant portion of PWH face barriers in accessing care. The HIV workforce is strained, hampered by a growing population of patients, a dwindling pipeline of providers, and burdens that are forcing some out of practice. As the HIV population ages and faces an increasing burden of chronic comorbidities, support is needed to ensure that practicing clinicians have the resources needed to provide holistic primary care. To achieve the goal of EHE in the United States, a concerted effort will be needed to inspire and invigorate a new generation of HIV providers. Financial incentives, such as loan repayment and improved compensation, will be needed to attract trainees to the field of HIV. Intentional programs will have to be developed to ensure that we are recruiting and supporting a diverse workforce that can practice in the areas of greatest disparity. And innovative models of care, which support interdisciplinary teams and make good use of technology, will need to be developed to reach our most complex and marginalized patients. Though challenges remain, the HIV workforce has never been closer to ending the HIV epidemic.

CLINICS CARE POINTS

- Early exposure to HIV clinical care may increase interest in the field and competency in managing patients with HIV (PWH). Health professions schools and training programs should consider increasing opportunities for learners to encounter and care for PWH.

- The HIV workforce will be reliant on an expanded pool of clinicians. Health systems should support expanded training in the care of PWH for pharmacists, PAs, and NPs.
- Clinician diversity will be critical in increasing access to HIV care for marginalized communities. HIV clinical training programs should seek out diverse applicants from those traditionally unrepresented in medicine.
- To recruit a new generation of providers, the field of HIV Medicine must ensure that it communicates the positives of providing HIV care to young trainees. Despite noted difficulties, there is much room for optimism as we incorporate an increasing array of treatments and technologies into routine care. The values of the field remain rooted in social justice and healthy equity, which may align with newer generational values.

DISCLOSURE

The authors report no disclosures relevant to the content of this study. Dr K. Promer reports honorarium from ViiV Health care for producing educational content unrelated to this work. Dr D. Wooten has served on the ViiV Healthcare advisory board. All authors contributed meaningfully to the development and authoring of this content. All authors had access to the final draft prior to submission.

REFERENCES

1. Person AK, Armstrong WS, Evans T, et al. Principles for Ending Human Immunodeficiency Virus as an Epidemic in the United States: A Policy Paper of the Infectious Diseases Society of America and the HIV Medicine Association. Clin Infect Dis 2023;76(1):1–9.
2. Gandhi RT, Bedimo R, Hoy JF, et al. Antiretroviral Drugs for Treatment and Prevention of HIV Infection in Adults: 2022 Recommendations of the International Antiviral Society–USA Panel. JAMA 2023;329(1):63.
3. About the Ending the HIV Epidemic in the U.S. Initiative. Ending the HIV Epidemic in the U.S. (EHE). Available at: https://www.cdc.gov/endhiv/about-ehe/index.html. [Accessed 22 September 2023].
4. Armstrong WS. The Human Immunodeficiency Virus Workforce in Crisis: An Urgent Need to Build the Foundation Required to End the Epidemic. Clin Infect Dis 2021;72(9):1627–30.
5. Marcus JL, Leyden WA, Alexeeff SE, et al. Comparison of Overall and Comorbidity-Free Life Expectancy Between Insured Adults With and Without HIV Infection, 2000-2016. JAMA Netw Open 2020;3(6):e207954.
6. Trickey A, Sabin CA, Burkholder G, et al. Life expectancy after 2015 of adults with HIV on long-term antiretroviral therapy in Europe and North America: a collaborative analysis of cohort studies. Lancet HIV 2023;10(5):e295–307.
7. Smit M, Brinkman K, Geerlings S, et al. Future challenges for clinical care of an ageing population infected with HIV: a modelling study. Lancet Infect Dis 2015; 15(7):810–8.
8. Mayer KH, Loo S, Crawford PM, et al. Excess clinical comorbidity among HIV-Infected Patients Accessing Primary Care in US Community Health Centers. Public Health Rep Wash DC 1974 2018;133(1):109–18.
9. Weber MSR, Duran Ramirez JJ, Hentzien M, et al. Time Trends in Causes of Death in People with HIV: Insights from the Swiss HIV Cohort Study. Clin Infect Dis 2024;12:ciae014.

10. Sullivan PS, Satcher Johnson A, Pembleton ES, et al. Epidemiology of HIV in the USA: epidemic burden, inequities, contexts, and responses. Lancet 2021; 397(10279):1095–106.

11. Centers for Disease Control and Prevention. Estimated HIV incidence and prevalence in the United States, 2017–2021. HIV Surveill Suppl Rep 2023 2023;28(3). Available at: http://www.cdc.gov/hiv/library/reports/hiv-surveillance.html. [Accessed 3 September 2023].

12. Kamitani E, Johnson WD, Wichser ME, et al. Growth in Proportion and Disparities of HIV PrEP Use Among Key Populations Identified in the United States National Goals: Systematic Review and Meta-analysis of Published Surveys. JAIDS J Acquir Immune Defic Syndr 2020;84(4):379–86.

13. Centers for Disease Control and Prevention. HIV in the Southern United States. 2019. Available at: https://www.cdc.gov/hiv/pdf/policies/cdc-hiv-in-the-south-issue-brief.pdf. [Accessed 30 September 2019].

14. Adimora AA, Ramirez C, Schoenbach VJ, et al. Policies and politics that promote HIV infection in the Southern United States. AIDS 2014;28(10):1393–7.

15. Reif S, Safley D, McAllaster C, et al. State of HIV in the US Deep South. J Community Health 2017;42(5):844–53.

16. U.S. Health and Human Services. America's HIV Epidemic Analysis Dashboard. 2019. Available at: https://ahead.hiv.gov/. [Accessed 30 November 2023].

17. Dasgupta S, Tie Y, Beer L, et al. Barriers to HIV Care by Viral Suppression Status Among US Adults With HIV: Findings From the Centers for Disease Control and Prevention Medical Monitoring Project. J Assoc Nurses AIDS Care 2021;32(5): 561–8.

18. Dombrowski JC, Ramchandani MS, Golden MR. Implementation of Low-Barrier Human Immunodeficiency Virus Care: Lessons Learned From the Max Clinic in Seattle. Clin Infect Dis 2023;77(2):252–7.

19. Armstrong WS, Evans T, Tookes HE. To End The HIV Epidemic, We Need To Reach Unsheltered Homeless Populations. Health Aff Forefr 2023. https://doi.org/10.1377/forefront.20231018.878582.

20. Gilman B, Bouchery E, Hogan P, et al. The HIV Clinician Workforce in the United States. HIV Spec 2016;2–9.

21. Weiser J, Beer L, West BT, et al. Qualifications, Demographics, Satisfaction, and Future Capacity of the HIV Care Provider Workforce in the United States, 2013-2014. Clin Infect Dis 2016;63(7):966–75.

22. Sinsky CA, Brown RL, Stillman MJ, et al. COVID-Related Stress and Work Intentions in a Sample of US Health Care Workers. Mayo Clin Proc Innov Qual Outcomes 2021;5(6):1165–73.

23. Rotenstein LS, Brown R, Sinsky C, et al. The Association of Work Overload with Burnout and Intent to Leave the Job Across the Healthcare Workforce During COVID-19. J Gen Intern Med 2023;38(8):1920–7.

24. Nelson J. Pathways to Achieve Diversity in the HIV Workforce. Presented at: health resources and services administration (HRSA), HIV/AIDS bureau (HAB) virtual technical expert panel presentation; 2023.

25. Lakshmi S, Beekmann SE, Polgreen PM, et al. HIV primary care by the infectious disease physician in the United States - extending the continuum of care. AIDS Care 2018;30(5):569–77.

26. Joseph A. Limits of 'Fauci effect': infectious disease applicants plummet, and hospitals are scrambling. STAT News; 2022. Available at: https://www.statnews.com/2022/12/07/infectious-disease-fellowship-drop-in-applicants/. [Accessed 5 October 2023].

27. Prasad R, D'Amico F, Wilson SA, et al. Training family medicine residents in HIV primary care: a national survey of program directors. Fam Med 2014;46(7): 527–31.

28. Adams J, Chacko K, Guiton G, et al. Training internal medicine residents in outpatient HIV care: a survey of program Directors. J Gen Intern Med 2010;25(9): 977–81.

29. Barakat LA, Dunne DW, Tetrault JM, et al. The Changing Face of HIV Care: Expanding HIV Training in an Internal Medicine Residency Program. Acad Med J Assoc Am Med Coll 2018;93(11):1673–8.

30. Fessler DA, Huang GC, Potter J, et al. Development and Implementation of a Novel HIV Primary Care Track for Internal Medicine Residents. J Gen Intern Med 2017;32(3):350–4.

31. Budak JZ, Volkman K, Wood BR, et al. Building HIV Workforce Capacity Through a Residency Pathway: Outcomes and Challenges. Open Forum Infect Dis 2018; 5(12):ofy317.

32. Bono RS, Dahman B, Sabik LM, et al. Human Immunodeficiency Virus–Experienced Clinician Workforce Capacity: Urban–Rural Disparities in the Southern United States. Clin Infect Dis 2021;72(9):1615–22.

33. Andrews HS, Chirch LM, Luther VP, et al. Analysis of the Infectious Diseases Fellowship Program Directors Postmatch 2023 Survey. J Infect Dis 2024;229(3): 630–4.

34. 7,700 resident physicians placed into fellowship training positions through the NRMP's medicine and pediatric specialties match. National Resident Matching Program (NRMP); 2023. Available at: https://www.nrmp.org/about/news/2023/11/7700-resident-physicians-placed-into-fellowship-training-positions-through-the-nrmps-medicine-and-pediatric-specialties-match/. [Accessed 30 November 2023].

35. Schmitt SK. IDSA statement on 2023 ID fellowship match. Infectious Disease Society of America; 2023. Available at: https://www.idsociety.org/news-publications-new/articles/2023/idsa-statement-on-2023-id-fellowship-match/. [Accessed 30 November 2023].

36. Blyth DM, Barsoumian AE, Yun HC. Timing of Infectious Disease Clinical Rotation Is Associated With Infectious Disease Fellowship Application. Open Forum Infect Dis 2018;5(8):ofy155.

37. Bonura EM, Lee ES, Ramsey K, et al. Factors Influencing Internal Medicine Resident Choice of Infectious Diseases or Other Specialties: A National Cross-sectional Study. Clin Infect Dis 2016;63(2):155–63.

38. Marshall AA, Wooten DA. An HIV Primary Care Rotation Improved HIV and STI Knowledge, Enhanced Sexual History-Taking Skills, and Increased Interest in a Career in Infectious Diseases Among Medical Students and Residents. Open Forum Infect Dis 2021;8(6):ofab207.

39. Marcelin JR, Brosnihan P, Swindells S, et al. The Value of a Longitudinal Human Immunodeficiency Virus Track for Medical Students: 10-Year Program Evaluation. Open Forum Infect Dis 2022;9(7):ofac184.

40. HIV clinical fellowship opportunity. Available at: https://www.hivma.org/professional-development/hivma-clinical-fellowship/. [Accessed 15 November 2023].

41. Training opportunities. Available at: https://aahivm.org/training-opportunities/. [Accessed 15 November 2023].

42. Bolduc P, Day PG, Behl-Chadha B, et al. Community-Based HIV and Viral Hepatitis Fellowship Evaluation: Results from a Qualitative Study. J Prim Care Community Health 2022;13. 21501319221138193.

43. Budak JZ, Sears DA, Wood BR, et al. Human immunodeficiency virus training pathways in residency: a national survey of curricula and outcomes. Clin Infect Dis 2021;72(9):1623–6.

44. Weddle AL. Position of the Infectious Diseases Society of America and the HIV Medical Association on Team-Based Infectious Diseases Care and the Role of Advanced Practice Providers and Clinical Pharmacists. Clin Infect Dis 2024. https://doi.org/10.1093/cid/ciae265.

45. Greenberg AE, CDEIPI Consortium. Centers for AIDS Research (CFAR) Diversity, Equity, and Inclusion Pathway Initiative (CDEIPI): Developing Career Pathways for Early-Stage Scholars From Racial and Ethnic Groups Underrepresented in HIV Science and Medicine. JAIDS J Acquir Immune Defic Syndr 2023;94(2S):S5–12.

46. Magnus M, Segarra L, Robinson B, et al. Impact of a Multi-Institutional Initiative to Engage Students and Early-Stage Scholars From Underrepresented Racial and Ethnic Minority Groups in HIV Research: The Centers for AIDS Research Diversity, Equity, and Inclusion Pathway Initiative. JAIDS J Acquir Immune Defic Syndr 2023;94(2S):S13–20.

47. Quinn KG, John SA, Hirshfield S, et al. Challenges to meeting the HIV care needs of older adults in the rural South. SSM Qual Res Health 2022;2:100113.

48. Swartz TH, Aberg JA. Preserving the future of infectious diseases: why we must address the decline in compensation for clinicians and researchers. Clin Infect Dis 2023;77(10):1387–94.

49. Mohareb AM, Brown TS. Medical Student Debt and the US Infectious Diseases Workforce. Clin Infect Dis 2023;76(7):1322–7.

50. HELP Act Information and Resources. Available at: https://www.hivma.org/policy–advocacy/help-act/. [Accessed 1 November 2023].

51. Bio-Preparedness Workforce Pilot Program. Infectious disease society of America. Available at: https://www.idsociety.org/policy–advocacy/bio-preparedness-workforce-pilot/. [Accessed 1 November 2023].

52. The ryan white HIV/AIDS program. Kaiser Family Foundation; 2022. Available at: https://www.kff.org/hivaids/fact-sheet/the-ryan-white-hivaids-program-the-basics/. [Accessed 30 November 2023].

53. Person AK, Terndrup CP, Jain MK, et al. "Do We Stay or Do We Go?" The Impact of anti-LGBTQ+ Legislation on the HIV Workforce in the South. Clin Infect Dis 2023;ciad493. https://doi.org/10.1093/cid/ciad493.

54. Goldschmidt RH, Graves DW. The National HIV Telephone Consultation Service (Warmline): a clinical resource for physicians caring for African-Americans. J Natl Med Assoc 2003;95(2 Suppl 2):8S–11S.

55. Waldura JF, Neff S, Dehlendorf C, et al. Teleconsultation improves primary care clinicians' confidence about caring for HIV. J Gen Intern Med 2013;28(6):793–800.

56. Sherman EM, Cocohoba JM, Neff SE, et al. Health care provider satisfaction with telephone consultations provided by pharmacists and physicians at the National HIV/AIDS Clinicians' Consultation Center. Ann Pharmacother 2011;45(12):1499–505.

57. Osei-Twum JA, Wiles B, Killackey T, et al. Impact of Project ECHO on Patient and Community Health Outcomes: A Scoping Review. Acad Med J Assoc Am Med Coll 2022;97(9):1393–402.

58. Wood BR, Bauer K, Lechtenberg R, et al. Direct and Indirect Effects of a Project ECHO Longitudinal Clinical Tele-Mentoring Program on Viral Suppression for

Persons With HIV: A Population-Based Analysis. J Acquir Immune Defic Syndr 1999 2022;90(5):538–45.

59. Ramirez JA, Maddali MV, Nematollahi S, et al. New Strategies in Clinical Guideline Delivery: Randomized Trial of Online, Interactive Decision Support Versus Guidelines for Human Immunodeficiency Virus Treatment Selection by Trainees. Clin Infect Dis 2021;72(9):1608–14.

60. Tookes HE, Bartholomew TS, Suarez E, et al. Acceptability, feasibility, and pilot results of the tele-harm reduction intervention for rapid initiation of antiretrovirals among people who inject drugs. Drug Alcohol Depend 2021;229(Pt A):109124.

61. Bailey ZD, Feldman JM, Bassett MT. How Structural Racism Works — Racist Policies as a Root Cause of U.S. Racial Health Inequities. In: Malina D, editor. N Engl J Med 2021;384(8):768–73.

62. Committee on the Review of Federal Policies that Contribute to Racial and Ethnic Health Inequities, Board on Population Health and Public Health Practice, Health and Medicine Division, National Academies of Sciences, Engineering, and Medicine. In: Burke SP, Polsky DE, Geller AB, editors. Federal policy to advance racial, ethnic, and tribal health equity. National Academies Press; 2023. p. 26834.

63. Place of Service Code Set. Centers for Medicare and Medicaid Services. 2023. Available at: https://www.cms.gov/medicare/coding-billing/place-of-service-codes/code-sets. [Accessed 30 November 2023].

64. U.S. Government Accountability Office. Substance Use Disorder: Medicaid Coverage of Peer Support Services for Adults. 2020. Available at: https://www.gao.gov/products/gao-20-616. [Accessed 1 November 2023].

Moving?

Make sure your subscription moves with you!

To notify us of your new address, find your **Clinics Account Number** (located on your mailing label above your name), and contact customer service at:

Email: journalscustomerservice-usa@elsevier.com

800-654-2452 (subscribers in the U.S. & Canada)
314-447-8871 (subscribers outside of the U.S. & Canada)

Fax number: 314-447-8029

Elsevier Health Sciences Division
Subscription Customer Service
3251 Riverport Lane
Maryland Heights, MO 63043